Psychodynamic Approaches to the Experience of Dementia

Psychodynamic Approaches to the Experience of Dementia: Perspectives from Observation, Theory and Practice demonstrates the impact of healthcare approaches that take into account not only the practical needs but also the emotional experience of the patient, their partners, families and friends, lay carers and professional staff.

Currently there is no cure for dementia, but the psychosocial and therapeutic approaches described in this volume have appeared to help people, both patients and carers, feel more contained and less lonely and isolated. Psychoanalytic theory provides a disciplined way of thinking about the internal world of an individual and their relationships. Each author provides their own commentary on the personal and interpersonal effects of dementia, endeavouring to understand behaviours and emotions which may otherwise seem incomprehensible. The subject is approached from a psychodynamic perspective, considering the unconscious, previous and current experiences and relationships, including those between patients and staff.

Psychodynamic Approaches to the Experience of Dementia illustrates the practical and theoretical thinking of clinicians from a wide range of disciplines who are engaged in the care of people in late life with a diagnosis of dementia. It will be essential reading for mental health and health professionals in practice and training in the field of dementia.

Sandra Evans has been an NHS psychiatrist, teacher and trainer for over 30 years. Sandra is a group analyst also in private practice with GANLondon.

Jane Garner has over 30 years clinical experience in the NHS using psychodynamic ideas to inform psychiatric practice and teaching, particularly in the areas of old age and dementia services, continuing care, institutional abuse, sex and relationships.

Rachel Darnley-Smith is a music therapist and senior lecturer at Roehampton University, UK. She has worked with people with dementia over many years, mostly in the NHS and published widely on music therapy, aesthetics and psychoanalysis.

'This excellent book is a refreshing and valuable contribution to our understanding of the challenges faced by people with dementia and how we might help. By shining the different light of psychodynamics on dementia, the authors and the editors reveal novel insights and opportunities into dementia and how to improve the quality of care provided. The editors, Sandra Evans, Jane Garner and Rachel Darnley-Smith have done a fantastic job in commissioning and writing a set of chapters that will enable readers to challenge their assumptions and by doing so to think and act differently for the benefit of those with dementia.'

– **Sube Banerjee**, Professor of Dementia and Deputy Dean,
Brighton and Sussex Medical School

'I would highly recommend this multi-authored book which brings a psychodynamic understanding to dementia care. This beautifully perceptive and insightful book helps the reader (both professional and lay) develop a greater understanding of the emotions encountered as the illness progresses.'

– **Amanda Thompsell**, Old Age Psychiatrist at SLAM and
Chair of the Faculty of Old Age Psychiatry at the
Royal College of Psychiatrists

'This is an essential and unique book which courageously explores the subjective world of dementia. So many find too terrifying to contemplate and yet with this book as a guide, clinicians, but also families and carers, will come closer to understanding how the world impacts on the mind of an individual suffering from this disease. It also helps with insights in relation to how the experience of dementia in someone close to them impacts on their experience of the world. This is an extraordinarily helpful and long-awaited book, which will be welcomed by professionals as well as those effected by this illness.'

– **Peter Fonagy**, OBE, Professor of Contemporary
Psychoanalysis and Developmental Science,
University College London

'This unique, much needed book movingly and intelligently reflects upon the experience of people living with dementia and their families and carers through a new lens. Collectively, drawing upon psychodynamic and psychoanalytic theories; psychiatrists, analytic psychotherapists, psychologists, arts therapists and counsellors provide new meanings for those living with dementia, their families, carers and therapists. This rich multi-disciplinary perspective will appeal to professionals and family members and carers.'

– **Professor Helen Odell-Miller**, OBE, Director,
Cambridge Institute for Music Therapy,
Anglia Ruskin University

Psychodynamic Approaches to the Experience of Dementia

Perspectives from Observation, Theory and Practice

Edited by Sandra Evans, Jane Garner and Rachel Darnley-Smith

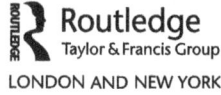

LONDON AND NEW YORK

First published 2020
by Routledge
2 Park Square, Milton Park, Abingdon, Oxon OX14 4RN

and by Routledge
52 Vanderbilt Avenue, New York, NY 10017

Routledge is an imprint of the Taylor & Francis Group, an informa business

British Library Cataloguing-in-Publication Data
A catalogue record for this book is available from the British Library

Library of Congress Cataloging-in-Publication Data
A catalog record for this book has been requested

ISBN: 978-0-415-78664-5 (hbk)
ISBN: 978-0-415-78665-2 (pbk)
ISBN: 978-1-315-16022-1 (ebk)

Typeset in Times New Roman
by Apex CoVantage, LLC

Contents

Figures and illustrations

Contributors

Daniel Anderson

Dr Daniel Anderson is a consultant psychiatrist and group analyst. He works part-time at The Christie NHS Foundation Trust in the field of psycho-oncology and also works in private practice in Manchester and Chester. He specialises in the mental health care of older adults including dementia care. He is imminently due to submit his PhD thesis to the University of Manchester, which is an ethnographic study using discourse analysis of group process notes as they relate to gender and sexuality, and the consequent pedagogical issues for the training of group analysts.

Andrew Balfour

Andrew Balfour studied English Literature before training in clinical psychology at University College London. He went on to train as an adult psychoanalytic psychotherapist at the Tavistock & Portman NHS Trust whilst working in a staff post there. He subsequently trained as a couple psychotherapist at Tavistock Relationships (formerly Tavistock Centre for Couple Relationships). For more than10 years he was Clinical Director and he is now Chief Executive there. He has published widely and teaches both in Britain and abroad. With Mary Morgan and Christopher Vincent, he co-edited *How Couple Relationships Shape our World: Clinical Practice, Research and Policy Perspectives* (Karnac, 2012). He has a longstanding clinical and research interest in dementia and has developed an intervention for couples living with dementia (*Living Together with Dementia*, Balfour, 2014). His latest book is Engaging Couples: New Directions in Therapeutic Work with Families, which he edited with Christopher Clulow and Kate Thompson (Routledge, 2018).

Juliette Brown

Juliette is a consultant psychiatrist of adults and older adults in East London. She was a Darzi Fellow in Clinical Leadership, is a member of Association for Psychoanalytic Psychotherapy in the NHS and Clinical Network for Dementia Leadership Group, NHS England. She has research interests in application of psychoanalytic theory, shared decision making, service improvement, trauma-informed care and the cultural and philosophic basis of psychiatric illness and treatment. She has peer reviewed for BJ Psych Bulletin and Psychoanalytic Psychotherapy.

Angela Byers

Angela Byers has worked for 25 years as a registered art therapist, mainly in NHS psychiatric services but also in social services' residential homes for older people, and as a visiting tutor to the art therapy training at Goldsmiths College. Angela's publications about her work with people with dementia describe non-verbal communications in an art therapy group, the creative sorting of art therapy materials and the retention of aesthetic pleasure in dementia. She has also conducted an ethnographic study of a residential home for older people in Cape Town, South Africa, as well as assisting a colleague to undertake a qualitative study of residential homes and community centres for older people there.

Rachel Darnley-Smith

Rachel Darnley-Smith is a music therapist and independent researcher. She has worked for many years with older adults, mostly in NHS mental health settings. She holds a PhD in music from the University of Durham and her research interests and publications continue to range across themes arising from the practice of music therapy concerning aesthetics, recognition theory, music and psychoanalysis. Recent publications include 'Jung and the Transcendent Function in Music Therapy' in Music – Psychoanalysis – Musicology, ed. Samuel Wilson, Routledge (2018). In 2019, she was guest editor for a special edition of the British Journal of Music Therapy (Sage) on Music and Psychoanalysis. Since 1999 she has been an active member of the Association for Psychoanalytic Psychotherapy in the NHS Older Adults Section. Rachel currently lectures part-time in the Department of Psychology at Roehampton University and is a Governor of the Music Therapy Charity.

Sandra Evans

Sandra Evans is Deputy Head of Academic & Pastoral Office, Barts & the London School of Medicine and Dentistry and ex-officio Chair of the Association for Psychoanalytic Psychotherapy in the NHS Older Adults Section. Sandra has worked in NHS psychiatry for over thirty years as a clinician, a teacher and trainer and more recently in senior leadership roles. She trained and qualified as a Group Analyst in 1998 and has since deepened her interest in and understanding of psychoanalytic approaches to aging through further study and engagement with academic and learning communities.

Adrienne Freeman

Adrienne Freeman is lead Music Therapist for the Older People's In-patient Therapies team within the Enfield sector of Barnet, Enfield and Haringey Mental Health NHS Trust. Experienced in multiple areas of mental health, her clinical specialism is in dementia, on which she lectures, presents and publishes. She is an experienced external examiner to Music Therapy training programmes. Currently chair of the Training and Education Committee for the British Association for Music Therapy (BAMT), she is also a Trustee and has for many years been on BAMT's Supervision and Consultation Register.

Her most recent publication is 'Fathoming the constellations: Ways of working with families in music therapy for people with advanced dementia.' British Journal of Music Therapy, 31(1), 43–49.

Jane Garner
Consultant in Old Age Psychiatry, leading a team in North London for many years. Consultant seeing students at University College London. Previously a number of honorary positions at the Royal College of Psychiatrists including Deputy Chief Examiner and Secretary of the Old Age Faculty, Regional Adviser, Regional Tutor. Founder member and Honorary Secretary of the Older Adult Section of the Association for Psychoanalytic Psychotherapy in the NHS. Academic, clinical and authorial interests in psychotherapy with older adults, institutional abuse, continuing care in dementia, use of psychodynamic ideas in psychiatric practice. Coeditor with Sandra Evans of 'Talking Over the Years: a handbook of dynamic psychotherapy with older adults'. Currently retired from clinical practice.

Matthew Hagger
Matthew Hagger is a Consultant in Liaison Psychiatry at the Royal Free hospital, London. He works with both older and younger adults and has worked in liaison psychiatry in a variety of settings. He has maintained a long standing interest in psychodynamic approaches in working with patients, carers and staff and also teaching general hospital staff about mental health. He is a member of the Older adults section of the Association of Psychoanalytic Psychotherapy in the NHS.

Neil Jeyasingam
Dr. Neil Jeyasingam is a psychogeriatrician and psychotherapist in private and public practice as a fellow of the Royal Australian and New Zealand College of Psychiatrists. He holds a double masters in health administration and psychiatry, and has over 40 publications in fields including psychotherapy and ageing. A former Clinical Director and Maudsley Research Scholar, he is one of the founding members of the Faculty of Psychotherapy, and contributes to its teaching program on old age psychotherapy.

Susan Maciver
Susan Maciver began her professional life as an English teacher but trained as a counsellor thirty years ago. She now works as a psychodynamic counsellor and organisational therapist. With Chris McGregor and Tom Russ she is a member of the Working with Older People Group at Human Development Scotland.

Chris McGregor
Christine McGregor is a psychodynamic counsellor, accredited by BACP and a member of Human Development Scotland. She was formerly the Social Work Commissioner for The Mental Welfare Commission of Scotland and the Vice Convenor of Alzheimer Scotland. She also served on the Board on Alzheimer Disease International. She is currently in private practice working with elderly people and is a founding member of HDS Working with Older People group.

Stephanie Petty
Stephanie holds a Doctorate in Clinical Psychology (ClinPsyD), with chartered membership of the British Psychological Society (BPS) and is a registered Practitioner Psychologist with the Health and Care Professions Council (HCPC).

Stephanie is employed as a Senior Clinical Psychologist at The Retreat, York, within the Specialist Older Adult Services. She is completing a PhD with the Institute of Mental Health, Division of Psychiatry and Applied Psychology, University of Nottingham, researching the emotional experiences of individuals with dementia, notably when in hospital. Additionally, Stephanie is an Associate Lecturer at the University of York within the Department of Psychology.

Michelle Potts

Michelle Potts is a Social Worker registered with the Health and Care Professions Council (HCPC). She completed an undergraduate degree in Psychology at the University of Liverpool and worked at The Retreat Hospital as an Assistant Psychologist, firstly in a therapeutic community and later with individuals with dementia. This sparked in her interest in emotional experience and dementia, which led her to write the reflective journal for the study included in this chapter. Whilst completing a Masters in Social Work at the University of York, Michelle's research focused on how scarcity can influence a persons' ability to make long-term beneficial decisions. This research relates to her wider interests in social policy and poverty and their impact on those most vulnerable in society.

Louis Resnick

At the time of writing Louis was a fourth year medical student at the University of Edinburgh with an interest in person-centred care. His chapter began life as a student selected research project supervised by Drs Tom Russ and Neill Anderson. Since publication Louis has graduated and now works as a locum doctor in Glasgow. He plans to defer further training in pursuit of higher education.

Tom C. Russ

Tom Russ is a consultant psychiatrist in old age psychiatry and director of the Alzheimer Scotland Dementia Research Centre at the University of Edinburgh. He divides his time between clinical practice in the NHS and research on environmental risk factors for dementia and music as a non-pharmacological intervention for people with dementia. He has always been interested in psychoanalysis and worked at the Tavistock Clinic as a junior doctor.

Julia C. Segal

Julia Segal is a Fellow of the British Association for Counselling and Psychotherapy. She trained with Relate and since 1983 has been counselling people with neurological conditions (particularly multiple sclerosis), and members of their families, using the ideas of Melanie Klein to understand and illuminate everyday experience. She has written extensively on the way illness impacts on relationships within the family as well as with healthcare professionals, most recently in *The Trouble with Illness* (Jessica Kingsley, 2017). Julia is best known for her books which include *Phantasy in Everyday Life* (Penguin books 1985; Karnac 1995), *Melanie Klein: Key Figures in Counselling and Psychotherapy* (Sage Publications 1992) and *Helping Children with Ill or Disabled Parents* (Jessica Kingsley 1996). She has a website http://thetroublewithillness.com.

Foreword

Nori Graham

When I became Chair of the Alzheimer's Society over 30 years ago, public awareness of dementia hardly existed. It seems hard to believe nowadays, but at that time, most people, even members of the educated part of the population, had no idea what Alzheimer's Disease might be. Now, as a result of people living longer, the hard work of the Alzheimer's Society, advances in research and, perhaps above all, the appearance of characters suffering from dementia in popular soaps on television, everyone knows about Alzheimer's. It has become the number one dread for those in advancing years.

There have been major advances in our understanding of dementia. Neuroscientific studies have explored the role of amyloid and other substances in the brain. An increasing number of genes transmitting vulnerability are being explored. Imaging of the brain has shown the major loss of brain tissue that occurs in the disease. Revisions to the classification system have highlighted different types of dementia and epidemiological studies have demonstrated the various courses of the disease depending on diagnosis. Life-style factors have become key in approaches to prevention. Psychosocial studies have shown the high prevalence of depression and anxiety in the carers of people with dementia. There is the beginning of a recognition that each person with dementia is just that, a person, with a human experience of themselves, their relationships, life itself. With that recognition comes approaches to managing mental and emotional disorder in dementia and helping people continue to live a meaningful life.

Changes have occurred in the way advocacy on behalf of those with Alzheimer's is achieved. Forty years ago, no one would have dreamed of the possibility that people with Alzheimer's themselves would play an active part in advocacy. Nowadays audiences at virtually all conferences on the topic of dementia are addressed also by people with the condition, generally those who have benefited from earlier diagnosis and have been fortunate to respond, even if only temporarily, to drug treatment.

One of the most important advances in psychosocial care is the introduction of approaches that are person centred. Typified by the work of the late Tom Kitwood, person-centred care is built around the needs of the individual and depends on coming to know the affected individual through the development of an interpersonal relationship. It is only natural that the next step should be, as exemplified in this excellent book, the introduction of lessons learned from psychoanalysis to person-centred care.

Psychoanalysis is used as a treatment for many disorders, though not for dementia. It is, however, also a theory for understanding and as such can be used, not instead of, but to complement existing treatments. The close attention given by psychoanalysts to the minutiae of language and behaviour is a technique from which we can all learn. There is a sense in which psychiatry with clinical psychology, social work and the therapies is the medicine of communication. If effective communication and, especially, effective listening is the key to success in helping manage mental health problems such as depression, anxiety, obsessional and psychotic states, how much more is it the way forward in relating to people with dementia whose loss of memory and verbal skills may seem like such a barrier? We can lose the fluency of our communication when we meet someone with the diagnosis, that combined with the cognitive difficulties of the person with dementia often leads to extreme poverty of interaction. This book discusses some ways forward for primary and secondary care and the third sector.

In this book, Sandra Evans, Jane Garner and Rachel Darnley-Smith with the multidisciplinary authorship have brought their psychodynamic experience to bear on all aspects of clinical practice with people with dementia, those who are close to them as well as the professionals involved. They look closely at the way, for example, people with dementia may feel unwanted when staff in residential homes are totally task-orientated. They examine the possibilities that all those involved in the process, the one with dementia, staff and family members, may be helped by having their attention drawn to emotional aspects of changing relationships – changes involving disappointment, loss, fear for the future, anxiety, disruption of bonds of attachment as well as the possibility of enduring hope and love. For the staff, working with people who are not going to get better requires different skills, understanding and resilience.

The case vignettes with which the points are illustrated bring to life the way clinicians can use the concepts outlined. Policy makers, all professionals involved clinically and lay people will find this work of direct value to them adding meaning to the feelings evoked by the disease for which there is yet no cure.

Acknowledgements

Without the enormous privilege of being allowed to enter peoples' lives, often at times when they are at their most vulnerable, we, the editors of this book would not have had an opportunity to develop our thoughts.

It is in the hope that this shared experience, from patients, their families and their professional and lay carers, will be of benefit to others, that we have written this book.

That is certainly the essence of the generosity of our patients – that others might benefit from their experience. We might add that there were also exchanges of joy and it is essential that these too are shared.

Acknowledgments are also due to the authors of individual chapters, who generously agreed to contribute their clinical experience and expertise to this volume through spending many hours writing and responding to our queries. This has enabled us to produce a volume that is far reaching in scope and one that we hopefully anticipate will set standards of good practice in the care of elderly people for many years to come.

Editorial staff at Routledge have supported us throughout the process, through their own expertise and encouragement. In particular we thank Joanne Forshaw for her support of the project from the outset.

Finally we thank our friends and colleagues who are past and current members of the Older Adults Section of the APP (Association of Psychoanalytic Psychotherapy in the NHS) who have over many years been a source of stimulating discussion and inspiration, sparking ideas together in moments for articles, books and conferences and who have contributed ideas, and in some cases chapters to this latest project, especially as it has taken shape in recent months.

Introduction

Sandra Evans, Jane Garner and Rachel Darnley-Smith

We are urged to think about dementia by politico-demographic imperative and by our personal and clinical experiences. Approximately 800,000 people in the UK have dementia and, thanks to the National Dementia Strategy 2009, more people now know their diagnosis (Department of Health, 2009). This raising of awareness has made it possible for dementia to emerge from the shadows, for people to talk about their hopes and their fears and to access much needed help and support. The UK seems to be mirroring the socio-medical experience of addressing cancer some 40 years ago, with increasing emphasis on early diagnosis, ideas for prevention and hopes for finding a cure.

There is currently no cure for dementia, but there are things that can be done to alleviate suffering. Formal support that is task-based, or provides respite from stressful situations is usually essential but the more informal inter-personal strategies seem equally helpful; the ones based on sharing painful feelings, listening to anxieties or expressions of frustration and anger or just learning that there are others with similar experiences. Understanding seemingly incomprehensible behaviours or emotions can assist partners and families find a way to communicate with the person with dementia, even if it is momentary. This enables people, both patients and relatives, to feel less lonely and isolated.

The current absence of an effective treatment for dementia does not remove the responsibility of our society to look for ways to prevent or halt the disease process: money and resources need to be found to assist with that programme. However, given the number of people with dementia, other treatments and management strategies must be funded too. More than twice the number of people with dementia are affected by the illness as partners, families and friends become involved in the inexorable decline and increased dependence. It is estimated that many more than two million people are touched by dementia each year.

Psychoanalysis is not only a treatment. It is a disciplined way of thinking about a problem which focusses upon the internal world of the individual in the context of both early and later psychosocial experiences. Psychoanalysis may assist in facing all emotions, including the darker side of the human psyche. As a theory it examines thoughts and feelings about life and death. Freud wrote about sex, incest, violence and anxiety. Thinkers and clinicians who came after him considered the mother/infant bond, the early maternal environment where parents of whatever gender and interpretation foster feelings for their children and provide the environment in which they learn or not, to face challenges and adversities throughout their lives.

Psychoanalysis, through the development of group and social theories, is also able to examine the macro environment: family structures, friendship and social groups, institutional structures – funded and underfunded governments – local and national, policy makers and the media and the social media. All these influence the way we think and feel about a disease process which robs us and those we love of their autobiography, their confidence and their ability to think. None of these factors, those we are living through, those we are working with, occurs in a vacuum. As clinicians, if we can build some understanding, intrapersonal and interpersonal, of the nature of these influences, both at a micro and at a macro level, we may be able to interpret feelings and behaviours, including our own. We can walk alongside those affected by dementia and feel less daunted.

The authors are clinicians drawn from a wide variety of disciplines, all of whom have worked with and thought about people with dementia. The book will reflect our daily contact with the illness itself. Training and experience across the clinical disciplines represented here has included neurobiology, the diagnostic process, the interpretation of results and the likely outcomes of treatment/management. Experience will have been gained in the planning of services, the allocation of funding, and the use of decision-making tools in health and social care. Psychoanalytically informed clinicians endeavour to work intuitively with a notion of the unconscious.

Throughout this volume we have concerned ourselves with factors which we believe clouds clear thinking, which may direct funding and resources away from older people with dementia: the impact of 'the unconscious at work' (Obholzer and Roberts, 1994). The authors have made the care of older people and those with dementia their particular concern. In all, the purpose of the volume throughout is to describe and translate their experience of working from the point of view of their individual training: each chapter offers thoughts, information and ideas recognising that dementia affects us all.

References

Department of Health, Living Well with Dementia: A National Dementia Strategy (London: HMSO, 2009).

Obholzer, A. & Zagier Roberts, Vega (1994). *The Unconscious at Work: Individual and Organisational Stress in the Human Services*. London: Routledge.

Chapter 1

Encountering dementia

Louis Resnick

It was a fruitful afternoon on urology. I had come to work: taking histories; examining patients.

An elderly gentleman, smartly dressed in crisp white shirt, green tie and tweed blazer was pacing up and down the corridor. He periodically stopped, looking lost before journeying on. Was he alright? Did he need help?

He was kempt, thin wisps of white hair combed into a side parting. He smiled and nodded when I offered to accompany him. Polite conversation ensued. He spoke with charm and intelligence of his service in the Second World War and the successes of his three children.

However, something was wrong. He told me the floors we walked on used to belong to an army barracks where he was stationed after the War. He made vague references to a hotel, the other patients as guests and me, a member of staff. He mentioned his wife who would pick him up soon.

After a few laps of the corridor I wanted to get back to work. He was pleasant but keeping me from learning opportunities. I steered him towards his bed, into his armchair and drew conversation to a close.

Flicking through the gentleman's notes – Alzheimer's Disease – I felt a twinge of sadness to read that his wife had died two years previously. Overall I felt I had "done well"; demonstrating appropriate and sensitive engagement with a person with dementia. I returned to work.

Before long the gentleman appeared at the office doorway. He tried to gain my attention: 'I'm sorry, Sir, I have work to be getting on with, I will see you in a while'. This failed to placate. Lingering turned into pestering and polite refusal turned into ignoring. Entering the office he tapped me on the shoulder. Feeling a boundary had been crossed, I got up, ushering him from the room. He stopped me in the corridor and grabbed my forearm.

He was angry, explaining that for the past two hours I had been keeping him waiting for the hotel manager. I responded with 'But Sir I was with you only five minutes ago . . .' Alas our realities were not reconcilable. Hostility ensued. He insisted I account for my actions, I persisted I had done no wrong. Irritation replaced patience. I no longer liked this man, I wanted him to go away. I played my last card, apologetically informing him that, far from being a guest at a hotel, he was in hospital with "memory problems". He looked pained, replying with indignation:

'Do you expect me to believe that? I'm an intelligent man!'

I felt guilty, helpless and spent of strategy. I announced my resignation:

'I'm sorry, Sir, but I don't know what else to say to you.'

A nurse came to my rescue. Breezy and pacifying, she took the man by his arm and persuaded him to sit down for a cup of tea. I watched as anguish melted from his face. Leading him back to his chair she turned round and mouthed a supportive "Don't worry".

Returning to the office, my feelings were of uselessness and embarrassment. Uselessness because I had experienced a communicational dead end, and embarrassment at how quickly I had come to resent him. Earlier feelings of pride at a successful interaction were replaced by scorn. In the moment I hated him. A charismatic chap who delighted in telling me of his service during the war had become an angry customer deliberately antagonising me and distracting me from work.

What had just happened? Why had my gentle enquiry and supportive listening failed to appease? Why was I left without tools to reconcile our realities?

I took a few minutes to cool off, then went back to work.

Introduction

There can be no knowledge without emotion.

Arnold Bennett, 1867–1931

I can find dementia difficult. Experience has seen me engage with patients with whom communication has been a real challenge. With this powerful emotions have emerged: sadness, anxiety, resentment and even fear. These feelings can be difficult and I am unsure how to process them. This project represents my desire to understand and learn how to better manage these experiences.

As a medical student there is seldom space for emotional expression. Johanna Shapiro's work (2011) on medical alexithymia resonated with me. She suggests doctors are subscribed to a profession that extols virtues of openness whilst tacitly encouraging an ethic of detachment and objectivity. Therefore I write as a medical student stranded in something of an emotional hinterland; although theoretically aware of the important role emotion can play in the doctor-patient relationship I am also unsure of its acceptability. Am I allowed to feel sad, angry, annoyed?

With this in mind I undertook a series of observations in this personally provocative area – dementia care – to reflect and gain insight into thoughts and feelings aroused. Dementia is challenging in many ways: diagnostically; physical demands of dependency; the presentation of psycho-behavioural disturbances (mood lability, agitation, aggression, nighttime wakening etc.), the latter of which, if present, correlate with higher levels of caregiver stress (Donaldson et al., 1998). This project allowed me to experience the illness from the perspective of both patient and caregiver and to discuss the theoretical underpinnings of associated feeling states.

The project

I spent six hours directly observing care of patients with dementia on a short-stay dementia ward at a psychiatric hospital: five 1–1.5-hour-long observations over the course of four consecutive weekdays.

Ward consultants were supervisors for the project. The charge nurse gave information to the nursing team and introduced me to all the patients before the first observation.

Observations were loosely based on the psychodynamic method outlined by Davenhill (2007). During the observations I wore an identity badge and sat in an armchair in the communal lounge. I had a diary to record sound bites when appropriate, however left the bulk of the write up until after each observation. I tried to remain as unobtrusive as possible and limited interaction with patients although sometimes this was unavoidable (for example when it concerned patient safety).

Time not formally observing was spent helping with nursing tasks, principally feeding patients at dinner time. On the last day I also joined an Occupational Therapy craft session. Although this time was not strictly observation, I still recorded my thoughts and feelings.

Consent was gained from next of kin via telephone and followed up by a project proposal letter. Permission was sought through introductions with each patient before the first observation.

Although I undertook the observations primed with relevant theory, I was not looking for particular themes to accord with this experience. It was more important for me just to 'be' and reflect upon my experience in the moment. Notes taken during the observation are here recorded in italics.

Findings

I experienced two main senses during the observations. The first was a feeling of *unwantedness* when healthcare staff were performing tasks and not spending time with patients. The second feeling was one of *connectedness* experienced when staff were with patients free from undertaking tasks. These states will be illustrated using examples from my observational diary.

Key to understanding these feeling states was a contrast in perspective gained through formal observation (enjoying a patient's perspective) and when engaged in other activity on the ward (enjoying a nurse's perspective). These two perspectives will be referred to as 'patient' and 'nurse' (because most healthcare workers observed were nurses the term 'nurse' will be used synonymously with 'staff').

Feeling unwanted: nurses performing tasks

A significant extent of observation saw nurses undertaking 'tasks'. This was experienced as a patient:

> Medication round. It is apparent this is another 'job' for nurses. Meds (sic) are dished out like military roll call.

And the multiplicity of pressures discussed with nursing staff:

> . . . stresses and strains of bureaucracy and paperwork. Not being able to spend enough time just 'with' patients, feeling rushed to do other things when they are.

It was noticed that a substitute for quality time spent with patients took the form of snippets of interaction with patients whilst moving between jobs:

> I notice that staff walk briskly across the lounge to the staffroom. Most will engage with patients en route. Bits of banter, lots of "are you alright?". It almost feels like addressing someone you meet in the street but don't want to stop to talk to.

When I was a nurse I felt these snippets were helpful, striking a balance between task and patient. However, when experiencing them as a patient I felt unattended to:

> The insight into how patients are doing is very different when one is sat in a goldfish bowl [the office] surrounded by notes and a ringing telephone. I had such a positive impression of the liveliness of patients when I was a nurse. Walking from the kitchen to the office and saying 'hi!' to a patient before locking myself away for an hour creates an impression that all is well. As a patient I experience the slow burn of tedium. When a member of staff walks by I feel like a dog waiting outside the supermarket for its owner: the expectation, elation felt when the doors slide open followed by the disappointment when they walk past.

These fragments did provide a momentary surge in activity in an otherwise unstimulating environment:

> There is no stimulation, no life, no excitement. Literally nothing is happening . . . The tiniest of moments became a spectacle: a door opening; a patient adjusting in his seat.

However, these parings, often coinciding with the symbolic exit of staff through a security door, ultimately left me feeling unwanted:

The moment they get out their keys to unlock the door is a powerful moment. The keys are sturdy so the sound of unlocking cuts through the room. It is a signal that the interaction has ended.

Therefore as a patient there was a palpable sense that one was secondary to practical jobs.

Feeling connected: nurses being 'with' patients

However, there were instances I felt the warmth of connection with a member of the team, when nurses spent time just being 'with' patients seemingly free from tasks. For example:

In response to moments of aggression or distress:

Afterwards the patient is sat down. [The Occupation Therapist] crouches on the floor and holds his hands. Lovely image seen through the doorframe. Like a crystallised scene in a stained glass window.

When providing company to patients:

James is being led round by a young nurse. He is zombie-like, jaw agape . . . Nurse looks at him lovingly, almost longingly. "What's the matter, David?" She understands his world. They look as though they are dancing together, like a couple in the corner at a party. She hugs him. "Is that what you were wanting?" . . . They are intimately close; it almost looks as though she is going to kiss him. She looks into his eyes and then away as they continue to dance.

I experienced this myself when I fed dinner to a particular patient every day:

I enjoy being with him. It is peaceful and I feel there is a common understanding between us.

Of these two feeling states, the more common feeling was of unwantedness when not in the company of healthcare staff.

The discussion will explore the feeling of unwantedness in an effort to understand why nursing staff appeared preoccupied with tasks instead of spending time with patients.

Discussion

There may be many reasons why staff seem to dedicate so much time to tasks in favour of spending time with patients. Some ideas are explored in this section. An important driver of this discussion was the contrast in feelings of 'all is well' when in the role of nurse compared to the unmet need I experienced as a patient. I offer four reasons for this. Two are pragmatic: a lack of time and the fact that engagement with some patients with dementia is effortful. And two are psychological: Menzies Lyth (1959) suggested that nurses use task-orientation as a social defence mechanism and Steven Sabat (2006) argues staff malignantly position patients.

Lack of time

A theme emerged that nurses simply did not have time to complete all the tasks. Therefore, time just 'to be' with patients became a scare resource.

Jones (1992) found dementia care workers with a shortage of time felt pressurised to "become task-orientated rather than communication-orientated" (p. 86). The deleterious effects of this time pressure are profound considering the amount of time a patient with dementia might need to communicate effectively.

As a compromise for quality interaction I experienced bitty communication from staff which, if anything, compounded feelings of unwantedness. Goldsmith (1996) agrees with this notion, arguing that this compromise can be "counterproductive" and leave patients "psychologically damaged" (p. 80). Staff too can be left frustrated with this fragmentary interaction.

Why was the nursing team so pushed for time? Two reasons seemed obvious. The first is an under-resourced work force. At the time of the observation there were a high number of staff absences due to illness.

Another reason was administration constraining nursing activities with unwanted paperwork. This was articulated by a member of the team:

> Feels like for everything you do you have to record it three times in three separate places.

Kontos and Naglie (2007) theorise that one of the side effects of striving for top-down efficiency in healthcare is creating a system wherein the measure of care "lies with the physical task rather than the quality of human interaction" (p. 550). This idea accords with the pressure felt by nurses to evidence care rather than deliver it.

This resonates with my experience as a medical student. Medical school curricula are lengthy and time on attachment brief. There is a culture that values gaining harder (more examinable) skills over spending unstructured time with patients. On the urology ward I was there to "do work" and became restless when distracted by an interaction with a patient. This encounter saw me value being with the patient free from agenda secondary to doing things.

Effort-laden

Another consideration is that spending time with patients with dementia can be effort-laden. Therefore, nurses might shy away from opportunities to communicate.

Goldsmith (1996) acknowledges that a caregiver must make a decision to provide "extra energy and input into the communication if it is to be a meaningful one" (p. 77). This marries with my experience with one particular patient:

> Stilted conversation. Extreme word-finding difficulties.

It saddening to learn how patients who are self-aware of the extra effort required to communicate might experience this as burdensome, as one patient shared: "People haven't got the time to talk to me now because it takes such a long time" (Goldsmith, 1996, p. 80). Such a feeling might compound any pre-existing experience of isolation or unwantedness.

Such encounters can be also be abasing. Goldsmith comments on the 'humbling' effects of interaction with some persons with dementia by drawing us "into a world in which we recognise the limitations of our own power" (p. 10). I share this sentiment, recalling the awkwardness and embarrassment when I lacked the tools required to really understand a patient's reality:

> Took a seat next to a coffee table and a patient in a wheelchair wearing a flat cap who makes 'blahblahblah' noises. I'm unsure whether it is meaningful.

We hope that the training and expertise of all healthcare workers equips them with tools necessary to enjoy spending time with patients with communication difficulties. However, observation of people in the staffroom or leaving the hospital on break demonstrates that time spent with patients is in some way more effortful or less enjoyable than the company of themselves or other workers.

Social defence mechanism

A third explanation for the amount of time nurses appeared occupied with tasks is offered by Menzies Lyth (1959). She conducted an empirical study of the nursing service of a large general hospital. She noted that the nursing role demanded repeated exposure to "people who are physically ill or injured" leading to "high levels of tension, distress and anxiety" (p. 439). In response to these anxieties, unconscious defences shield staff from emotional trauma. Some of these defence mechanisms are initiated by the individual (including dropping out of training, frequent changes of job, sick leave) whereas others were initiated by the system (excessive movement of nurses, insufficient staff, threat of crisis).

One of these social defence mechanisms includes "the attempt to eliminate decisions by ritual task-performance". Menzies Lyth observed student nurses ritually committing to tasks despite it not being "objectively necessary" (p. 446). She theorised that deference to task lessened anxiety by removing the number and variety of decisions affecting patient welfare out the sphere of individual responsibility.

In considering the root of these anxieties Menzies Lyth mentions the psychodynamic tensions between life-giving and death-giving phantasies experienced as an infant. Being involved with the suffering of others gives humans a painful reminder of their own mortality. We devise social strategies to deny or avoid these feelings.

Such theorising may be esoteric but the idea of caregivers establishing defence mechanisms in response to emotional trauma is quite widespread (Weil, 1951, p. 67). One contributor to Goldsmith disregards excuses of lack of time as a "greatly over-used excuse" by some nurses who "appear to feel safer if not involved with the feelings and needs of the client with dementia (Goldsmith, 1996, p. 80). Dunham & Cannon (2008) suggest "caregivers do not intend to be malicious"; however they "adopt these strategies because they are often overwhelmed by the demands of the disease" (p. 46).

An example of this was my experience of a nurse squirting foul-tasting medication into a patient's mouth whilst in the middle of his dinner:

> "Open up, Frank!" Horrible. Feel embarrassed, ashamed.

Such detached efficiency could be seen by Menzies Lyth as a picture of a nurse so allegiant to task that the patient is morphed into a means by which to complete the drug round.

As an observer I witnessed staff committed to doing tasks. A motivation for this might be subconscious defence mechanisms obviating anxieties associated with exposure to the infirm. I write aware that feelings aroused in me when spending time with patients with dementia could be colouring my thoughts about the motivations of others. However Menzies Lyth's study looked at over 500 nurses, 150 of whom were speciality trained, so even the most experienced healthcare worker is not immune to powerful emotional impulses. The observer cannot say whether it was staff on the ground or higher forces that expressed preference for 'doing' – it may well be that nurses deferred to task against their will.

Malignant positioning

The final explanation draws on the theory of malignant positioning (Sabat, 2006) which associates the "primary social personae" of persons with dementia as that of "patient" (p. 271). As a result, persons are positioned as inferior and their ability to meaningfully communicate diminished. Key to this process is negative stigmata of dementia and lessened value of interaction. Therefore opportunities for connection with patients are overlooked. Through this Sabat describes how the diagnosis of dementia "sets the stage" (p. 289), with potentially meaningful behaviour disregarded.

I realised I was guilty of this process overtly:

> One patient paces up and down the ward every fifteen minutes or so . . . He's done this every day since I have been here. I've lumped this into the "crazy" category. This is some repetitive action explained by dementia. I ask the nurse why he does that. "To keep fit . . . he used to be a physiotherapist."

And implicitly:

> On the way from the lounge to the staffroom a softly spoken man asks me for the time. He apologies for his short term memory problems. "How is your observation going?" he asks. This pleasantly surprises me. I should have more faith.

Following on from this Sabat argues that this positioning opens the door for malignant social psychology. Malignant social psychology describes social processes that compound symptoms of dementia by encouraging the creation of narratives that confirm the initial positioning (Kitwood, 1998, p. 46). An example is the objectification of the person. This was witnessed when the care of someone was discussed in close proximity to another patient:

> A relative goes up to one of the nurses to share his concern about why his relative [is] sleeping so much. They discuss him and the other patients almost directly over Bob, who is slumped in a chair in between them.

Other examples included infantilisation. For example, during the tea round:

NURSE: "Do you want a plain or chocolate biscuit?"
PATIENT: "Chocolate one."
NURSE: "Chocolate one? I'll give you one of each, ey?"

And ignoring:

> Patients come and tap on the window. Doors shut in their face. They avoid eye contact.

Additionally I noticed staff's preoccupation with quelling 'challenging behaviours' (for example, shouting, swearing, aggression and wandering). Staff made a case for these behaviours presenting a threat to the wellbeing of the person with dementia and other patients on the ward. In many ways this is fair. For example, when a patient wanders there is a risk that he or she might fall.

However there is much to be said for challenging behaviour representing a valid response to the way the world might be perceived by the individual. Hussain (1982) revealed that 93% of all wandering journeys seem to lead to a logical destination. This understands challenging behaviour as something we (healthcare workers, relatives etc.) are challenged by and not as something that is inherently challenging. Patients "attract labels like difficult or noncompliant" that confirm the "hidden bias of their helpers". Patients who are "happy and quiet" are rewarded with benign paternalism from staff, whereas those presenting "challenging behaviours" are deemed "naughty" or "doing it on purpose" (Goldsmith, 1996, p. 38).

I noticed how nurse preference for passivity could be seen as serving the emotional wellbeing of staff, not patients. For example, plying patients with hot drinks:

> Sitting down, drowning patients in tea, coffee, biscuits.

And the insistence on sitting:

PATIENT: "When is my daughter getting here?"
NURSE: "Around quarter past one."
PATIENT: "Am I just supposed to sit here?"
NURSE: "Yes, you sit there."

This idea echoes Main (1957) writing on the use of sedatives in hospital "only at the moment when [the nurse] had reached the limit of her human resources and was no longer able to stand the patient's problems without anxiety, impatience, guilt, anger, or despair" (p. 130). His comment that "it was always the patient and never the nurse who took the sedative" (p. 130) reflects the almost prescription-like administration of hot drinks and biscuits at times of turbulence or distress.

Nurses spending so much time away from patients can be explained by disregarding the need for interaction secondary to malignant positioning. Important to this understanding is the guilt associated with my own positioning of patients that began almost immediately as I arrived on the ward. As a result of this positioning examples of malignant social psychology were observed. Of particular note was the prescription of pseudo-sedative measures in an effort to tolerate the anxiety evoked by challenging behaviours.

Conclusions

The aim of this project was for me to gain insight into the feelings evoked when interacting with patients with dementia. Suspicion about the acceptability of my emotions pushed me to investigate their origins in a bid to improve my understanding of both patients and myself.

I undertook a short series of observations in a dementia ward. The result was an experience of two major feeling states: unwantedness and connection. The feeling of connection came about through interaction with healthcare workers. A feeling of unwantedness arose when health workers appeared task-orientated. I thought about this 'unwantedness' in an effort to understand why the ward left patients lacking a feeling of connection. Reasons cited were shortage of time and difficulties in finding the effort required to spend time with persons with communication problems. I also explored the role of social defence mechanisms lessening anxiety experienced by confrontation with suffering, and staff distancing patients by way of malignant positioning.

My experience in urology involved a difficult interaction with a patient with dementia. I experienced feelings of resentment and abasement. Intrinsic to the arousal of these feelings was my preference to engage in tasks on the ward and limit time spent with patients. The observations I later undertook allowed me to gain the view of both the patient and the healthcare provider. Contrasting these viewpoints enabled me to speculate on why caregivers ostensibly preferred task completion to patient contact. I offered two groups of reasons: pragmatic and subconscious.

Pragmatic issues of poverty of time and communication difficulties reduce patient contact. As a patient I experienced unwantedness yet as a healthcare professional I was ignorant of this unmet need. Despite me *knowing* that patients might be yearning for connection I was disinclined to offer it. This disinclination cannot be explained by pragmatics alone – tasks need to be done but not at the cost of placating suffering. Efforts to obviate emotional grief manifested as preoccupation with tasks. I was also guilty of employing distancing strategies and witnessed examples of malignant positioning.

In short, unconscious processes drive healthcare professionals' distance from patients in a way that is not sufficiently considered and influence our behaviour more than we care to realise.

Final thoughts

This project taught me a great deal, most of which has not come in the form of tidy conclusions.

Taking on the role of patient has taught me the value of human connection. I experienced a profound feeling state of unwantedness; a need only quenched by genuine human interaction. One of the most powerful insights into the value of this connection was through regular time spent with one of the patients on the dementia ward. I will share that here.

The man was an ex-factory worker in his mid-sixties. He suffered dementia as a result of both alcohol misuse and previous strokes. In addition to hemiplegia, his most striking symptom was expressive dysphasia. In spite of his best efforts, he could not express much of what he tried to say. Over the week I spent time at lunch helping him with his meal and discussing his life.

Initially conversation was limited to "ayes" and shakes of the head. He was frequently frustrated, quickly ending efforts to answer questions with dejected sighs. I was nervous, stuck for conversation, finding it difficult to balance helping a dependent adult while not babying him. Over time I became more relaxed. A bond developed. By the end of the week we were laughing over stories shared. Remarkably his dysphasia seemed less and his self-expression improved. Now he was able to speak short sentences and react to things happening around him. One time I spilled soup on his lap, he responded: "You're not very good at this, are you?" He had more lucid moments, as if for a few seconds he was dementia-free. One of these came through reflection on a life well lived: "I have no regrets. Absolutely none. Why regret when you can live?"

It is reassuring to know that quality time spent with a patient – listening, sharing, encouraging, laughing, holding – can be demonstrably healing. For this man his symptoms were relieved before my eyes. This and the lessons learned make me confident that future practice will see me less likely to fall back on excuses of time, instead trusting its value as a healer.

I am pleased to state that dementia no longer frightens me (as much). I used to feel distance when faced with a disease I believed robbed the person of so much. Now I enjoy a calm curiosity to understand the person behind a condition that leaves far more than it takes away.

References

Davenhill, R. (2007). Assessment. In R. Davenhill (ed.) *Looking Into Later Life: A Psychoanalytic Approach to Depression and Dementia in Old Age*. London: Karnac, 50–61.

Donaldson, C., Tarrier, N., and Burns, A. (1998). Determinants of carer stress in Alzheimer's disease. *International Journal of Geriatric Psychiatry*, 13, 248–256.

Dunham, C.C., and Cannon, J.H. (2008). They're still in control enough to be in control: Paradox of power in dementia caregiving. *Journal of Aging Studies*, 22, 45–53.

Goldsmith, M. (1996). *Hearing the Voice of People With Dementia: Opportunities and Obstacles*. London: Jessica Kingsley.

Hussain, R. (1982). Stimulus control in the modification of problematic behaviour in elderly institutionalized patients. *International Journal of Behavioural Geriatrics*, 1, 33–42.

Jones, G. (1992). A communication model for dementia. In G. Jones and B.M.L. Miesen (eds.) *Care Giving In Dementia: Volume 1 Research and Applications*. London: Tavistock/Routledge.

Kitwood, T. (1998). *Dementia Reconsidered: The Person Comes First*. Buckingham: Open University Press.

Kontos, P.C., and Naglie, G. (2007). Bridging theory and practice: Imagination, the body, and person-centred dementia care. *Dementia*, 6, 549–569.

Main, T.F. (1957). The ailment. *British Journal of Medical Psychology*, 30, 129–145.

Menzies, I.E.P. (1959). The functioning of social systems as a defence against anxiety: A report on a study of the nursing service of a general hospital. *Human Relations*, 13, 95–121. My source was a shortened version of the original paper. Find at www.modern timesworkplace.com/archives/ericsess/sessvol1/Lythp439.opd.pdf [accessed 6 February 2015].

Sabat, S.R. (2006). Mind, meaning and personhood in dementia: The effects of positioning. In J.C. Hughes, S. Louw, and S.R. Sabat (eds.) *Dementia: Mind, Meaning and the Person*. Oxford: Oxford University Press, 287–302.

Shapiro, J. (2011). Does medical education promote professional alexithymia? A call for attending to the emotions of patients and self in medical training. *Academic Medicine*, 86, 326–332.

Weil, S. (1951). *Waiting on God*. London: Routledge and Kegan Paul Limited.

Chapter 2

Where lies the expert?

Jane Garner

I know nothing except the fact of my ignorance.

Socrates

The Oxford English Dictionary defines expert as a noun 'one whose special knowledge or skill causes him to be an authority' and as a verb 'to experience, to know by experience'. Experts have recently been belittled, notably by politicians campaigning during the build up to the Brexit referendum which resulted in Britain voting to leave the European Union. Perhaps the cult of the expert has collapsed with the populist backlash following the banking crisis of 2008 (Mallaby, 2016). The triumph of the expert is bound to be fragile unless knowledge keeps apace with the changing times. We live in a post-truth, alternative truth, false news world where facts and evidence apparently matter less than immediate feelings. Immediate feeling is important but often needs to be processed via the lens of evidence. This chapter will look at expertise in dementia. Does it lie with the patient, the family, the staff employed to care, the institutions or politicians? Is it possible to alter/manipulate the level of expertise wherever it lies? No one can know it all, what we wish to know may be unknowable. Life is uncertainty. 'Knowledge is proud that he has learned so much, wisdom is humble that he knows no more' William Cowper (1731–1800).

The word 'expert' has the same root as experience. Patient groups are pleased when we work with 'experts by experience'. Perhaps this takes on more importance and relevance in neuropsychiatric conditions where signs and symptoms affect all aspects of the person. The notion of the 'expert patient' was an initiative of the UK Department of Health (2001) reflecting trends in political philosophy, ethics and health service research. The hope was to change attitudes, expectations and practices in the care of patients with chronic illness so that they are encouraged to become more actively involved in decision making concerning their treatment to liberate them from 'medical paternalism'. Badcott (2005) suggests that the potential for success of the concept depends on whether the patient can be considered truly to be an expert and acceptance by the medical professions of a more equitable and positive role for patients. It tends to be about self-management of long-term conditions, models of peer support, physical illness and medication.

Even mental health research in this area is on improving the physical health of psychiatric patients via health action plans (Cormac et al., 2004). Edgar (2005) questions the Expert Patient Initiative – its over reliance on instrumental forms of reasoning. The patient is an expert in the hermeneutic sense – it is they who experience their illness. There can be a risk of confusing experience with expertise and it may not be possible to generalise this to others. Badcott (2005) wonders whether the notion is well meaning but a rather vacuous aspiration, Frank reminds us (1995/2013) that ill people are more than patients of medicine or victims of disease. They are wounded storytellers, telling stories to make sense of their suffering. Edgar (2005) drawing on Frank's work writes of narrative identity – part of who we are is also from stories, without them we feel fragmented. Illness may interrupt storytelling. These tales are culturally based but not dissimilar worldwide, perhaps due to our collective unconscious. Few stories are appropriate to the experience of chronic illness which may be a narrative of 'useless suffering' (Levinas, 1988). The tale of a battle is often invoked. It may be that the idea of an expert patient – a knight in the battle – encourages this.

Shared decision making is widely recommended as a way to support patients in making healthcare choices. Older patients tend to have multimorbidities, because of that and the progressive nature of a dementia, continuity of dialogue is required between professional and patient (Van de Pol et al., 2016). Professionals are accustomed to applying a biomedical, disease-oriented approach to care, patients request a person-centred approach. Expertise will be within the relationship. The patient may contribute as an expert in a number of ways. They are an expert in their own life story and the experience of the effect of the illness in their life.

Individuality

The diagnosis 'dementia' sounds unitary but each presentation is different. There may be different cognitive difficulties. Each patient brings their own unique history of previous experience of a dementing illness in a family member or friend or from the newspaper, previous experience of ill-health and of loss and their own life history, previous and current relationships and sociocultural situation. The diagnostic process may take longer than the patient expected. If pre-diagnostic counselling is available it may be helpful to explore fears, possible outcomes and implications, beliefs about dementia, and available psychological coping mechanisms. This may reduce 'shock' and facilitate some adjustment. Being given the diagnosis, hearing the word 'dementia' has been described as a relief after months of worrying 'what could be wrong' but also a shock, a blow, not unlike stepping off a cliff edge. The patient will bring all their previous experience, self-knowledge, self-deception, weaknesses and strengths to the encounter. The extent of distress may not be expressed at the time. Dementia can be seen as a catastrophic loss, an archetype of loss of self and identity. Brown (2017) considers this to be due to conscious and unconscious focus on the later years of the illness , the dread of the endgame, which undermines abilities to think about and use the intervening years.

Dementia with its progressive, inevitable deterioration in memory, language and skills causes us to consider the meaning of personhood and identity. We may think about why the patient would maximise or minimise symptoms. Simone de Beauvoir poses the question 'can I have become a different person whilst remaining myself?' Hughes (2001) sees the person as a 'situated-embodied-agent'. We are 'situated' in a familial, cultural and historical context with lives as narrative and shape which contribute to our identity. 'Embodiment' adds to the narrative through bodily perceptions and experience giving a psychobiological shape and unity. The patient may expand the idea of 'I think therefore I am'. Bodily memories, skills, preferences and relationships do not deteriorate to the extent that higher thinking does. Affectivity is retained long after thinking is impaired; rituals and movement may prompt some recall; the ability to recognise far outlasts the ability to recall (Garner, 2004a). The person continues to experience. That experience/expertise is unlikely to be communicated verbally in the later stages. Nevertheless an emotional life continues albeit unverbalised. One may not recall the name of the nurse or doctor at the level of cognitive skill, but staff elicit different and consistent affective reactions: this is the one who is warm and comforting; this is the one who upsets me as my sister did. Autonomy may be retained for some decisions while being lost for others. Despite these losses, personhood is not lost. The essential self, the singular self, is not lost although the extra coverings of self have been assaulted. One may not be thinking well with a dementing illness or even thinking at all, nevertheless 'I am' until I die (Garner, 2004a) and the patient at some level will 'know' their identity.

There are some firsthand accounts of the illness. Oppenheimer (2006) notes that some people appear unaware of any important alteration in themselves although changes are obvious to close others, to themselves they feel like the person they always were. Other people are very aware and frightened of the change, no longer really at home in their own minds with a feeling that 'me' is under threat.

Davis (1989), writing from the perspective of someone with dementia, knows how to establish a routine, including vigorous exercise in order to function at the top of his albeit 'limited capacity'.

In considering the expert, the concept of brain compensation, neuroplasticity and drawing on personal psychological reserves is available for some. Books by patients give particular stories, sometimes with more general points and advice. Individual readers will find resonance with at least some the stories (Garner, 2007). Most of these books support evidence that affective memory outlives cognitive memory. Fleming et al. (1996) found improved memory for emotional material in people with Alzheimer's Disease. Studies after the Kobe earthquake in Japan (Ikeda et al., 1998) reinforce the idea that people with severe dementia can be reached affectively long after they cease to be reached cognitively (Williams and Garner, 1998). Kitwood (1990) in writing of the 'malignant social psychology' which surrounds people with dementia, recognises that often functioning is at a worse level than that determined by the dementia in response to the behaviour and attitude of others. A psychosocial environment which belittles and undermines the person with dementia causes mood and functioning to be at a lower level than would be if attitudes were different. Affective tone is recognised and responded to long after other abilities are lost. There can be a stereotyping of people with dementia, an expectation they will fail/function badly. The notion of 'person-hood' is now recognised as one of the most important advances in dementia care throughout the course of the illness. The key factor is the relationship with and attitude of others. Potentially meaningful behaviour is often disregarded because the patient has dementia. A man's sense of his identity as a person depends on communication with other persons.

Emotional factors

There is no linear relationship between brain pathology (for example seen on scans) and levels of ability. An organic aetiology is not in question but biopsy-chosociocultural factors interact to produce the presentation and experience of dementia. All those who work with patients are aware that anger can temporarily unlock a flow of language and memory. Similarly, a therapeutic intervention, giving a feeling of being understood, may integrate the memory if only for a moment. Emotionally caused impairment is open to change. Organic impairment needs to be recognised and mourning take place for injured brain cells and lost abilities (Sinason, 1992). Solms (1995) is concerned that in contemporary psychiatry 'the brain is more real than the mind'. It is easy to attribute everything about a patient with a dementing illness to organically based impairment, but in doing so one misses the complexity and subtlety of human experience and interaction as well as the opportunity for psychotherapeutic intervention. When seeing a patient with a dementing illness the emotional quality of the relationship between therapist and patient needs particular attention. Freud (1914) emphasised that what the patient does not remember will be repeated in the transference relationship. He was referring to patients with repressed memories, but the same seems true for those with cognitive impairment. The relationship is still used for communication (Garner, 2006). An emotional life continues without language. It is easy to dismiss the patients continuing abilities. Psychotherapists can learn to use words in the individual's personal vocabulary to retell the person's individual stories (Hausman, 1992). At a later stage in the disease the therapist can operate as an auxiliary ego to facilitate the recall of memories otherwise forgotten. Recognition of empathy in the interviewer/therapist seems to act as a cue to the individual to recall emotionally important material (Williams, 1997). The present is meaningful because of connections with the past. Childhood memories remain vivid (Evans, 2009). Perhaps this brings together an understanding of mind and brain. Emotional memory is a mid-brain function (Van der Kolk and McFarlane, 1996) rather than cortical and so is retained for longer. Ability to maintain relationships persists. Even though verbal skills and conscious memories may diminish, the emphasis of psychoanalytic understanding on the unconscious, on non-verbal communication via transference and countertransference makes it a particularly useful paradigm to use with someone with a dementia (Garner, 2013).

Degree of cognitive impairment has little correlation with quality of life. People can retain the capacity for joy and enjoyment. Some delight in memories recounted by others if they have failed to recall them themselves. The social environment needs to be conducive to fun, i.e. safe and inclusive. Humour with playfulness, laughter, amusement can be a way of dealing with the serious challenge of dementia (Grierson, 2008). Hope is central to well-being. False hope and false promises are unhelpful and may be cruel. Realistic hope maybe for a meaningful end rather than for a cure. Erikson (1977) places hope within a developmental context, learned in infancy and evolving throughout life.

Future care

It will be important for the patient to discuss future care while they still have mental capacity. They will be an expert at that moment but perhaps not subsequently, or at least not able to discuss it although they may expertly navigate dependency if early experience was good enough. Advance directives may be made, it raises the question of whether one can change one's mind later. 'Mother said she would never wear trousers but a now she seems to prefer them' etc. However it seems to be important to discuss and record future wishes and preferences for care (see chapter 4).

Life review and development

The diagnosis may introduce a process of reflection which may include future care and as often happens with age, looking back on the life one has led with its successes and regrets. Life review, life story work, reminiscence, thinking of different paths they could have taken all have a part to play in this reflection. Some have found in 'life writing' in a supportive group, assisted by psychology students and the writing course tutor, a way of expressing themselves, also thinking about their lives with the message that people are not defined by dementia. Dementia does not disqualify people from productive activity, from personal and psychological development. The group in Canterbury have produced a book of their writings *Welcome to Our World* (Saints, M.J. et al., 2014). The eight contributors have a wide breadth of life experience with working lives as barrister, editor, traveller, translator, lecturer, policeman, driving instructor, lifeboat volunteer, merchant navy sailor, headmaster, au pair, carpenter, fruit picker, antiques restorer. There was mention of being born a disappointing gender for the parent, disagreement with decisions made about oneself as a child, having siblings, early boy/girl relationships, meeting future spouses, childbirth, family relationships, grandparents and great grandparents, war time experiences, regrets at losing touch with others, medical and psychiatric history, being a student protestor, recalling England winning the World Cup, childhood delights and games, foreign travel and the lasting pleasure of holidays.

Dementia was mentioned in different ways; the diagnosis came as a relief; the diagnosis came as a shock; the diagnosis prompted the devising of a battle plan; the experience of living with dementia is 'not a life sentence'; the difference between the professional saying 'dementia' easily in contrast to the upset being the one to receive the word. All contributors were in agreement that you are much more in life than your dementia. Beyond the life stories and memories was expert advice about aspects of dementia, e.g. how to embark on foreign travel; coping with the upset of not driving while looking at the positive aspects of bus journeys. These contributors had a positive attitude to their future from the group and from their writing. There is a literature on 'Living Well with Dementia' (Bryden, 2005). In some ways this must be applauded but there is a danger in this idea, a 'polyannaism' with little emphasis on emotions but on tasks, on positive aspects, ignoring the negative and perhaps minimising the different experience and expertise of those who feel they cannot live up to such positivity. Aspects of the negative may help us all understand something of shame as an emotion when expertise is crushed. Kohut (1972) writes of the 'catastrophic reaction' when anxiety is too great for defences. For Kohut this is a narcissistic rage against the shame and humiliation regarding a defect in the self (in the expertise of the self). It is a fear of ridicule, the response to failure, the failure to live up to the ego ideal. It calls into question our preconceptions about ourselves, the humiliation of a deteriorating mind. Confabulation in this context maybe a way of protecting the self from shame. This is not lying. The patient may say 'Oh yes, I'll get the bus there'. The member of staff does not know whether they can. One day they may be able to, not the next. The bus stop may be closed/changed. They were experts in this, perhaps not now. This sort of conversation raises the question of truth-telling in dementia. How far should one enter this different reality, respecting both the truth and the patient?

A number of writers expand the idea of growth and development throughout life and the psychological tasks to be undertaken in old age (Garner, 2004b). Fromm (1955) tells us that 'The whole life of the individual is nothing but the process of giving birth to himself; indeed we should be fully born before we die'. The capacity for growth may increase with adversity. The unconscious does not necessarily participate in the process of growing older (Grotjahn, 1940). Problematic emotional constellations may not fade away. People with dementia are adults usually nearer the end of life, by which time they will be a long way through the evolutionary process of the life cycle. It may be possible to use expertise, resilience and creativity garnered over the decades to help and understand the self with the illness. If earlier conflicts have not been resolved it may be more distressing and agitating. For some there is existential terror of losing the idea of self. How one deals with old age and further dementia depends on whether persecutory anxiety or depression is to the fore (Hess, 2004; Garner, 2013).

Further expertise

In addition to being an expert in oneself, one's illness and one's emotional memories, in a therapeutic relationship there are other ways to contribute knowledge and expertise. Peer support is helpful. A group of other patients may be able to advise better than family or staff and the possibility for resentment towards those without dementia will be avoided. Although the voices of people with dementia are increasingly being heard, the user movement is still in its infancy. For some years the Faculty of Old Age Psychiatry of the Royal College of Psychiatrists has had a consumer group including patients with dementia (Ong et al., 2007). Being a representative of others going beyond 'what I need' to 'what we need' is a complex task for all and if insight and understanding are becoming problems it is even more difficult. Dementia Engagement and Empowerment Project (DEEP) is run by Innovations in Dementia, a community interest company. It goes beyond people's own stories and encourages them to think about services. DEEP groups usually have a non-demented facilitator but not all. Involvement at a local level is not just about being consulted but provides opportunities for people to shape their own agenda.

There is a need for mechanisms to support people with dementia to carry on contributing as needs and abilities change so that the voices of those with more advanced dementia can be heard (Brainwaves Sept, 2015). This will be dependent on the empathy of others. Expertise here will be accessible via the understanding of transference and countertransference.

People who stand up to speak at a conference, volunteer to teach students, volunteer to be the expert may have an atypical dementia with, for example, the preservation of language skills or of confidence and so they may lose credibility as a representative, 'can they be talking about me, they are not like me'. The Alzheimer's society Dementia Friendly Communities Programme focusses on improving inclusion and quality of life for people with dementia. For it to be useful it requires the involvement and ideas of many of those with dementia.

Family as expert

Beyond and around the person with dementia are others who may be considered when thinking about expertise to contribute. They will be mentioned briefly without forgetting that the person on their own with no spouse/important other can fall through the system. Partners, family and close friends may all have something to offer. Over 60% of people with a dementia continue to live in the community. Health and social policy is directed to home treatment because it is cheaper but there is little available for the couple (Balfour, 2014). Expertise will be primarily about the person due to the shared experience over the years before dementia. They will be able to give a valuable collateral history. They must be seen on their own. Some feel the need 'protect' the patient and so diminish their description of the signs and symptoms. Moniz-Cooke (2008) suggests this is to protect the self-image of their partner. It is often a balance between protection and the need for a diagnosis; later a balance between protection and independence. Expertise and energy is involved in this balance, walking this tightrope.

People have different experiences as a partner/carer in these circumstances. Some find sharing in a support group helpful both as a contributor and in receiving others' ideas. Some have written or spoken of their experiences. John Bayley (1997) gave an interview to the *Telegraph* on his wife, Iris Murdoch's progressive loss of memory from Alzheimer's Disease 'It is rather like falling from stair to stair in a series of bumps'. There can be great fear in thinking of a change in the relationship from wife/lover etc. to carer. Waddell (2007) writes a moving story of a family dealing with dementia in which son and daughter seem emotionally expert. When there is a window of clarity for the patient then emotional contact is made. Whether emotionally expert or not, carers need their stories to be heard (Benbow et al., 2009). Their narrative needs to be understood, to have meaning attached/included. If the carer is understood they will be more able to understand the one for whom they care. They experience the conscious problems and burden of caring/coping and the unconscious conflict stimulated by this role and situation. One of the main reactions in the partner is a sense of loss (Garner, 1997 and see chapter 5). The sense of pain, anger and loss may feel overwhelming. Loss is the price of attachment. Human factors of faith, hope and object constancy can mean that the lost object is not irretrievably lost and can be found in the inner world. The spouse may need psychotherapeutic help to regain/retrieve expertise in the midst of this loss. There is likely to be depression for what is lost and anxiety thinking about losses to come (Freud, 1917).

The family carer may have expertise and well-being enhanced by psychological intervention. Livingstone et al. (2014) showed an increase in clinical effectiveness, decrease in depression and anxiety, increase in quality of life and cost effectiveness at 8 months and again at 24 months using the START intervention (Strategies for Relatives). The relative needs understanding and meaning as well as more practical competence. Health workers are well aware that the anger and hostility associated with the grief of having a family member with dementia may be directed towards staff (Garner, 1997). Relatives will be expert in some areas but the guilt associated with needing help to care for the patient or with letting them be admitted to a long stay facility may cause relatives to be hypercritical of staff.

Staff as expert

The expert not only has examination success/credentials but also experience which is acknowledged by peers. Expertise is accrued not just by taking in data and mastering facts but also by assimilating information via teachers, mentors and peer review. Staff employed to care for patients with dementia between them will be knowledgeable in many areas: epidemiology, statistics, research methodology, genetics, radiology, neuropharmacology, sociology, psychology, human relationships etc. The staff should have access to a fund of knowledge, competence and the ability to assess 'evidence', but more particularly will have personal, psychological capacities. Individual staff need a nuanced understanding of the patient, of themselves, of colleagues and of the institution. Evans (1998) draws on the concept of malignant mirroring (Zinkin, 1983) to explain the poor services expected by and provided to older people: it reflects a psychopathology of diminishment and imperfection. Warmth is judged before competence. Warmth carries more weight in affective and behavioural reactions (Fisk et al., 2006). For example it is not helpful to undertake cognitive testing in a situation which feels as if it is pass/fail. The '*I' newspaper* (2014) wrote of the 'desperate shortage of support following insensitive consultations'. The professional needs to have such personal skills in communication that the patient does not feel worse following the appointment even if the news delivered is not altogether good.

Empathy and professional expertise

Medicine is a broad discipline, within it one can choose a specialism with more or less patient contact. Continuity of care is disappearing in the health service – seeing a different GP each time, juniors having patients scattered all over the hospital because of insufficient beds, the erosion of the 'firm' system. Reik (1948) wrote of 'listening with the third ear'. Intuitively one mind speaking to another, beyond words. Empathy has a cognitive/intellectual component and emotional empathy which leads to compassion. The only way to come anywhere near an understanding of what it may feel like to have a dementia is by close and empathic listening, fusing the horizons of physician and patient even when speech is failing. We underestimate the complexity of the inner life of the patient which can be drawn on for shared decision making. We must not 'mirror' the forgetting that occurs in the patient by assuming there is no activity remaining in the minds of people with dementia (Evans, 2008).

Training, modelling and supervision need also to be directed to the understanding of subjectivity, of an affective self (Yakeley et al., 2014). Managing your emotions is part of understanding human performance (Dawson, 2015). Delivering care is tiring and difficult work. Being cared for can be demeaning and infantilising. It is often easier for the staff to 'do' rather than to 'be'. It is necessary for the carer to have a non-judgemental, available mind to process, think and understand. The expert carer will have the capacity for containment (Bion, 1962), taking in and processing the experience of the patient then conveying back in a manageable, modified form. The carer needs to be able to bear 'not knowing' and to bear the painful reality of the experience (Sinason, 1992), in addition, to acknowledge that if the person is unwilling to accept care, not seeing themselves in need, that is a need in itself (Oppenheimer, 2006). and should be respected until risk in incapacity outweighs self-determination.

Expertise in wider politics

Beyond and above the patient, the family and the staff are the civil servants, the institutions and the politicians. We hear unempathic political dialogue. Post-modern promotion of self-reliance, competitiveness and the free market leaves little room for the chronic and multiple handicaps (including dementia) which accumulate for some in old age. We are frequently told that older people will overwhelm us with numbers and dependency. Some epidemiologists argue that current measures of population ageing are misleading and that the numbers of dependent older people have actually been falling (Spijker and MacInnes, 2013). Old people are seen as a group that 'takes' rather than individuals who have made life-long contributions. Despite an ongoing effort to create dementia-friendly communities, language at a personal level and in public discourse may contribute to the stigmatising of dementia. There is ageism even in global health policy (Lloyd-Sherlock, 2016). Institutional abuse of older adults, subtle and insidious, is widespread. Much of it occurs unwittingly (Garner and Evans, 2000). Guidelines are interpreted as tramlines/ rules, and insufficient attention is paid to the individual patient. The focus has been on numbers for early diagnosis, this has not been matched by attention to the need for post-diagnostic support (BPS, 2014). The politicians/department of health need to understand that staff are dealing with an increased complexity of care, enhanced patient/family expectations and that if NHS staff are not cared for, they will not be in a position to care for patients.

Conclusion

The expert has special knowledge or experience giving them authority. The patient brings into the consulting room social context, history, personal commitments, values and their self. They are an expert in these areas. People with dementia can share experience, knowledge and learning. They can effect change through collective action. While not necessarily remembering details of a meeting, they will remember how they were made to feel.

Staff and patients have more in common than usually thought. There is a giving and receiving both ways in the therapeutic relationship. Organic and psychogenic factors operate in us all. We struggle with the conscious manifestation of unconscious mental processes. Patients take into the senium and into dementia the strengths, internal resources and coping strategies they have used over the years. Staff need to be expert in the complex emotional state of each patient – the uniqueness of each that is retained in dementia. Although professionals are accustomed to applying a biomedical/disease-orientated approach to care, the more the patient is losing the capacity to think, the more the staff need to provide a thinking mind to process and understand this particular individual. The aim of all psychological interventions is to reduce emotional isolation. The person with dementia, also in the later stages, remains an emotional witness even when losing more concrete aspects of the expert. It is a privilege to enter people's lives, and care needs to be taken in the manner in which that is done. The staff 'expert' needs to be aware of their own emotional state and the extent of what they do not know. They need to care for individual patients and contribute positively to the culture of the unit/institution.

Politicians, too, need to set an empathic tone, be aware of the limitations of their knowledge and aware of their unconscious prejudice and bias. Welcome ideas, such as the 'Expert Patient', need to be carried through. It would seem from the Francis Report (2013) and the ongoing NHS difficulties that well-founded ideas fail without psychological understanding, moral strength and commitment. A further meaning of 'expert' is derived from 'ex' and 'pars' – having no part in. That position is too easy to take.

'Integrity without knowledge is weak and useless and knowledge without integrity is dangerous and dreadful' (Samuel Johnson, *Rasselas* [1759] chapter 41).

Acknowledgement

Some of the ideas in this chapter came from a conversation with Nada Savitch when she was a director of Innovations in Dementia.

References

Badcott, D. (2005). The expert patient: Valid recognition or false hope? *Medicine, Healthcare and Philosophy*, 8(2), 173–178.

Balfour, A. (2014). Developing therapeutic work in dementia care – The living together with dementia project. *Psychoanalytic Psychotherapy*, 28(3), 304–320.

Benbow, S., Ong, Y.L., Black, S., and Garner, J. (2009). Narratives in a users' and carers' group: Meanings and impact. *International Psychogeriatrics*, 21(1), 33–39.

Bion, W.R. (1962). *Learning From Experience*. London: Heinemann.

Brainwaves. (2015, September). *Innovations in Dementia*. Newsletter 90. www.innovationsindementia.org.uk/brainwaves

British Psychological Society. (2014). *Clinical Psychology in the Early Stage Dementia Care Pathway*. BPS Leicester.

Brown, J. (2016). Self and identity over time: Dementia. *Journal of Evaluative Clinical Practice*, vol 23(5), 1006–1012. http://doi.org/10.1111/jep.12643.

Bryden, C. (2005). *Dancing With Dementia*. London: Jessica Kingsley.

Cormac, I., Martin, D., and Ferriter, M. (2004). Improving the physical health of psychiatric patients. *Advances in Psychiatric Treatment*, 10(2), 107.

Cowper, W. (1785). *The Task, Book 6. The Winter's Walk at Noon 1. 96.*

Daily Telegraph. (1997). Interview with John Bayley, 8 February.

Davis, R. (1989). *My Journey Into Alzheimer's Disease: Healthful Insights for Family and Friends*. Wheaton, IL: Tyndale House.

Dawson, S. (2015). Human performance and medical error. *MPS Casebook*, 23(1), 6–7.

Dept. of Health. (2001). *The Expert Patient*. HMSO.

Edgar, A. (2005). The expert patient: Illness as Practice. *Medicine, Healthcare and Philosophy*, 8(2), 165–171.

Erikson, E. (1977). *Childhood and Society*. London: Paladine.

Evans, S. (1998). Beyond the mirror: A group analytic exploration of late life and depression. *Ageing and Mental Health*, 2, 94–99.

Evans, S. (2008). Beyond forgetfulness: How psychoanalytic ideas can help us to understand the experience of patients with dementia. *Psychoanalytic Psychotherapy*, 22(3), 155–176.

Evans, S. (2009). Where is the unconscious in dementia? In R. Doctor and R. Lucas (eds.) *The Organic and the Ivnner World*. London: Karnac.

Fisk, S.T., Cuddy, A., and Glick, P. (2006). Universal dimensions of social cognition: Warmth and competence. *Trends, Cognitive Science*, 11, 77–83.

Fleming, K., Maguire, G., Kim, S., et al. (1996). Memory for emotional stimuli in patients with Alzheimer's disease. *Alzheimer's Disease Clinical Abstracts*, 1, 8.

The Francis Report: Report of the Mid-Staffordshire NHS Foundation Trust Public Inquiry (2013) London HMSO.

Frank, A.W. (2013). *The Wounded Storyteller: Body, Illness and Ethics*, 4th ed. Chicago: University of Chicago Press.

Freud, S. (1914). Remembering, Repeating and Working Through. (Further Recommendations on the Technique of Psychoanalysis II). In J. Strachey (ed.) *SE XII*. London: Hogarth Press, 145–156.

Freud, S. (1917). Mourning and melancholia. In *SE XIV*. London: Hogarth Press.

Fromm, E. (1955). *The Sane Society*. New York: Fawcett Prier Books.

Garner, J. (1997). Dementia: an intimate death. *British Journal of Medical Psychology* 70, 177–184.

Garner, J. (2004a). Dementia. In S. Evans and J. Garner (eds.) *Talking Over the Years: A Handbook of Dynamic Psychotherapy With Older Adults*. Hove: Brunner-Routledge.

Garner, J. (2004b). Growing into old age. In S. Evans and J. Garner (eds.) *Talking Over the Years: A Handbook of Dynamic Psychotherapy With Older Adults*. Hove: Brunner-Routledge.

Garner, J. (2004c). Identity and Alzheimer's disease. In G. Leavey and D. Kelleher (eds.) *Identity and Health*. Hove: Brunner-Routledge.

Garner, J. (2006). Psychotherapy with older adults. In S. Bloch (ed.) *An Introduction to the Psychotherapies*, 4th ed. Oxford: Oxford University Press.

Garner, J. (2007). Reading about self-help books on dementia. *Psychiatric Bulletin*, 31(3), 118–119.

Garner, J. (2013). Psychodynamic psychotherapy. In T. Dening and A. Thomas (eds.) *Oxford Textbook of Old Age Psychiatry*. Oxford: Oxford University Press, 247–257.

Garner, J., and Evans, S. (2000). *Institutional Abuse of Older Adults*. London: RCPsychs.

Grierson, J. (2008). *Knickers in the Fridge*. Gt Britain: Lulu www.lulu.com (Print on demand).

Grotjahn, M. (1940). Psychoanalytic investigation of a seventy-one year old man with senile dementia. *Psychoanalytic Quarterly*, 9, 80–87.

Hausman, C. (1992). Dynamic psychotherapy with elderly demented patients. In S.G. Jones and B. Miesen (eds.) *Care Giving in Dementia*. London: Tavistock/Routledge, 181–198.

Hess, N. (2004). Loneliness in old age: Klein and others. In S. Evans and J. Garner (eds.) *Talking Over the Years: A Handbook of Dynamic Psychotherapy With Older Adults*. Hove: Brunner-Routledge.

Hughes, J.C. (2001). Views of the person with dementia. *Journal of Medical Ethics*, 27, 86–91.

Ikeda, M., Mori, E., Hirono, N., et al. (1998). Amnestic people with Alzheimer's disease who remembered the Kobe earthquake. *British Journal of Psychiatry*, 172, 425–428.

'I' Newspaper. (2014). Insensitive consultations. 2 July

Johnson, S. (1759). *The History of Rasselas; Prince of Abyssinia*. Printed by R. & J. Dodsley & W. Johnston. Now https://openlibrary.org/works/OL14862722W

Kitwood, T. (1990). The dialectics of dementia: With particular reference to Alzheimer's disease. *Ageing and Society*, 10, 177–196.

Kitwood, T. (1997). *Dementia Reconsidered: The Person Comes First*. Buckingham: Oxford University Press.

Kohut, H. (1972). Thoughts on narcissism and narcissistic rage in the search for the self. *Psychoanalytic Study of the Child*, 27, 360–400.

Levinas, E. (1988). Useless suffering in Bernasconi & Wood Eds *The Provocation of Levinas: Rethinking the Other*. Routledge, London, 156–67.

Livingstone, G., Barber, J., Rapaport, P., Knapp, M., et al. (2014). Long-term clinical and cost-effectiveness of psychological intervention for family carers of people with dementia: A single-blind, randomised, controlled trial. *The Lancet Psychiatry*, 1, 7.

Lloyd-Sherlock, P.G., Ebrahim, S., and McKee, M. (2016). Institutional ageism in global health policy. *British Medical Journal*, 354: i4514.

Mallaby, S. (2016, October 20). Cult of the expert and how it collapsed. *The Guardian*.

Moniz-Cooke, E. (2008). Assessment and psychological intervention for older people with suspected dementia: A memory clinic handbook perspective. In K. Laidlaw and B. Knight (eds.) *Handbook of Emotional Disorders in Later Life: Assessment and Treatment*. Oxford: Oxford University Press, 424–450.

Ong, Y.L., Benbow, S., Black, S., and Garner, J. (2007). Reflections on experience of involving users and carers in the work of the Faculty of Old Age Psychiatry. *Quality in Ageing – Policy, Practice and Research*, 8(2), 45–49.

Oppenheimer, C. (2006). I am: Thou art: Personal identity in dementia. In J. Hughes, S.J. Louw, and S.R. Sabat (eds.) *Dementia, Mind, Meaning and Person*. Oxford: Oxford University Press.

Reik, T. (1948). *Listening With the Third Ear: The Inner Experience of a Psychoanalyst*. New York: Grove Press.

Saints, M.J., De Frene, B., Jennings, L. (2014). *Welcome to Our World: A Collection of Life Writing by People Living with Dementia*. Canterbury: Forget-Me-Nots.

Sinason, V. (1992). The man who was losing his brain. In *Mental Handicap and the Human Condition: New Approaches From the Tavistock*. London: Free Association Books, 87–100.

Solms, M. (1995). Is the brain more real than the mind? *Psychoanalytic Psychotherapy*, 9(2), 107–120.

Spijker, J., and MacInnes, J. (2013). Population ageing: The time bomb that isn't? *BMJ*, 347, 20–22.

Van der Kolk, B.A. and McFarlane, A.C. (1996). The black hole of trauma. In: van der Kolk, B.A., MacFarlane, A.C., and Weisaeth, L. (eds) *Traumatic stress: the effects of overwhelming experience on mind, body and society*, 2–23. Guilford Press, New York.

van de Pol, M., Fluit, C., Lagro, J., et al. (2016). Expert and patient consensus on a dynamic model for shared decision making in frail older patients. *Patient Education and Counselling*, 99, 1069–1077.

Waddell, M. (2007). Only connect. In R. Davenhill (ed.) *Looking in to Later Life: A Psychoanalytic Approach to Depression and Dementia in Old Age*. The Tavistock Clinic Series. London: Karnac, 187–200.

Williams, D.D.R. (1997). The psychiatric interview: A different approach in the elderly. *Old Age Psychiatrist*, 7, 4.

Williams, D.D.R., and Garner, J. (1998). People with dementia can remember. *British Journal of Psychiatry*, 172, 379–380.

Yakeley, J., Hale, R., Johnston, J., Kirtchuk, G., and Shoenberg, P. (2014). Psychiatry, subjectivity and emotion – Deepening the medical model. *Psychiatric Bulletin*, 38(3), 97–101.

Zinkin, L. (1983). Malignant mirroring. *Group Analysis*, XVI, 113–126.

Chapter 3

Working with people with mild neurocognitive disorders (mild NCD) or mild cognitive impairments (MCI)

Julia C. Segal

> *Two elderly couples are chatting. One of the men says: "We went to a great restaurant last night." "What's it called?" asked his pal. He racks his brain, then he says: "What's that red flower you give to someone you love?" "A rose," his mate says. "Rose," calls the man, "what's the name of that restaurant we went to last night?"*
>
> *http://hahas.co.uk/alzheimers/*

We joke about memory loss, particularly as we get older and find ourselves having an increasing number of 'senior moments', but this joking is a response to real anxieties and real fear of future losses, not only for ourselves but also for those we love or care about. This chapter is about the work of psychodynamic counsellors or psychotherapists in the context of mild neurocognitive disorders or mild cognitive impairments.

Plan

To give context I look briefly at the literature about mild neurocognitive disorders (NCD), classified before 2015 as mild cognitive impairment (MCI). My main focus, however, is the experience of working with this group of people. Until fairly recently it was considered suspect to try to work with anyone who had any kind of cognitive problems: could they give 'informed consent', and was counselling a 'treatment' which required it? Freud famously considered anyone over 50 too old for psychoanalysis: Hanna Segal, working in the 1950s with a man of 73 (Segal H.M. 1958 and 1981, pp. 173–182) successfully challenged this assumption. In the 1980s and 1990s counsellors and psychotherapists exploring the possibilities and limits of their work found they could work effectively with people who had cognitive problems, even of a fairly severe kind, as reported for example by Sinason (1992, pp. 87–110), Segal J.C (2013) and Segal J.C. et al. (2010). This chapter is intended to encourage others to explore further.

Definition

In the DSM V (2015), diagnosis of mild neurocognitive disorder requires evidence of a modest decline from a previous level of performance in one or more cognitive domains. DSM-IV in 1994 distinguished mild cognitive impairment (MCI) from more serious dementias and opened up discussion about exactly what it meant, particularly in terms of prognosis towards dementia. DSM-V focussed on concern about cognitive capacities (whether the patient's, or someone else's), although objective measures were also advised. In addition, for the condition to be 'mild' it 'should not interfere with capacity for independence in everyday activities'.

The idea that 'independence' is an appropriate aim in the context of rehabilitation has been challenged by those who argue that 'interdependence' or 'mature adult dependence' are more appropriate goals for any adult who wishes to remain in a relationship, not only those with any kind of disability (e.g. Segal J.C., 2001). In terms of psychotherapeutic aims and concerns, this distinction can be important.

Epidemiology

Estimates of the prevalence of mild NCD in the USA range from 2% to 10% at age 65 and 5% to 25% by age 85, with greater prevalence amongst those who live in institutions (DSM-5, 2015). With a global prevalence rate estimated at around 6% (Sachdev et al., 2015), there are many possible underlying causes, including drug or alcohol abuse, medications and physical conditions including traumatic brain injury, hypertension, Parkinson's and multiple sclerosis. In spite of the new retroviral treatments, around 25% of people diagnosed with HIV still have fluctuating symptoms of mild NCD, although only 5% reach criteria for major NCD (DSM-V). An NHS booklet for General Practitioners (Barrett and Burns, 2014) suggests that around one third of people presenting with MCI improve, one third stay the same and one third go on to develop dementia of one kind or another. Prognosis and the meaning of symptoms for the future often concern clients and their families.

Co-morbidity

Unsurprisingly, depression and anxiety are common amongst those with changes in their cognitive capacities. Orgeta et al. (2015) looking at people with MCI found rates of depression between 36% and 63% and anxiety rates from 10% to 74%. They point out:

> Anxiety and depression have a substantial impact on outcomes as they decrease the ability to live independently, increase the risk of institutionalisation and result in higher caregiver burden. In people with MCI, early symptoms of depression can often be resistant to antidepressants, whereas both

depression and anxiety have been found to predict higher rates of progression to Alzheimer's disease.

(p. 293)

Cognitive problems may be more evident in the presence of depression, but it is not simple to differentiate clearly between depression, appropriate grieving responses to a loss (either current or anticipated) and symptoms of neurological impairment. In addition, it is unclear what part might be played by physical changes to the brain or the body in creating symptoms of depression such as lethargy or hopelessness concurrently with cognitive changes. Anxiety too may arise as a consequence of physical effects of cardiac problems, whether detected consciously or unconsciously, which also cause some decline in cognitive capacity (Garfinkel and Critchley, 2015). Depression or anxiety may also be responses to conscious or unconscious awareness of the onset of more serious dementia. These inter-connections may play a significant part in therapy or counselling as clients attempt to sort out how much of their problems are intractable and deteriorating, and how much can improve. Often there are underlying fears about who is responsible or to be blamed for symptoms. 'If I could be more positive I wouldn't have these problems'; 'I know it's not her fault but . . .'; 'I always thought God would take care of me'. Although researchers sometimes express a hope that addressing depression or anxiety could hold back progression from MCI to dementia, and clients may hope or believe that this could be the case, there is little evidence in the literature to support such beliefs.

Medical model: treatments

Many medications for neurocognitive deficits have been trialled, with very limited success. Currently there is no cure, although increased social activities and exercise, improvements to a poor diet, changes to prescribed medication or drug use (particularly abstention if the NCD is related to excessive alcohol or other recreational drugs) may have a beneficial effect for some people; diagnosis and treatment of an underlying physical health condition may also help. Computer-based 'brain training' unfortunately has not been found to carry over from the specific domains into other activities (Barnes et al., 2009; Rapp et al., 2010). Although high blood pressure is correlated with MCI, reducing levels through medication seems to have less effect on cognition than life-style changes (Goldstein et al., 2013).

Although clinicians are beginning to recommend that depression and anxiety in people with dementia or other NCDs be treated, pharmacological treatments seem to be largely ineffective (Banerjee et al., 2011; Bains et al., 2002) and often accompanied by side effects. By contrast, Orgeta's review (2015) of psychological treatments found evidence that psychological treatments can help with depression and anxiety for people with MCI and dementia, with no reports of any adverse effects.

Psychodynamic counselling and psychotherapy in the context of MCI/mild NCD

If counselling depended entirely on cognition, it would make sense to seriously question the value of offering it to someone who is cognitively compromised.

However, neither counselling nor psychotherapy simply depend upon thinking and talking: nor are they 'treatments'. Both depend on the experience of emotional contact, person to person; it is this which can change the way someone feels about themselves in the world. Being present, offering emotional availability and focussed attention can be powerful means of entering into another's world, understanding and acknowledging anxieties and fears; recognising, witnessing and, in some real, comforting sense 'knowing' the other – and in the process, perhaps, enabling the other person to regain contact with important, perhaps neglected, aspects of themselves. Words are one means to this end, but we communicate in many other ways, from the moment we are born until the moment we die.

Although communication itself may be under threat from cognitive deterioration, losses are piecemeal and much useful capacity remains even while some abilities are reduced or lost. In addition, counsellors and psychotherapists normally work with non-verbal as well as verbal communication and may be able to use their skills and time to make contact when others have lost patience. In a longer-term relationship, gesture may be sufficient to evoke certain shared knowledge and understanding.

The author has to confess that this was not clear to her until after she had begun offering counselling to people attending a multiple sclerosis clinic, which included those who were clearly compromised in some cognitive domains. It was here that she discovered that not only clients but also carers could value the contribution of counselling in helping people to live with mild (or less mild) neurocognitive deficits. Later, when working with people who had other neurological conditions, it became even more clear that, in spite of sometimes quite serious cognitive impairment in some areas, other areas of the mind can remain available. Families are sometimes aware of this: they see a member of the family who appears barely able to function at home, yet is apparently capable of keeping down a job. Different areas of the mind may be tapped by different tasks and different relationships, and psychodynamic work can benefit from this too.

Beatrice Allegranti (2016) writes about an educational film for people affected by dementia that 'aims to highlight embodied awareness and understanding of how to engage with and re-build the often fractured intimacy of relationships with self and others that can occur with the onset and development of dementia'. Even mild cognitive problems can give rise to 'fractured intimacy' and a sense of people 'losing touch' with each other, which can be addressed in counselling or psychotherapy.

What does psychodynamic counselling/ psychotherapy offer families affected by mild NCD?

Psychodynamic therapies work with meaning, with understanding and with the emotional contact of a one-to-one relationship. Mirroring our first relationships in this way, they offer a period of time in which attention is focussed on the individual and their relationships with others and with themselves.

The symptoms of neurocognitive disorders may be discussed in counselling or therapy. Observing and thinking about the true current impact of a cognitive deficit is not easy, coloured as it is by emotions, by memories, by fears and unrealistic assumptions. Other issues very quickly arise. There may be fears for the individual's own future, including the part they play in the lives of those they care for and who care for them. Past relationships may be evoked, with others in the family who suffered dementias, perhaps. With deteriorating memory and cognition, both speech and communication change; the past may come to play a bigger part in consciousness and different aspects of the personality, maybe buried for many years, emerge and challenge current, long-held assumptions. Racism, sexism or intellectual snobbery may appear in someone who held such attitudes in check throughout their adult lives. The balance of power within the family is altered, and possessions, home, living and sleeping arrangements, everything which made up a life worth living, may all be at risk. Anxieties about such issues can be difficult to share: the safety and confidentiality of a therapy session may be vital for allowing thoughts to be brought to a conclusion rather than (as turns out often to have been the case) truncated at their most disturbing point.

There are many specific ways in which psychodynamic thinking can help those affected by mild NCD, some of which I now consider separately.

Loneliness

Family members are not always aware of mild cognitive impairments, partly because they may be covered up. If people do become aware of some anomaly in a conversation, they may hesitate to mention it, and may find themselves cutting visits short. Gradually the person concerned may feel (or be) 'cut off'. Admitting to some kind of difficulty, or having it noticed, inevitably changes the way other people perceive someone and behave towards them. Hiding problems, however, brings loneliness, experienced often by partners as well as the person with mild NCD themselves. Sharing anxieties about dementia and 'losing their marbles' with a therapist, whose behaviour would not be altered as a consequence, reduces some of the loneliness – and may help facilitate appropriate sharing with others.

Normal feelings about loneliness in old age, or about losing people who matter, can be exacerbated by (realistic or unrealistic) fears that loss of cognitive capacities means loss of social status, rejection or abandonment (Segal J.C., 2017 discusses this in chapter 8); in addition, there are more psychological anxieties to do with an inner loneliness which can arise when memory begins to fail and past events and people can no longer be evoked at will. A counsellor or psychotherapist, interested in making real emotional contact, can help to reduce some of these anxieties. In addition, if memory is becoming unreliable, it may be particularly important that someone else is capable of holding onto memories which come and go: sometimes what needs remembering involves sensitive feelings or thoughts or events from the past (such as an abortion or child abuse) which are not willingly shared with current family members. When memories become muddled with dreams or hallucinations from periods of serious illness, access to another mind that knows the difference may also be valued.

Tolerating awareness of loss

Tolerating awareness of loss can be a huge problem in any health condition (cf. Segal J.C., 2017 Chapter 1.) Often people will fight to maintain 'normal' relations, taking no account of cognitive problems, in order to put off the moment when awareness is forced upon them. Recognition which would have practical as well as psychological consequences can be resisted, often with accusations which carry some of the anger that might more appropriately be directed at the fact of having to make changes. 'He only remembers what he wants to remember!' protects against the thought that the ability to remember or forget is now quite capricious – and that this has real consequences. 'He meant to make me feel bad'. 'She wet the bed on purpose, she knew I was in a hurry this morning and she wanted to keep me'. There are plenty of highly emotional interpretations which can be applied to behaviour that is influenced by cognitive deficits. Difficulties in following a conversation may be interpreted as aloofness or distraction or lack of interest. Failing to remember a medical appointment may signify 'ordinary' ambivalence about seeing the doctor; forgetting a partner's health problem may be a sign of lack of consideration. Sometimes these interpretations may be true: perhaps the man did allow himself to fall so that someone would have to help him off the floor. Shouting at someone who has missed something seems more natural than recognising that they are losing their sharpness for reasons which are uncomfortable to acknowledge: anyway, it might 'wake them up'. Such shouting (or hitting or punishing in some other way) can be followed by guilt, perhaps of a kind which allows someone to apologise, but often of a persecutory kind which makes everything worse.

Understanding the ways and the reasons why people avoid recognising the reality of loss (afraid it perhaps means: 'If my mother, the bedrock of my existence, can no longer join a normal conversation she is lost to me forever') can help to mitigate abuse of one kind or another. Some families may eventually reach these ideas themselves, but help from a professional can ease this process and reduce the damage caused along the way.

Handling changes

Once changes have been recognised, difficult questions are raised. How serious is this? Is it normal, temporary, long term? Is it 'just them', perhaps reacting to growing old or to a bereavement or to physical deterioration? Is it 'madness', 'losing it' or deliberate awkwardness? Is it the medication, or is it an illness? Emotions may not be far from the surface, confusing and biasing interpretations. Even sarcasm or mockery, if part of the liveliness of the deteriorating mind, may be missed. A mother suddenly becoming a 'sweet little old lady' from one visit to another may leave her daughter feeling bereft of the caustic, sharp voice she grew up with; and perhaps a little scared of her own ambivalence, if she now has power over her mother's life.

There are also decisions to be made. At what point does one let the children or professionals know? Will they interfere, take away a life which is still (just) manageable? Will they impose controls, lock doors, take away the key? Once others know, there is no going back. But while they do not know, other people may make painful assumptions: 'Why don't you make more effort to visit? Don't you care about us?' or 'What do you do all day? You are lucky to have time to yourself, I don't', which may be very hard for a carer who spends the day covering up their partner's increasingly disabling loss of cognitive capacity. Talking to a professional may be easier than talking to a friend.

Understanding

People can feel very guilty (and angry) when they realise they have misinterpreted behaviour: guilt can then be denied and converted to accusation: 'it was your/ his fault, NOT MINE!' They can be taken by surprise by their own reactions to weakness: expecting kindness, they may find themselves being cruel; expecting affection, they may see only rejection – or vice versa. Character failings may be judged more harshly because any threat to life can bring to the fore primitive defences of splitting, denial and idealisation while weakening the capacity to hold two contradictory thoughts in mind at once, necessary for more subtle, complex judgements (Segal J.C., 2017, ch.2).

The understanding and clear-eyed compassion of a good therapist has something in common with the value of a good confessor: helping people understand, recognise and forgive their own and others' faults.

Difficult feelings evoked in others

Psychodynamic therapists are trained to 'pick up' other people's feelings by questioning their own. They learn to pay attention to their own feelings and to develop a subtle capacity to distinguish between feelings which truly belong to themselves and feelings which are a communication from their clients. This capacity can be very helpful in a context where words are no longer available. Suicidal feelings, for example, can often be conveyed non-verbally. So too can irritation, a sense of uselessness, or a desperate, wordless need for help. Peace, contentment and happiness can also be conveyed in this way.

'Projective identification' is a concept therapists find useful (see, for example, Segal J.C., 1992, p. 36). It refers to a process which happens when feelings become unbearable. When people cannot bear a particular feeling, they may evoke it in someone else as part of an attempt to deny that it affects them: 'YOU're upset (or worried, or jealous or frightened), NOT ME!' These powerful feelings bring with them a sense that they cannot be spoken, that they belong entirely and convincingly to the 'recipient' while the person 'projecting' the feeling appears completely unaffected by them. In fact, recognising that the feelings are shared often turns out to be a relief for both. Relatives and carers often find themselves experiencing extreme feelings or thoughts of one kind or another, and in counselling it can be possible to help them to consider the extent to which these belong entirely to themselves and to what extent they might be shared with (even evoked by) the person they are caring for. A counsellor or therapist may be able to understand an individual or family by using this mechanism; it is sometimes possible to help other family members to use it too.

Fantasies and fears

Counsellors and psychotherapists often find that their clients have quite unrealistic fantasies about the world which can easily be modified once they are discussed and compared with reality: this applies to clients with mild cognitive problems too. Anxieties about losing love and affection are often related more to the past than a realistic view of the future; there may be specific fears about letting out a shameful secret if the mind continues deteriorating. Working through anxieties and distressing memories with a therapist can change perception of present and future problems until they eventually become less disturbing. Even practical changes can sometimes be made once some of the fears of admitting to cognitive impairment have been reduced.

Grief work

Grieving for lost mental capacities, for lost relationships and for future losses is hard: there is always something more urgent to do. A therapist offers time to think, to feel, to weep. There is reassurance in being in the presence of someone who will not judge but is equally not afraid to recognise past mistakes or bad behaviour for what they are.

In one case, a client worked through the loss of a lover, unknown to his wife but vividly alive to him, in five weekly counselling sessions. Referred for 'constantly being in a bad temper', not once did he know who his counsellor was, nor what she had come for. But he talked movingly about his relationship with his now-deceased lover, and about how he had never been able to discuss her passing with anyone before. By the end of his sessions his wife confirmed that his bad temper had disappeared. It seemed that grieving for a past loss is possible even when current memory and awareness is compromised.

Relationships with family members

During the early stages of cognitive impairments, relationships can be at risk. Mild impairments easily lead to misperceptions or misinterpretations, causing minor or more serious family conflicts. Without a diagnosis the offender is judged by normal social or family criteria, which may be harsh or accusatory. Where there has been a change families are challenged to wonder about the past: was my father always so unkind about small children? Was my picture of him wrong? Or was I always 'well-behaved' in order to avoid such digs myself? The idea that his current cruel dig at a small child's demands might arise from anxieties about the acceptability of his own demands might occur to a professional far more quickly than to a distressed daughter.

Daily life with someone whose mind is deteriorating can be irritating, eventually becoming wearing and soul-destroying. Even mild memory losses can be hurtful. Simply forgetting that their grandchildren did thank them for a present, that a partner did offer them a cup of tea or did inform them of an appointment which seems to have arrived out of the blue can be upsetting. Watching a previously proud parent or partner recognise they have made an elementary mistake can also be excruciatingly painful. A teenager said that what made her most angry was 'people refusing to admit they are in the wrong when they are', but unfortunately this is exactly the combination produced by some forms of mild NCD; being obviously, glaringly, in the wrong and being quite unable to acknowledge it. Amongst the most painful accusations are 'you don't care!' to someone who has given up significant aspects of their own lives to provide care. A particular vulnerability is created when cognitive impairments accompany more serious physical disabilities. Refusal to take precautions against incontinence (because the problem is denied) may be particularly distressing for carers who have to clear up without being certain whether the person could or could not have helped themselves.

Distress at the reality of losses can make people angry (sadness may come later) while at the same time very conflicted over whether or how to express their angry feelings. Many try simply to suppress them, with the risk of a dangerous build-up leading to some kind of explosion. Physical attacks, whether punching, hitting, denying physical assistance or simply putting food or drink or medication out of reach, are not uncommon when a partner has been driven to distraction by unjust accusations. It may be horror at realising some aspect of behaviour has gone beyond the bounds of the acceptable which triggers requests for counselling. If the carer's shame (or, for others, bravado, or blaming the victim) can be overcome sufficiently to talk to a counsellor or therapist, better ways of dealing with their anger may emerge.

Where counselling or psychotherapy is acceptable to carers, they can be grateful for the opportunity to share their feelings and anxieties about their relationship. Carers identify with those they care for and about, and, particularly in a long-term relationship, it may be hard for a carer to allow themselves to think clearly if the person they are caring for cannot. In order to think, a carer may have to leave the room – and yet, even wanting to be alone can feel like a betrayal. Having to separate and to let go of identifications with the mind of a lifetime partner (or parent) means reorganising one's whole view of the world and one's place in it.

Carers often find themselves feeling guilty for having capacities which their partner is losing; for being able to 'get away' when the partner cannot; for being more healthy or capable, and for being unable to make their partner better, for having stopped loving them or even for caring desperately about the loss of aspects of their partner's (or parent's) mind. They may try to suppress their 'selfish' feelings, as if self-preservation was sinful. On their own, carers may admit to distressing guilt at moments of wanting the end to come, and may not have considered that their cared-for partner might also wish this sometimes and be equally unable to express it. It seems that having someone else knowing your blackest, guiltiest thoughts, without judging, can be reassuring.

While there can be great relief for a carer to see a therapist on their own, couples counselling can also benefit some who would feel too guilty to talk 'behind their partner's back'. The conflict between the desire to let the other know what is going on for the carer, while not wanting to make a partner feel blamed or worse themselves, can be agonising, and often results in carers simply keeping quiet while resentment builds dangerously. Talking to friends may be impossible, partly because guilt about their feelings is so strong, as is their desire not to betray a loved partner, and also, perhaps, a desire to 'forget' while in the presence of someone who might not understand – or if they did, might no longer want to offer their company. Grief for losses already incurred, and for those to come, can be shared in couples counselling: the presence of a therapist or counsellor may enable mutual affection to be held in mind while more distressing feelings are expressed in a way which clarifies their aim. Blame and accusation may be more accurately focussed on the condition rather than the person; old argument styles or dead-ends be modified by the therapist; irritation and anger may be expressed and recognised as real but partial aspects of the relationship; behaviour resulting from cognitive deficiencies may be discussed and modified; interpretations of speech and behaviour may be modified in the light of new knowledge.

Counselling may be particularly helpful when people have to consider their capacity to care for someone else or for themselves and to make painful decisions about seeking help.

Child carers and young children

Sometimes parents of young or adolescent children can suffer from mild cognitive deterioration; this is a particular problem if the parent is single. These children may be the first to detect problems but may find it hard to obtain the attention, information and help they need. Other adults are reluctant to interfere, and the parent may be able to cover up their deficiencies. One such teenager's concerns about his mother's mind were not taken seriously until brought to a counsellor because he had mugged another child. These issues are discussed in both *The Trouble with Illness* (Segal J.C., 2017) and 'Helping children with ill or disabled parents' (Segal J.C., 1996).

Working through diagnosis

In the early stages of cognitive decline, it may be hard to obtain recognition from the medical profession. Just as relatives may not want to know about deteriorating capacities, doctors too may prefer to reassure rather than take seriously complaints of loss of memory from someone whose problems could be explained perhaps by a bereavement or by another health condition. Mild cognitive impairments may not show up on rapid psychological tests, particularly for those with higher intelligence or education. The comfort and sense of control which a patient can obtain from understanding their own body and its vicissitudes may be underestimated. If a patient feels their worries are not taken seriously, anxieties, based on little or mis-information, can grow in the dark.

Complex psychological assessments are unlikely to be offered in the early stages of NCD although they can be helpful in clarifying symptoms. Processing the meaning of the results may take a longer time (and need more repetitions, perhaps) than the psychology service can offer, particularly if speed of comprehension is affected. Family members may have to help the affected person to remember and think about what they have been told. Such assessments may also enable family members to understand, for example, why someone can continue to place bets on horses, while being quite unable to remember how to put the washing machine on, and can help make sense of difficult or strange behaviour.

Endings

Counsellors or therapists who work with people at the end of their lives sometimes think about the length of time a client has left; is it worth working with someone who is about to die? This may seem a harsh thought, but it is a thought which occurs, and not only to Healthcare Managers who control a budget. However, the way someone dies remains in the mind of those who care about them for a very much longer time; in particular, children remember how their parents died. Such memories affect the grieving process; they influence attitudes not only to death and health in general but to life itself. Friends and other relatives are also affected. Anxieties about having failed someone who dies suddenly are very common, and opportunities to prepare for a death can be important. Healthcare professionals of all kinds also find satisfaction in helping people achieve a 'good death'. This is a comforting concept, which feeds into a sense of the world being a good place.

Conclusion

Working with people with mild cognitive impairment is possible and rewarding, both for the client and the counsellor or therapist. Working with members of their families or other carers, particularly if the deterioration continues over a long period, can make the difference between someone being able or unable to continue caring, and can have a positive effect on grieving processes.

References

Allegranti, B. (2016). Dementia and embodied psychotherapy. *Therapy Today March*, pp. 8–12.

American Psychiatric Association (August 2015). *DSM-5 Update Supplement to Diagnostic and Statistical Manual of Mental Disorders* Fifth Edition. Arlington, VA: American Psychiatric Association Publishing.

Bains, J., Birks, J., and Dening, T. (2002). Antidepressants for treating depression in dementia.*Cochrane Database Syst Rev.* 2002 Oct 21; (4):CD003944.

Banerjee, S., Hellier J., Dewey M., Romeo, R., Ballard, C., Baldwin, R., et al. (2011). Sertraline or mirtazapine for depression in dementia (HTA-SADD): a randomised, multicentre, double-blind, placebo-controlled trial. Lancet; 378: 403–11.

Barnes, D., Yaffe, K., Belfor, N., Jagust, W., DeCarli, C., Reed, B., and Kramer, J. (2009, July–September). Computer-based cognitive training for mild cognitive impairment: Results from a pilot randomized, controlled trial. *Alzheimer Disease and Associated Disorders*, 23(3), 205–210. http://doi.org/10.1097/WAD.0b013e31819c6137.

Barrett E., and Burns A. (2014, July). *Dementia Revealed: What Primary Care Needs to Know*. A Primer for General Practice Version 2: November 2014 Prepared in partnership by NHS England and Hardwick CCG with the support of the Department of Health and the Royal College of General Practitioners NHS England. Available at www.england.nhs.uk/wp-content/uploads/2014/09/dementia-revealed-toolkit.pdf

DSM-5 Update Supplement to Diagnostic and Statistical Manual of Mental Disorders Fifth Edition August 2015 American Psychiatric Publishing: A division of American Psychiatric Association, Washington DC, London England. (2013)

Garfinkel, S.N., and Critchley, H.D. (2016, January). How the heart supports fear processing. *Trends in Cognitive Sciences*, 20(1), Special Focus on Emotion. Opinion: Threat and the Body. http://doi.org/10.1016/j.tics.2015.10.005 © 2015 Elsevier Ltd.

Goldstein, F., Levey, A., and Steenland, K. (2013, January). High blood pressure and cognitive decline in mild cognitive impairment. *Journal of the American Geriatrics Society*, 61(1), 67–73. http://doi.org/10.1111/jgs.12067.

Orgeta, V., Qazi, A., Spector, A., and Orrell, M. (2015). Psychological treatments for depression and anxiety in dementia and mild cognitive impairment: Systematic review and meta-analysis. *The British Journal of Psychiatry*, 207(4), 293–298. http://doi.org/10.1192/bjp.bp.114.148130.

Rapp, S., Brenes, G., and Marsh, A. (2010). Memory enhancement training for older adults with mild cognitive impairment: A preliminary study. *Aging & Mental Health*, 5–11. Published online: 9 June. http://doi.org/10.1080/13607860120101077.

Sachdev, P. et al. (full list of authors: Perminder S. Sachdev, Darren M. Lipnicki, Nicole A. Kochan, John D. Crawford, Anbupalam Thalamuthu, Gavin Andrews, Carol Brayne, Fiona E. Matthews, Blossom C.M. Stephan, Richard B. Lipton, Mindy J. Katz, Karen Ritchie, Isabelle Carrière, Marie-Laure Ancelin, Linda C.W. Lam, Candy H.Y. Wong, Ada W.T. Fung, Antonio Guaita, Roberta Vaccaro, Annalisa Davin, Mary Ganguli, Hiroko Dodge, Tiffany Hughes, Kaarin J. Anstey, Nicolas Cherbuin, Peter Butterworth, Tze Pin Ng, Qi Gao, Simone Reppermund, Henry Brodaty, Nicole Schupf, Jennifer Manly, Yaakov Stern, Antonio Lobo, Raúl Lopez-Anton, Javier Santabárbara) Cohort Studies of Memory in an International Consortium (COSMIC). (2015, November 5). The prevalence of mild cognitive impairment in diverse geographical and ethnocultural regions: The COSMIC collaboration. *PLoS One*. http://doi.org/10.1371/journal.pone.0142388. Available at www.cfas.ac.uk/files/2015/11/Prevalence-of-Mild-Cognitive-Impairement-in-Diverse-Geographical-and-Ehnocultural-regions-The-COSMIC-Collaboration.pdf

Segal, H.M. (1981). Fear of death: Notes on the analysis of an old man. In *The Work of Hanna Segal*. New York and London: Jason Aronson. Originally published *International Journal of Psychoanalysis* (1958), 39 (Parts II–IV): 178–181.

Segal, J.C. (1992). *Melanie Klein: Key Figures in Counselling and Psychotherapy*. London: Sage Publications.

Segal, J.C. (2001). Counselling people with multiple sclerosis. In K. Etherington (ed.) *Rehabilitation Counselling in Physical and Mental Health*. London and Philadelphia: Jessica Kingsley Publishers.

Segal, J.C. (2013). Caring for a partner with cognitive impairments due to multiple sclerosis: A psychodynamic perspective. *Neuropsychoanalysis; An Interdisciplinary Journal for Psychoanalysis and the Neurosciences*, 15(1), 87–99. ISSN:1529-4145/; E-ISSN: 2044-3978.

Segal, J.C. (2017). *The Trouble with Illness: How Illness and Disability Affect Relationships*. London: Jessica Kingsley.

Segal, J.C., Baker, S., Koerber, E., and Arbiser, E. (2010). Working with brain damaged clients. *Therapy Today March*, 22–26. ISSN: 2045-4244.

Segal, J.C., and Simkins, J. (1996). *Helping Children With Ill or Disabled Parents: A Guide for Professionals*. London: Jessica Kingsley.

Sinason, V. (1992). *Mental Handicap and the Human Condition: New Approaches From the Tavistock*. London: Free Association Books.

Chapter 4

Prognosis and planning

Advance care planning through a psychoanalytic frame

Juliette Brown

> *But, for the unquiet heart and brain,*
> *A use in measured language lies;*
> > *Alfred, Lord Tennyson, In Memoriam A.H.H., Canto 5*

Introduction

Advance care planning is a process of discussion and planning for future care in the context of a life limiting illness. It can include any and all of the following: discussion on likely progression, making advance statements of one's wishes, recording a refusal of specific treatment, and transferring decision making capacities to a proxy. It requires an ability to comprehend 'certain possibilities' about one's future (Sinclair et al., 2016). In dementia, it is a provocation to engage in thought about one's future with dementia and to consider a time when one loses the ability to communicate one's wishes and thoughts. It requires some consideration of what it may mean to have a diagnosis of dementia.

It *is* possible to talk with people with dementia about the course of the illness, its effects, and what these might mean. As simple as this sounds, it is also remarkably controversial, and is not by any means a standard practice in the psychiatry of older adults. Ethical, philosophical, legal, practical, social, and psychological issues attach themselves to the process, and reflect the difficulties we all face in conceiving our own futures, which contain little of certainty other than some form of decline and death. Despite this, there is renewed focus on how we can best support people with dementia after diagnosis (DoH, 2016), on advance care planning (Dening et al., 2011), and on attention to process in the delivery of diagnosis and discussion of prognosis (Dooley et al., 2015), in a broader medical context that recognises its failure adequately to engage people in the decisions that affect their care (Elwyn et al., 2012).

Psychoanalytically informed psychiatry can improve the quality of care that we offer. When we prepare for a discussion on prognosis and planning, psychodynamic approaches are most valuable. They help us avoid potentially harmful discussions, appreciate the importance of structure to the discussion, and provide some insight into what might emerge. We become better aware of what is communicated, both explicitly and less consciously, and better able to respond in ways that are helpful. In this work, individuals with dementia may bring to the surface unexamined fears. They may bring material that speaks of loss, grief, missing parts, anxiety and unease, fear and denial, damaged self-esteem, trauma, persecution, and a sense of personal failure. In acknowledging the fact of the illness and its effects, we are often asking people to think differently about themselves and their illness, with the aim of depriving the disease of some of its power. We can appreciate, through psychoanalytic theory, just how difficult this might be.

My aim with this chapter is that clinicians offering a discussion on prognosis and planning have a structure, a frame, in which to do so, and can understand the importance of that frame. I would also like clinicians to be able to apply psycho-analytic theory to make sense of the material that may emerge. I'll use – under headings 'frame' and 'material' – clinical illustrations from my own practice – as a psychiatrist working with adults who have been diagnosed with dementia in the NHS. The vignettes are 'distorted in fact' to borrow Bion's phrase. Each is an anonymised amalgam of particular responses, which serve to link the lived experience of people with dementia exposed in these discussions to an analytic understanding.

Frame

Clinicians repeatedly speak of uncertainty about how to approach discussion on prognosis and planning, recognising the potential harm of proposing difficult thinking about the future without adequate preparation. Advance care planning takes place, even as early as diagnosis, in the context of diminished cognitive reserve and an increasingly unreliable external world. The dangers are manifold (Sampson and Burns, 2013). Richard Cheston in his 1996 review of the literature on psychotherapeutic work in dementia noted that 'any intervention which aims to increase levels of insight must proceed with caution' (p. 214). For many, the challenge of a diagnosis combined with diminished cognitive reserves triggers defences of denial. Insight into the illness and its prognosis may simply add to depressive and persecutory anxieties, and the capacity and desire to face the reali-ties of dementia must be continually gauged to avoid exposing individuals to realities they cannot tolerate.

Drawing on the psychoanalytic framework, we begin with a form of assessment for suitability, attention to setting, to time, to pragmatics, and to expectations. Practically, this involves thinking about the referrer and the referral and gleaning knowledge of the individual patient and their situation. It requires planning an initial meeting and making some contact. My preference is for written contact initially with an appointment that is confirmed verbally through phone contact and for home visits, which can prompt a greater depth of thought about the mean-ing of dementia for the individual in the personal context. I use an appointment letter that references recent contact with the service (memory clinic) and extends an invitation to a discussion about what this diagnosis might mean and what plans can be made. The written invitation suggests that involving significant others in the discussion can be useful, and the tone is one of invitation rather than exhortation. The individual will have consented to be contacted to start a discussion, but may have little recall of that process of consent. They may also not recall (or want to recall) their diagnosis. At diagnosis, individual awareness of the illness and recall of the diagnosis will vary and will need to be assessed from referral and at first meeting.

Clinical illustration

I was referred a white British woman in her early 60s, formerly fit and active, working as an architect, with a partner and children who were young adults nearing college age. Her diagnosis of an uncommon subtype of dementia followed a number of years of difficulties with word finding, recognition of objects, and recall. The referral letter described a discussion about lasting power of attorney, and her willingness to be supported in further discussion on prognosis and planning. Preparatory work included some specific research and consultation on the prognosis in this subtype, phone contact to establish a convenient appointment time, and a brief discussion on who might be involved in the meeting. I was conscious of my immediate responses to a rare, younger onset dementia in a woman with a young family, presuming the need for a complicated mourning for the expectations she might have had for her life at that age.

We meet at her home, and following introductions, I tell them that this is not the only time we can meet. Indeed, we can meet as many times as is necessary. I check what their expectation of the meeting is and begin by reviewing her understanding of the diagnosis. Practically this means asking initially if she is comfortable to talk about the diagnosis. Having established her permission to do so, I remind her that she met clinicians in the memory service who reviewed her experiences, the account of people close to her, and a series of investigations, and found that the difficulties she was experiencing were due to a dementia of this particular subtype. I come close to using the word 'concluded' rather than 'found' in relation to the diagnosis, and then realised that this is a clinical perspective. Of course, her experience hardly concludes with the diagnosis, although something of her expectations of herself and her future may. In the course of this part of the consultation, one is gauging a cognitive capacity to take part in the discussion, and a level of psychological readiness to think about the facts of and the meaning of dementia.

I found a woman who was able to deliver her own narrative of the development of the disease, recall aspects of the process of diagnosis, who was able to describe the difficulties she was having, and had already, with the support of her partner, conducted a fair amount of mourning for a future together that had been markedly changed. She was intelligent, articulate, and used to managing complex situations, all of which disposed her to want to manage the impact of the illness. Most importantly, she possessed a facility to reflect on the experiences she was having and the effect on those around her. As the dementia had progressed at a relatively slow rate, she had some time over which to adjust, and had, with the help of her partner and a support group, achieved a level of acceptance. Clare (2001) describes how people with dementia can manage the integration of dementia into their self-concept in a variety of ways, including a spectrum of reactions from minimising the changes wrought by dementia, to adapting them to the existing self. Despite this work, and their involvement with the support group, she and her partner sought further information on the likely course of the illness.

In the second part of the discussion I explained, with caveats about individual variation, the possible course of her illness in three broad stages. The first stage described is one in which she may increasingly experience difficulty of the kind she is already having. At some point more marked changes may occur including difficultly recognising friends and family, her reactions to her environment may be altered due to misrecognition, her interpretation of her surroundings will be affected, and she may need support for many aspects of daily life. She may become distressed at home and loved ones may find this difficult to cope with. In the later stages she may require help with more fundamental aspects of self-care, including eating and drinking, may need to be fed, may become bedbound, may not be able to communicate her wishes verbally, may need help with toileting and personal care, may be incontinent, may in the final stages have problems with swallowing, and may develop life threatening physical health conditions such as infections. Throughout this explanation I continue to judge from her responses (physical and verbal) her willingness and ability to tolerate the information given, and both seek and offer clarification.

We know that people with dementia often seek information and guidance about the disease (Pinner and Bouman, 2003; Menne-Heather et al., 2002), as, of course, do carers, and that there has been a significant shift toward disclosure of diagnosis in the last 15 years, parallel with work on diagnosis rates and on the quality of and access to specialist memory services. Disclosures around prognosis have been less common (Dooley et al., 2015). People with dementia can benefit from psychological support. It is effective (Cheston et al., 2003; Burns et al., 2005; Knight, 1986) and can reduce the need for other treatments including medication and hospitalisation (Fossey et al., 2006), but it is frequently denied to them (Murphy, 2000). From Kitwood's work on personhood (1990) followed an appreciation of the psychotherapeutic qualities of good dementia care (Cheston, 1996). Explicit mourning liberation can be a focus for work with older adults (Pollack, 1982), but psychological therapy for people with dementia may need to be more supportive (Junaid and Hegde, 2007).

She tells me she hadn't realised all of this. How does she feel about it? She is not worried that she won't be taken care of. She worries about the family. They need to think about how they will manage. She is processing new information. Her partner had experience with dementia in his family, but had struggled to achieve with her a degree of shared understanding about prognosis and the possible effects of her illness. He says that without this explicit, facilitated discussion, neither the shared understanding of what the future may look like, nor the understanding of the value of planning ahead would have been possible.

Lund et al. (2015) describe advance care planning as a rite of passage. It cannot meaningfully take place without a shift in awareness. It requires structures that facilitate the transgression of social norms around conceiving of and discussing one's own death. These discussions contribute to adjustment to the diagnosis (Sinclair et al., 2016).

In the next part of the discussion we move on to the options with regard to advance care planning. The focus here is on introducing three rather different elements in terms that are both straightforward and also accurate. I explain that she can if she wishes appoint a proxy to make decisions on her behalf should she lose the ability to communicate her wishes. This is a legal process that can be largely completed online. She and her partner have already begun the application and have rightly discovered that they don't need a solicitor for this, as the Office of the Public Guardian have set up a site to make the process possible without legal advice. They plan an LPA for both health and for finances. I ask about any discussion they may have had about her wishes. Often people feel their loved ones inherently know what they would want. Evidence suggests this is not so, and assumptions are commonly made (Dening et al., 2013). Only through making these expectations and assumptions conscious, through discussion and reflection, can these be addressed. At subsequent meetings, I'll act as a witness to their LPA document and formally assess her capacity to sign the document.

I tell them about advance decisions to refuse treatment. I remind her that people are always provided with supportive care, and, with pain relief, and there can be no active intervention to end life. With this is mind, and in the circumstance of the later stages, assuming she has lost capacity, does she have views on life prolonging treatments? This is something she has considered. She feels strongly that she would not want her life prolonged actively were she not able to recognise loved ones, and not in a position to care for herself. I look for depressive symptoms and for particular anxieties that might be driving her decision, and assess her legal capacity to make this decision.

Narratives around planning often reference autonomy and choice, but practically one finds the fear of being a burden to others is a common motivation (O'Kelly et al., 2015) that demands explicit exploration. Advocates of shared decision making recognise the interpersonal dynamics behind all autonomous decisions (Elwyn, 2012) and account for them. In a subsequent meeting we will review the legal implications of an advance decision, the need to be specific about what is being refused, and use a website designed for the purpose to produce an advance decision to refuse treatment. At that meeting, she will say 'It feels like this is something I don't have to worry about anymore'.

Lastly I explain advance statements, an opportunity to document who and what is and has been important. This discussion raises thoughts from her about her children, who won't, in future, have the chance to talk with her about her life. I offer a template that we use to do this with a series of prompts, which they accept. I have the sense, even in someone who has given her illness considerable thought, of someone facing questions she is unprepared for, making real time adjustment to the realities she faces. We review what has been done and said in this meeting and plan for a further meeting in a month's time.

Advance care planning may 'provide an opportunity to consider existential and relational aspects of impending loss of self' (Lund et al., 2015). We can expect that some of the work is in establishing parallel narratives – an illness narrative and a personal narrative – that preserves the person as distinct from the illness. Some of this work, thinking of Klein's notion of reparation, will be restorative work to fuse complicated feelings about oneself as someone with dementia, and oneself within a set of significant relationships in which dementia has its impact on all aspects of relational life. The discussion provides immediate opportunities to process dementia and bring to conscious awareness the work of mourning being done.

Through Klein we understand that from the earliest experience of external reality, contradictory emotions constitute our object relations, our internal perception and experience of important objects and parts as experienced in phantasy and reality. Guilt associated with aggression toward the object not only leads to defensive splits and to persecutory anxiety but also to a desire to repair and restore that can manifest in a manic reparatory activity or in true reparation in which the risks associated with love and desire, namely loss, are managed psychically (Segal, 1973). While manic reparation contains the object in a controlled and disparaged state, true reparation enables the lost object again to be felt as loveable, and under the tolerable threat of aggressive urges. Anxiety about such precarious contradictions is reduced by repeated loss and restoration. In disease states in which some good aspects of the self are lost, and diseased parts felt as bad and persecutory, work to reconcile contradictory feelings toward the diseased self can be reparative.

Dementia affects our capacity to retain and integrate narratives important to selfhood and identity (Brown, 2016), and renders the individual subject to 'narrative dispossession' (Baldwin, 2008). Describing the use of narrative theory as applied to dementia, Baldwin describes a process of making sense of self and external reality through narrative, the creative act of imposing coherence on disparate experience. Working with people with dementia, we will likely need to attend to fragments of narrative to preserve their capacity to co-author, and to retain some authority over the illness.

Philosophic perspectives on the self in dementia increasingly recognise the relational nature of our selves, often described in notions of post-personhood, notions wholly compatible with object relations, which explains the early and ongoing determining part played by real and hallucinatory relations between self and others in forming the experience of the self and in framing our thoughts and actions (Gomez, 1997). In the work on prognosis and planning, we navigate people who are both individual and relational, whose views and wishes are influenced by relations both real and phantasy, and by patterns of relating and thinking derived from object relations and from external experience.

As part of the framework in which these discussions take place, we also need to consider the stance of the facilitating clinician. There is a danger in assuming a desire for knowing or a desire for not-knowing. Clinically, we need to invoke a psychoanalytic stance of abstinence and repeatedly test the capacity to tolerate reality, without imposition. As clinicians, we may struggle to hold knowledge back, and invoke ethical imperatives around autonomy, weighing autonomy over the equally valid obligation to avoid harm. At the same time, we can avoid difficult discussions under the guise of beneficence. We can assume that there are cultural differences that preclude discussions on death and dying, or render them unnecessary, while evidence and clinical experience suggests that these differences are negligible, and assumptions about other cultures can be particularly unhelpful.

Health professionals bring unconscious wishes and fears to their work, and need to be supported to reflect actively on their motivations and on the personal impact of the work (Ballatt and Campling, 2011), intervening in a positive way into 'compulsive care-giving' (Bowlby, 1978). We may experience destructive feelings of failure and seek inappropriate reparation in our work. There is a greater potential for counter-transference responses in dementia, including paternalistic, infantilising attitudes and enacting fantasies related to one's own parents and grandparents (Cheston, 1996) and to one's own imagined future (Garner, 2004). Unexamined internal drives and conflicts are a risk to our selves and our patients. This type of work should not be 'delegated' to staff that are untrained, unsupported, unsupervised, or unwilling to engage with the psychodynamics and the social and psychological impact of a terminal and debilitating neurological disease.

In this work, we explicitly invoke the ideas of self and future at a time when the sense of coherent time and self-concept is challenged by cognitive impairment, and offer a discussion that can help process emotional experience and help transform dementia into a thing with a shape and form that can be better tolerated. Attention to the structure and frame of the discussion is critical to the containing function.

Material

A psychodynamic understanding of dementia can help us make sense of the material exposed in a discussion on prognosis and planning, and can improve our ability to respond appropriately to the material we face.

Mourning

Responses to a dementia diagnosis include those consistent with a state of mourning – denial, repression, withdrawal, regression, and affective responses including depression and anxiety. Good internal objects are menaced and, with them, the capacity to be alone (Evans, 2008). One is mourning former and future selves that appear lost or no longer accessible, and the threat of disintegration of the present self.

Clinical illustration

I meet with a Barbadian woman in her late 70s with a diagnosis of vascular dementia. The discussion on planning stalls. She had received my reminder of her diagnosis gratefully, as if she had been waiting for an explanation. She needed someone to hear her experience of dementia. 'I'm not sure what's happening to me. I can't hold on . . . '. I wait for her to say what it is she can't hold on to, but there is nothing specific. She just can't hold on. I hold back from a response. I'm not sure I have one, other than to sit with her experience. After a moment or two she says, 'I'm not all there but I'm not all gone'.

There is some sadness in her, some bewilderment, and surprise. I am aware of a desire to bolster her sense of identity, and security, in some way, and I ask her who is around now, who is important, who was around when she grew up. She speaks for a while about her childhood. Suddenly, she breaks into song. She sings the title line from Nina Simone's 'Don't let me be misunderstood', over and over a few times. I think of the rest of the song – of course, a poignant piece about apology, attempts to connect and preserve relationships in the face of regret. She seems only to recall this one line, for the moment. She asks me if I know the song. Yes, I know the song. She smiles, says that 'the song goes on after the singer'. She knows there are other lines, there is a complete song somewhere, that others have access to, even as she recalls just a part of it. After this we are able to talk about her situation now and her wishes for the future.

Listening to the experience of dementia, one hears repeatedly of loss. Old age, the end of life, and a diagnosis of dementia produce the same fundamental challenge – of destruction without creative renewal, finality, loss without apparent gain, prompting the need to mourn for the self (Garner, 2002). This means working through the kinds of conflicts that prevent us from existing as beings in time, where relationships and people have endings. Identification with the lost object complicates mourning. We can retain attachment to lost objects (including cherished parts of the self) but often at terrible cost (Freud, 1917).

Anxiety

Primitive defences as described by Klein (1935) are seen in older adults as a means to protect against annihilation anxieties (Davenhill, 2004). In dementia, splitting may occur relatively early in relation to perceived losses. Changes taking place in the brain are experienced as failures of the external world to perform reliably. Anxiety may follow a fear of dependence, an 'existential fear' about what the future holds (Bryden and Friedell, 2001; Burns et al., 2005). As Richard Cheston noted 'the starting point for empathic work with people with dementia is the awareness of the existential terror of a loss of being (however this is construed)' (Cheston, 1996, p. 213)

In this context, both attachment theory and object relations illuminate a complex dynamic with dependence. We each have an existence predicated on care from early, important others, experienced in reality and in phantasy, a foundation for growth that if incompletely performed is also a site of immanent loss, abandonment, and consequent annihilation (Bowlby, 1969). From early inadequate care and from persecutory anxiety that is the subject of excessive defence stem a lack of basic trust, which can translate in adult relations as a fear of dependence that is particularly corrosive in old age (Martindale, 1998). In many people, internal objects cannot withstand the attachment demands that are revived by a diagnosis of dementia. In this context, both significant others and the services that support them are called upon to provide a secure base that can tolerate projection and projective identification. This depends on adequate resourcing, support, appropriate value ascribed to the work, time, space, and a culture of kindness (Ballatt and Campling, 2011), but we work in wider cultures in which need is politically pathologised, and taking responsibility for one another is problematised (Fraser, 2013). Where value is determined by productivity, being dependent on others can be felt as shameful. Clinically we see a dynamic in which people with dementia project that shame, an inability to tolerate bad, or suffering parts, into the external world, which is experienced as persecutory, further fuelling annihilation anxieties.

Fraser (2013) helpfully subverts those values that link uselessness, dependence, and shame, asserting his desire to be a burden on loved ones, and thus signifying his faith in loving relationships that can tolerate the 'badness' of illness and change alongside feelings of love.

Clinical illustration

A former bus conductor with vascular dementia and a stoma was referred for discussion on prognosis and planning. He is well kempt and polite, but describes feeling tired, unmotivated, uneasy and anxious. He forgets his children's names, whether he has eaten. He was previously a more garrulous man. His speech is slowed, and not spontaneous. According to his son, he is furious with them at times and uncharacteristically aggressive. He is particularly 'resistive' to personal care. When we begin a conversation alone about his experience of dementia, we talk about what is troubling him most now. He tells me that he has concealed the fact of his stoma from his family for ten years. He is unsure why he did this and speaks of his desire for privacy and dignity. Now he has dementia and needs their help, it is no longer possible to conceal his stoma. I mention the word 'shame' and he turns his gaze from the middle distance for the first time to meet my gaze. I am thinking of the social effects of ill health, the association between illness and shame, and the corrosive effect of secrets on relational bonds. I say 'sometimes people feel better when you share the things you are ashamed of, they feel closer to you. It shows that you trust them'. He takes this in, and we spend some time sitting in silence. When I see him once more, he has talked to his family about the stoma, his children are giving him the help he wants, and he is accepting care.

Waddell (2007) links the extremes of age, both disposing to states in which a containing, thinking mind is needed to transform the unprocessed affect and experience of another (Bion, 1967). In the case of the infant, the apparatus for thinking has not yet been called into being. In cognitive impairment, the apparatus for higher thinking is subject to acquired injuries. Supporting people with dementia demands something of Bion's alpha function to transform painful experience. In Hanna Segal's description of psychodynamic work with the developing minds of young children, a process of naming and narration is actively engaged: 'The real help I was able to give her was in naming the different feelings inside her, helping her to know them, to differentiate them and, therefore, to feel more able to control them' (Segal, 1973, p. 100).

Esteem

As clinicians we can tend to focus on loss of function and 'forget' the ego losses, loss of esteem, self and identity, and the profound relational losses that explain the impact of dementia on the wider network. The functional losses of the dementias diminish the ability of the individual to sustain developmental gains. Dementia can be perceived socially as a cultural failure (Hughes, 2006). In narcissistic defences, external validation stands in for the healthy ego and its capacity to love (Kernberg, 1975), and the kind of threat to status provoked by dementia may prove a particular humiliation, leading to defensive projection of part objects. Anger and helplessness are common responses to the insult to one's sense of competence, disposing to the kind of narcissistic rage that defends against shame (Kohut, 1971).

Clinical illustration

A woman in her mid-70s with an Alzheimer's Disease diagnosis agreed to meet to discuss prognosis and planning for the future. She had worked until relatively recently as a classical musician. Her children steered the conversation gently toward her limitations, she gently steered it back toward her competencies, and we became stuck in a tug of war. To achieve any progress in the consultation, I needed to reflect on the narcissistic insult of a neuro-degenerative disease that affects thought, personality, and motor function in a woman of her experience and skill.

Clinical illustration

Another woman with the same diagnosis complained bitterly that her daughter was trying to move her bed to the front room to prevent her from falling down the stairs. The front room, in which we sat to contemplate this problem, was filled with the best furniture and with graduation and wedding photos of grandchildren and great-grandchildren. I suggested that this is where she presents herself to the world. To give up on her front room would be experienced as a drop in self-esteem more painful than a tumble down the stairs. She looks around at the photos, and says 'everything good is here, it's what I worked to achieve in this country'. 'It's your legacy?' I suggest, 'You want it preserved?' 'Well'. She smiles, looking at her daughter. 'I suppose she is my legacy'. 'And the others, and the grandchildren'. I think how important it must feel, that one's contribution is not forgotten, especially as one becomes aware of one's own forgetting, and leave the two of them looking through photographs together.

We must acknowledge that dementia can be experienced as a complex and chronic trauma (Bryden, 2001). Trauma calls for difficult work of the witness (partner, family, clinician), the establishment of safe spaces – actual and psychic – and counter narratives against shame (Herman, 1997). Trauma disposes to fragmentation as 'faced with situations where external reality confirms inner terrors, the result is a grave difficulty in distinguishing between them' (Bell, 1998, p. 170). In the face of trauma we make use of denial and avoidance, effectively abandoning the traumatised person to their traumatised state, and marking their distress as intolerable – too shameful, humiliating, and dreadful to be faced (Bryden and Friedell, 2001). The full implications of the diagnosis arrive at a time when denial might be the most useful defence (Bahro et al., 1997). Families are also experiencing their own separate related trauma in relation to the diagnosis. Naming this can help relieve tension and restore relationships. There are also families in which pre-existing trauma and complex dynamics further complicate the caring role, and we may also need to acknowledge that, and respect the limits of reparative work.

Coda

'We suggest that the physical healing of our dementia is not as important as our emotional healing, Our spiritual healing is the most valuable, as it lets us search for final meaning and to transcend loss' (Bryden and Friedell, 2001).

Our experience of self depends on persistence over time (Heidegger, 1927). We characterise ourselves by what can be most coherently narrativised in our past, present, and future experience (Schechtman, 2014). This coherent self-concept relies on a grasp of self over time that is challenged in dementia. Insults to the brain have an effect on the workings of the mind (Damasio, 1994). Developmental analyses of infancy (Winnicott) explain the coming into being of a sense of independent self in the glow of continuous, reliable care, and minimal frustrations. The maternal function creates the conditions for successful being, including the experience of an embodied self in time and space. Equally, reliable, attentive, attuned, and consistent care and facilitating environments help us (including people with dementia) maintain a sense of persistence over time (Verwoerdt, 1981; Kitwood, 1990). Caring services that respond to rage without retaliation enable the ego to be strengthened by undamaged internal objects (Garner, 2004).

In the context of the myriad losses of dementia, including those of self over time, and the difficulty of imagining one's own disintegration, we can begin to appreciate the importance of activity that supports people with dementia to retain authority over the illness and a sense, however transitory, of persistence over time.

A diagnosis of dementia propels one into a process of mourning, for a lost self, is an insult to one's sense of self mastery and a challenge to the work of art that is any given life narrative. When we abandon people with dementia to their unconscious fears, we are contributing to the illusion that there is no life between diagnosis and death, and no further role one can play in one's own story. Advance care planning invites us to process dementia. Thinking about the future by its nature involves some difficult thinking about the disease, the disease process, and the personal meaning to the individual of decline and death – thinking that is also difficult for the clinician, but locates the person with dementia firmly in mind. Interventions that acknowledge psychological need help us to deliver an appropriate response to dementia. Naming pain, anger, and sadness implies that these are acceptable and tolerable, and that some sense of agency can be restored (O'Kelly et al., 2015; Hausman, 1992).

Psychoanalytic thought exhorts us to listen better to experiences of loss and trauma. In recognising dementia in these terms, we can begin to understand the anxieties that are manifest, and develop thinking services that better reflect psychological need. Advance care planning is a process that demands a structure, and an ability to attend to the material that may emerge. We invite those who are able to bring to consciousness their psychological need, to gain a sense of control and freedom in the present moment, to understand what is difficult in dementia, and to rob it of some of its power.

References

Bahro, M., Silber, E., and Sunderland, T. (1997). Psychodynamic treatment in Alzheimer's disease. *Revue Medicale de la Suisse Romande*, 117, 659–661.

Baldwin, C. (2008). Narrative(,) citizenship and dementia: The personal and the political. *Journal of Aging Studies*, 22(3), 222–228.

Ballatt, J., and Campling, P. (2011). *Intelligent Kindness: Reforming the Culture of Health Care*. London: RCPsych Publications.

Bell, D. (1998). External injury and the internal world. In C. Garland (ed.) *Understanding Trauma: A Psychoanalytical Approach*. London: Gerald Duckworth & Co.

Bion, W.R. (1967a). *Second Thoughts*. London: William Heinemann.

Bowlby, J. (1969). *Attachment and Loss*, Vol. 1. Attachment. London: Pimlico.

Bowlby, J. (1978). Attachment theory and its therapeutic implications. *Adolescent Psychiatry*, 6, 5–33.

Brown, J. (2016). Self and identity over time: Dementia. *Journal of Evaluation in Clinical Practice*, 23 (5), 1006–1012.

Bryden, C., and Friedell, M. (2001). *Dementia Diagnosis – "Pointing the Bone"*. Conference presentation at the National Conference of the Alzheimer's Association Australia in Canberra. Available at http://morrisfriedell.com/Bone.htm [accessed 12 February 2016].

Burns, A., Guthrie, E., Marino-Francis, F., et al. (2005). Brief psychotherapy in Alzheimer's disease. Randomised controlled trial. *British Journal of Psychiatry*, 187, 143–147.

Cheston, R. (1996). Psychotherapeutic work with people with dementia: A review of the literature. *British Journal of Medical Psychology*, 71, 211–231.

Cheston, R., Jones, K., and Gilliard, J. (2003). Group psychotherapy and people with dementia. *Aging and Mental Health*, 7, 452–461.

Clare, L. (2001). Managing threats to self: Awareness in early stage Alzheimer's disease. *Social Science & Medicine*, 57(6), 1017–1029.

Damasio, A. (1994). *Descartes' Error*. New York: Grosset/Putnam.

Davenhill, R. (2004). Old and new: Freud and others. In S. Evans and J. Garner (eds.) *Talking over the years, a handbook of dynamic psychotherapy with older adults*. London: Routledge.

Dening, K.H., Jones, L., and Sampson, E.L. (2011). Advance care planning in dementia: A review. *International Psychogeriatrics*, 23(10), 1535–1551.

Dening, K.H., Jones, L., and Sampson, E.L. (2013). Preferences for end-of-life care: A nominal group study of people with dementia and their family carers. *Palliative Medicine*, 27(5), 409–417.

Department of Health. (2016). *Joint Declaration on Post-Diagnostic Support*. Policy Paper (Online). Available at www.gov.uk/government/publications/dementia-post-diagnostic-care-and-support/dementia-post-diagnostic-care-and-support [accessed 5 July 2017].

Dooley, J., Bailey, C., and McCabe, R. (2015, August). Communication in healthcare interactions in dementia: A systematic review of observational studies. *International Psychogeriatric*, 27(8), 1277–1300.

Elwyn, G., Frosch, D., Thomson, R., et al. (2012). Shared decision making: A model for clinical practice. *Journal of General Internal Medicine*, 27(10), 1361–1367.

Evans, S. (2008). 'Beyond forgetfulness': How psychoanalytic ideas can help us to understand the experience of patients with dementia. *Psychoanalytic Psychotherapy*, 22(3), 155–176.

Fossey, J., Ballard, C., Juszczak, E., et al. (2006). Effect of enhanced psychosocial care on antipsychotic use in nursing home residents with severe dementia: Cluster randomised trial. *British Medical Journal*, 332, 756–761.

Fraser, G. (2013, May, 3 Friday). Assisted dying. *The Guardian*.

Freud, S. (1917). *Mourning and Melancholia*, Standard ed., Vol. 14. London: Hogarth Press.

Garner, J. (2002). Psychodynamic work and older adults. *Advances in Psychiatric Treatment*, 8(2), 128–135.

Garner, J. (2004). Dementia. In S. Evans and J. Garner (eds.) *Talking Over the Years, a Handbook of Dynamic Psychotherapy With Older Adults*. London: Routledge.

Gomez, L. (1997). *An Introduction to Object Relations*. London: Free Association Books.

Hausman, C. (1992). Dynamic psychotherapy with elderly demented patients. In G. Jones and B. Miesen (eds.) *Care-giving in Dementia*. London: Routledge.

Heidegger, M. (1962, c.1927). *Being and Time*, translated by John Macquarrie and Edward Robinson. London: SCM Press.

Herman, J. (1997). *Trauma and Recovery*. New York: Basic Books.

Hughes, J.C., Louw, S.J., and Sabat, S.R. (2006). Seeing whole. In J.C. Hughes, S.J. Louw, and S.R. Sabat (eds.) *Dementia: Mind, Meaning, and the Person*. Oxford: Oxford University Press.

Junaid, O., and Hegde, S. (2007). Supportive psychotherapy in dementia. *Advances in Psychiatric Treatment*, 13, 17–23.

Kernberg, O.F. (1975). *Borderline Conditions and Pathological Narcissism*. New York: Aronson.

Kitwood, T. (1990). Psychotherapy and dementia. *Newsletter of the Psychotherapy Section of the British Psychological Society*, 8, 40–56.

Klein, M. (1935). A contribution to the psychogenesis of manic-depressive states. *The International Journal of Psychoanalysis*, 16, 145–174.

Knight, B. (1986). *Psychotherapy With Older Adults*. Thousand Oaks, CA: Sage.

Kohut, H. (1971). *The Analysis of the Self: A Systematic Approach to the Psychoanalytic Treatment of Narcissistic Personality Disorders*. New York: International Universities Press.

Lund, S., Richardson, A., and May, C. (2015). Barriers to advance care planning at the end of life: An explanatory systematic review of implementation studies. *PLoS One*, 10(2), e0116629.

Martindale, B. (1998). On ageing, dying, death and eternal life. *Psychoanalytic Psychotherapy*, 12, 259–270.

Menne-Heather, L., Kinney-Jennifer, M., and Morhardt-Darby, J. (2002). 'Trying to continue to do as much as they can do'. Theoretical insights regarding continuity and meaning making in the face of dementia. *Dementia: The International Journal of Social Research and Practice*, 1, 367–382.

Murphy, S. (2000). Provision of psychotherapy services for older people. *Psychiatric Bulletin*, 24, 181–184.

O'Kelly, A., Howarth, G., Richards, G., et al. (2015, March/April). Advance care planning for end of life care. *The Journal of Dementia Care*, 23(2).

Pinner, G., and Bouman, W.P. (2003). What should we tell patients about dementia? *Advances in Psychiatric Treatment*, 9, 335–341.

Pollack, G. (1982). On ageing and psychotherapy. *International Journal of Psychoanalysis*, 63, 275–281.

Sampson, E.L., and Burns, A. (2013, May). Planning a personalised future with dementia: 'The misleading simplicity of advance directives'. *Palliative Medicine*, 27(5), 387–388.

Schechtman, M. (2014). *Staying Alive: Personal Identity, Practical Concerns, and the Unity of a Life*. Oxford: Oxford University Press.

Segal, H. (1973). *Introduction to the Work of Melanie Klein*. London: Karnac Books and the Institute of Psycho-analysis.

Sinclair, J.B., Oyebode, J.R., and Owens, R.G. (2016). Consensus views on advance care planning for dementia: A Delphi study. *Health and Social Care in the Community*, 24(2), 165–174.

Tennyson, A. (1850). *In Memoriam A.H.H.* In The Works of Alfred Lord Tennyson (1899). Cambridge: Riverside Press.

Verwoerdt, A. (1981). Individual psychotherapy in senile dementia. In N. Miller and G. Cohen (eds.) *Clinical Aspects of Alzheimer's Disease and Senile Dementia*. New York: Raven.

Waddell, M. (2007). Only connect: The links between early and later life. In R. Davenhill (ed.) *Looking Into Later Life: A Psychoanalytic Approach to Depression and Dementia in Old Age*. Tavistock Clinic Series. London: Karnac.

Winnicott, D.W. (1965). *Maturational Processes and the Facilitating Environment: Studies in the Theory of Emotional Development*. London: Hogarth Press.

Chapter 5

The experience of loss in dementia; melancholia without the mourning?

Sandra Evans

Rose leaves, when the rose is dead,
Are heap'd for the belovèd's bed;
And so thy thoughts, when thou art gone,
Love itself shall slumber on.

Percy Bysshe Shelley, 1839

Introduction

Freud's seminal1917 paper, "Mourning and Melancholia" written more than a century ago, gives us the image of the "Shadow of the Object". This is the person-shaped void left by the lost loved one, who has died or left us. The bereaved are impacted by this emptiness which is experienced as a part of themselves in the shadows an which often diminishes their sense of self and the essence of life: the shadow falls "upon the ego". Giving up the "object-shaped" shadow (Bollas, 1998) is as painful as it is necessary to re-experience wholeness once again. Painful because it represents giving up that final attachment, the investment Freud calls cathexis, which represents the profound connection with the lost person.

We are by now used to understanding the experience of loss for the carers and partners of people with dementia and familiar with concerning ourselves with how they might feel. We are less confident when it comes to considering the experience for the person with a dementia diagnosis. Dementia is a process, not an absolute leaving straight after diagnosis. When a loved person has dementia, they do not disappear all at once but change in a way that is often experienced by the observing partner as losing them; they suffer a real-time grief at this loss and an anticipatory grief at their inevitable demise (Garner, 1997). This chapter will explore how Freud's forensic analysis of loss, depression and grief work helps us to think about, not only carers and families of people with dementia, but also those persons with dementia. Of significant importance is managing feelings, supporting carers and thinking about and containing difficult responses alongside the person with dementia. This is and has to remain, the essential part of the care package delivered to people with a new diagnosis.

Potential for institutional denial

There is no cure for this horrible illness. Purchasers of NHS care who fund not only diagnostics, which used to be aimed solely at starting people on a useful but not curative disease-modifying drug treatment, realized that this was not enough. A responsible Clinical Commissioning Group (CCG) would consider the potential risk of harm of an early diagnosis and look to offer support. As time has progressed since the National Dementia Strategy of 2009 (Banerjee, 2009), there is an absence of evidence of harm from early diagnosis. In fact, people seem to want it and are being referred to memory clinics in increasing numbers.

Limited investment into such services (which are patchily delivered across the UK) might signify a collective failure to mourn and therefore properly to address the problem of an incurable (so far) illness on behalf of society itself. One might argue that funding research into potential cures is a better use of money. What is problematic however is that we too are in denial. We have not yet grasped the reality; which is that once the damage is done to neurological tissue, it is irreversible (Ritchie et al., 2017). Researching futile paths to improve cognitive function in people who are very ill diverts us from their pain and the reality that there is still no cure. It also allows us collectively to deny the problem for those who are currently suffering the indignities of dementia. It would seem that this in itself represents a poor use of resources and a failure of quality care. In Davenhill's (2008) description of institutional and local authority neglect of dementia, we recognize a continued absence of fully committed engagement with the needs of people with dementia and their carers (Garner & Evans 2000).

On a more optimistic note, people with dementia themselves are speaking out, participating in NICE guideline committees, contributing to "experts by experience" groups in NHS trusts, charities and on the Royal College of Psychiatrists Old Age Faculty Executive. Having a voice is important; representing the feelings of such a vast range of people and experience is a major challenge.

Mourning and melancholia: reactions to the diagnosis of dementia

In his opening paragraphs, Freud iterates the features of mourning and loss and defines its differences from melancholia. His paper reminds us that we treat mourning as natural and normal. We tend not to interfere with its process unless confronted with evidence of pathological grief, or the beginnings of melancholia. In the not so distant past there was a tendency not to give people a diagnosis (Pinner and Bouman, 2003) almost certainly to spare their feelings; practitioners were concerned with avoiding a "catastrophic reaction" (Haupt, 1997; Draper et al., 2010). A similar infantilizing of cancer sufferers occurred until twenty years ago. This tendency however, robbed people of their chance to mourn and particularly to mourn together with their families; and then to move on and make plans.

Since 2009, we have been systematically giving people with suspected dementia the opportunity to learn of their diagnosis – still a subject for discourse fifteen or so years ago (Pinner and Bouman, 2003). Commissioning and planning services (NHS London Commissioning Strategy for Dementia, 2010) suggested that we offered pre-diagnostic counseling, although exactly how this might look was never specified. It seemed logical at the time to anticipate a potential increase in suicides and therefore any strategy designed to offset a crisis was probably good. It was mooted by the author at a Royal College of Psychiatrists meeting aimed at dementia diagnosis that an earlier diagnosis might precipitate an acute adjustment disorder in people still competent enough to kill themselves. In fact, no such surge in suicides occurred (National Audit on Suicide. Personal Communication, 2012) and very few people appear to suffer a classical catastrophic response to their diagnosis.

One could accept this fact as evidence of the heterogeneous sample from which people with dementia are drawn; they are from a "normal"/Gaussian distribution of the population. By this I mean they are likely as a group to have less tendency to severe mental illness than the population from which those who seek psychiatric help are usually drawn and who are, by definition, more at risk of suicide. In a similar way, a diagnosis of terminal cancer does not often precipitate catastrophic suicidal ideas, unless there is an underlying mood disorder or similar mental or emotional instability.

Dementia is a truly democratic disease. It affects the wealthy, physically and mentally healthy alike as well as those with learning difficulties or who are intellectually gifted. In the spirit of enquiry and as Freud would have done, we might also conjecture upon alternative explanations for the absence of a significant increase in mood disorders or self-harm behavior in the face of such catastrophic news. As stated earlier, a reason might include sufficient personal self-esteem or contentment on the part of the sufferer. Another explanation may also include the loss or diminishment of awareness of the problem. This could arise as a result of either frank denial or the deterioration of the part of the brain responsible for self-awareness and insight.

Breaking bad news in a memory clinic

A National Standard to which all UK memory clinics are exhorted to aspire (MSNAP, 2011) considers as good practice, by way of pre-diagnostic counseling, at the outset of a memory assessment an enquiry of a number of key questions. The person undergoing assessment will be asked about their own suspicions about whether they have dementia and their willingness to undergo assessment. They will also be asked about their desire to know the outcome of the assessment and about their choice of people with whom to share the information.

At the time of a clinical diagnosis, even a very early stage, much intellectual function may already be lost. Alzheimer's Disease particularly, which preferentially attacks cortical areas in the temporal, occipital and frontal lobes, will have caused some impairment in a person's appreciation of changes (Turnbull and Solms, 2007). There will of course be denial too. The author has seen many people over a period of more than twenty years with a new diagnosis of dementia. Although not systematically quantified, only a small handful, perhaps twenty of those people, could have been identified as having had that catastrophic response to the news of their illness. The so-called catastrophic response to the feared diagnosis seemingly occurred in response to the news breaking their defence-mechanism of an active repression of reality. Their presentation was often fragile, brittle and seemingly abrupt with the clinicians, but the countertransference gave a sense of great anxiety – which was perhaps unfelt by the sufferer themselves, so divorced from their true feelings at the time. Those people had often lived through and witnessed a loved one suffering a similar illness. They were traumatized by the memory and terrified by the prospect of what they had imagined/empathized with. Having a dementia diagnosis would act as a major threat, putting them in touch with a terror that is unbearable.

Most people, however, could indeed bear reality; some could bear the disclosure of the diagnosis in part because their own reality-testing abilities were significantly impaired. In fact, they understood the words, the concept of dementia and what it is, but they could not accept or acknowledge at a deeper level that they were ill. This is illustrative of the layered essence of insight. It is not absolute: present one minute and not the next. It is like dementia: a process of realization and acknowledgement. At the disclosure meeting, people would often ask "I know I have dementia but I'm not that bad really – am I"? It would appear that awareness and insight are not static either, once achieved. This is an essential consideration when assessing capacity and discussing choices.

Denial

Denial (Freud, 1936) is an active repression of knowledge (Freud, 1914) in the service of the protection of the ego. Literally, as Anna Freud saw it, a part of the ego actively hides the dreadful knowledge from the self in a repressive manner. It takes mental energy to finesse denial, and therefore to some extent deprives the mind of other aspects of its range of functions. In this act of self-preservation, the repressing ego may further deplete memories, which may have been useful to the person. One sees this phenomenon in Post-Traumatic Stress Disorder where the loss of memory of the traumatizing events also obscures associated memories that may themselves trigger remembering and are therefore dangerous to the integrity of the self-preservation strategy (Freud, 1914). Denial may be essential to the person's overall mental health and ability to carry on, and, as we know, is a normal and expected part of a grief response. (Anna Freud was building on her father's established work of a topographical map of the mind and work he had started with "Mourning and Melancholia" but was later described in 1918 after the First World War when he described the anxiety states caused by the trauma of shell shock.)

Reality-testing has shown that the loved object no longer exists, and it proceeds to demand that all libido shall be withdrawn from its attachments to that object. This demand arouses understandable opposition – it is a matter of general observation that people never willingly abandon a libidinal position.

Freud (1917)

In the denial of dementia, people may be partly and fearfully aware of the process of a loss of their own treasured intellectual functioning, or they may be only too aware of memories of what had occurred when their parent or grandparent had become demented. We may be witnessing an unwillingness to abandon a libidinal position, or we may equally be witnessing an avoidance of revisiting an earlier trauma: that of a parental institutionalization or other unpleasant experience, such as extreme dependence in an unsafe and unheld setting (Martindale, 1989).

We are also aware that denial is a flimsy structure and that people in denial may appear rigid but brittle. They demonstrate their vulnerability by perhaps contradicting their clinicians and jeopardizing their relationships with loved ones. They will defend their right to hold on to their version of reality with vigorous strength. Occasionally patients angrily walk out of memory clinics, leaving their exasperated families reeling and racked with guilt. They should of course be free to exercise this right always and until it becomes apparent that they lack capacity to make the decisions which will keep themselves, or others, safe.

People with dementia as yet formally undiagnosed may involve their families in a collusion of refusal to face facts, which naturally (although denial as part of the bereavement process is important and integral to the natural progression of the process and leads to a position of resolution or acceptance) is time-limited. The longer it continues beyond a certain point, the more problematic denial becomes and can, just as with grief, take on a pathological hue.

An importance question at this point might be whether denial is the same in dementia; even if there is a more ordinary repeated forgetting from the memory loss process itself (Freud, 1901). Can people with dementia overcome their denial? The answer most definitely is yes but people need time; precisely because insight and changing awareness is a process that can be guided and assisted. In dementia the person may need more time or a more concerted effort to process the grief and the denial. In a way for some, they have to *learn* that they have dementia. For others, it is important to have support in order to integrate the new situation and revised version of themselves – as a person with dementia. The author, also a group analyst by training as well as by philosophy sees the healing potential of groups, whether they are family or stranger groups of one's peers. A family gently reiterating what has been said by the clinician in the Diagnostic Memory Clinic confirming the dementia, while taking care not to diminish confidence nor point out the person's failings, can be enormously helpful in countering denial – producing a narrative that assists with acceptance and integration of the diagnosis into planning for the future (Benbow and Kingston, 2014). Similarly a group of one's peers, ideally others with a new diagnosis of dementia, who come together to learn about each other and their illness can facilitate a move from denial to increased awareness (Watkins et al., 2006). Chapter 13 in this book also describes such a group.

The relevance of the consideration of this dual aetiology of *not-knowing* when patients have dementia is in the pursuit of understanding something about mental functioning in dementia. The author is unaware at this point of research in the area so that clinical observation and experience are the limits of our knowledge, however the loss of awareness is a relatively early phenomenon in some dementias, particularly in Alzheimer's Disease.

Unlike Alzheimer's, the vascular-related dementias affect the brain in a different manner due to a more random assault on the millions of tiny blood vessels supplying nutrients to different areas of the brain. In vascular dementia one may see less loss-of-awareness directly due to brain deterioration and more scope for the application of active ego-defences such as repression and denial. This is not just an academic conjecture, however.

The clinical relevance of etiology is of great importance. Denial can be tackled and is potentially reversible. Agnosia or not knowing is much less likely to be so since it is more likely to be caused by brain disease itself damaging the frontal lobes: those parts attributed with sense of self, moderating influences and awareness (although may yet be assisted with new learning) Evans, S. (2006). The absence of awareness of loss can lead to increased risk to the person with dementia. Being unaware of how disabled one is by illness can lead to carrying on regardless for one's personal safety.

Loss of awareness

In patients who have a significant loss of awareness, the capacity to mourn their loss will also be impaired. As Mark Solms (1995) demonstrated through his work on a stroke unit, patients who had sustained significant physical losses through stroke disease (cerebrovascular accidents that caused specific and discrete functional impairments) subsequently produced emotional states which were often surprising and counter to the expected response. For example, in a right-sided stroke which caused a left-sided weakness and agnosia (loss of awareness of the affected limb), the patient appeared not to be distressed or disturbed despite profound loss of function (Solms, 1995). The patient simply did not know what he had lost and consequently could not begin to mourn it. In a similar way, a person with Alzheimer's Disease may be less aware what they have lost and is therefore less distressed but also is less able to mourn and process the changes (Evans, 2008).

Diminished awareness and carer stress

Most people with dementia are supported by partners, family and friends.

Reduced awareness will increase the risk of stress in the supporting carer; augmenting any feeling that they and the person with dementia are not on the "same page". This can induce feelings of isolation in both patient and partner or increase the risk of conflict between them. On many occasions the denial of illness can be every bit as strong in the healthy carer and this can also be influenced by the strength of feelings towards the person with dementia; both positive and negative.

Clinical illustration

An elderly woman and her daughter are seen in the memory clinic where the older woman is given a diagnosis of dementia. Her daughter, who has suffered many years of bullying behavior from her mother, is catastrophically affected by the revelation. She cannot accept it and is now faced with the prospect of her mother continuing to behave cruelly towards her but yet now with apparent diminished responsibility. This places the daughter in a more responsible position and with her own need still to resolve some issues with her mother before the older woman loses all capacity for understanding. It is hard for the daughter to accept the diagnosis (although at some level she might have known), as she has had to harden herself towards her mother's behaviour. She had become convinced that the bad behavior and abusive language was due to ongoing conscious malign intent as it always had been, even when it has worsened more recently.

In order to accept the fact of her mother's illness, she will need to come to terms with a new interpretation of her mother's recent swearing and her own retaliatory behaviour.

For this couple to be able to continue to function through the illness in a more positive way it will be relevant to offer them some mediation and counseling.

The carer perspective

Because people with dementia are ill but remain alive and still need us (in fact need us more and more), some grief work cannot begin. Those feeling bereft of the person that they used to know and love who may have changed in their illness cannot take back that part of themselves (ego) that is invested in the loved one in order personally to regroup and recover. The bereaved must continue as though the person with dementia is still the same and relate to them in a way that will not cause them additional anxiety; and yet as carers in the dual sense of the word, they are experiencing loss. The *carers still care*; by this I mean they are still hugely emotionally invested in the person with dementia as well as having to attend increasingly to their needs. At the same time, they are experiencing a relatively rapid loss of their sense of who that loved person used to be. If the person with dementia has lost awareness of their disability, the partner may be left even more isolated in their bereft state: holding on to a reality of their disappearing partner in an experience that cannot be shared. It takes great courage and emotional maturity to manage both.

In most dementias, this process will continue over many years. The carer and family of a person with dementia does not generally cut off from them, but will divide their attention increasingly between the person with dementia and the prosaic demands of everyday life. All the while, they will be experiencing a loss.

Attending to their own needs will often become secondary; this is not like a definitive bereavement when a person dies or leaves forever.

Caring for the carer

As a familiar theme in this book, it is often said that there is more than one sufferer in dementia and yet, finding the time to manage the needs of the main carer can be difficult within a clinical service. It is extraordinary that we do not routinely build this requirement into the business plan for a service. Why do we forget such an important element of the person with dementia – their carer, particularly when many carers of people with dementia are old themselves. We know that they still participate actively in their own and others' care (O'Neil and McGee, 2007).

There still exists a stereotype that older people and those with dementia are passive recipients of care whereas in fact many; over 8% of the oldest old in one Irish longitudinal study (O'Hanlon et al., 2004), were found to be primary carers for a family member. This stereotype is a huge barrier *even to the possibility of thinking* about funding needs. Every stereotype holds only a partial truth. The reality contradicts a propaganda convenient to successive governments and promulgated by a coarse and undisciplined media that older people and those with dementia are and will continue to be a huge strain on health and social services (Oliver, 2015).

People deal with the work of caring in various ways. So much depends on cultural factors which will include expectations (particularly the role of women in society as carer's of their children, their parents and their elderly in-laws Garner & Evans, 2018), financial position, and geographic proximity to the person with dementia. The final arbiter though in the author's experience is the relationship with the person with dementia and this is an area fraught with dynamics (Garner & Evans, 2000) and which is dealt with in greater detail in the chapter on attachment and couples.

Clinical illustration

Jools, a retired nurse is diagnosed with Alzheimer's Disease in her mid-eighties. She is an unusually able person who has worked at senior levels in the NHS and who faces her illness bravely, wishing to be armed with facts no matter how stark, in order to made plans and shoulder the responsibility for her own care. Her son Mark continues to support her in this endeavor, allowing her continuing independence but also at times emotionally needing her to be the same person as ever before. He is identified as her main carer, but the two increasingly develop a dyadic partnership in which her medical knowledge and experienced mind combines with his problem-solving and calm healthy brain. He has found a way to help her while coping with the loss of his clever, independent mother as she becomes increasingly muddled.

Discussion

In this touching illustration, the role of the carer is shared between Jools and her son. They have found a way to co-create a good-enough functioning mindful carer by merging both their minds' skills. Jools is still caring, as is her lifelong habit, both for herself and for Mark by holding on through her libidinal investments to the nursing professional part of herself. This is a part of her that Mark is also reluctant to give up and so he supports increasingly this professional part of his mother.

The loss for both of them may be even greater when finally even this will be hard to maintain. It is hoped that anticipating this loss by facing that reality and assisting Jools with planning for her own future in a pragmatic and honest way may avoid disaster.

Depression in dementia

> In mourning it is the world which has become poor and empty; in melancholia it is the ego itself.
>
> Freud (1917)

We are aware that dementia causes losses to all aspects of mental functioning (memory, problem-solving etc.) and can have a profound effect on the personality. The person may lose their sense of self; in dementia, the ego itself becomes impoverished as in Freud's 1917 distinction of melancholia from mourning. Should we say therefore that depression is a natural sequel of dementia? The author thinks not; however it does seem hard to countenance such profound losses in a person's life without an ensuing reactive downturn in mood. Perhaps it is the "loss of awareness" which protects against the profoundness of a melancholy for most people. After all, in the absence of awareness, the dementia sufferer may be left unaware of what and how much they have lost. If reduced awareness impairs the capacity to mourn, does this risk a later melancholia or is this experienced by the close family of the individual, unable to mourn.

In the dementias associated more with cerebrovascular disease, Evans (2004) describes a change in mood which predates and heralds the onset of cognitive symptoms. People often experience anxiety and sometimes depression alongside early symptoms of forgetfulness. We know that depression often causes difficulty remembering, even in much younger people who don't have degenerative brain diseases. Anxiety, distraction and rumination make it hard for the mind to take in new information and harder still for this information to be recalled. It has been mooted that the awareness of difficulty with remembering and the consequent feeling of vulnerability might contribute to a sense of anxiety and impending danger in those who have an "increased ischaemic burden" – i.e. a significant number of small vessels which are blocked, thereby starving the brain of vital nutrients. The association of these vascular changes seen on brain scans and the incipient anxiety and depression experienced by the person, aware that they can no longer think logically or remember easily, may signify different causal links. One is explained by neurobiology and the other is explained by the experience of the person whose brain is being assaulted by disease process (Evans, 2006).

The neurobiological model may find its causal pathways in the disruption of affect regulation through brain damage. This is not an unbalanced view but it describes the phenomenology entirely in terms of neuro-degeneration. It would appear more robust if there were a stronger association between late life depression and anxiety and the onset of vascular dementia – the so-called vascular depression hypothesis. As it stands, not all people who suffer depression and anxiety in late adult life go on to develop a vascular dementia in the next two to five years. If that were the case, the incidence of dementia would be nearer 50% after age 70 rather than in the region of 10% of the older population.

In a patient-centred, psychoanalytic model we think of the person whose brain is undergoing the assaults of early dementia. That person's mind has developed over many years and is influenced by experiences and memories and fears. The differences between peoples' responses to finding themselves less resourceful, less competent and less able that normal for them will depend on the *meaning to them of vulnerability, loss of independence and loss of abilities.*

> [In Melancholy . . .] We see how in him one part of the ego sets itself over against the other, judges it critically, and, as it were, takes it as its object.
>
> Freud (2017)

As Freud describes, the critical part of the mind – the super-ego – may be accepting and forgiving or it may be a harsh, introjected parental imago, berating the self for failure and causing anxiety and self-doubt. This harsh and critical agency may precipitate a depressive episode, pouring blame onto the person with dementia who will suffer shame at their losses. They may feel increasingly burdensome and worry that they do not deserve care or continued existence. Many older people, but in particular those with dementia are caught suggesting to their families that they be "put down" or "put out of their misery".

> The distinguishing mental features of melancholia are a profoundly painful dejection, cessation of interest in the outside world, loss of the capacity to love, inhibition of all activity, and a lowering of the self-regarding feelings to a degree that finds utterance in self-reproaches and self-revilings, and culminates in a delusional expectation of punishment.
>
> Freud (1917)

Many family members and professional carers have reported such utterances from the people they care for. They may fear that the person is suicidal. While it is conceivable that this is the case, it is not common. There has not been the predicted great increase in suicidal behaviour, or completed suicides since the National Dementia Strategy (Personal Communication with National Confidential Enquiry on Suicide). Despite its latest target figures of 75% of people with a diagnosis, we should be less concerned that people will kill themselves and more concerned that they may die sooner than they ought, or in a state of unhappy neglect and under-stimulation (see Chapter 15 on boredom).

> The disturbance of self-regard is absent in mourning; but otherwise the features are the same. . . . It is easy to see that this inhibition and circumscription of the ego is the expression of an exclusive devotion to mourning which leaves nothing over for other purposes or other interests.
>
> Freud (1917)

The author's interpretation on speaking to many persons with dementia themselves when they express these ideas is that it is more likely a seeking of reassurance that they are not a burden. They may be struggling to reality-test and wish to find out what others are thinking. Some do really consider themselves burdensome and will be less inclined to attend social venues or activities at which they can no longer keep up as before. Shame and humiliation can be avoided with a supportive, thoughtful and collaborative auxillary mind: that of carer (professional or family or friend).

Primary process thinking

As dementia progresses, there is a return to primary process thinking. This has been described elsewhere as a "middle" stage dementia in which logical thought becomes more difficult and the reality-testing function breaks down (Evans, 2008). The unconscious processes come to the fore in more evident wish fulfillment as well as the emergence of more problematic ego-preserving strategies. Wish fulfillment may manifest itself in the forgetting that certain key people are in fact deceased, calling an end to reactive mood problems as everything once more becomes possible. Anxiety and depression may diminish as dementia progresses because of deterioration in the integrity of the ego. We are reminded that an intact ego is required to experience anxiety.

Magical thinking as part of primary process thinking may rid the mind of its super-ego functions, causing fewer worries about social gaffs and functional abilities. Other examples of magical thinking can be positive but will be less so if internal objects are malign. The fear of thieves and belief that even family members are capable of taking one's property is compounded by the person losing items they have themselves hidden away for safe-keeping. Mind functions may return to the paranoid/schizoid and away from the depressive position (Klein, 1946).

The denial and unease of the diagnosing physician

During an exploration of the psychoanalytic in memory services one is invited to reflect on the clinician. We are aware that in the breaking bad news scenario, the clinician is alert also to the feelings of the patient to whom a disclosure of dementia can be made. Feedback clinics can be quite painful for staff as well as for patients (Bailey et al., 2018). The need for empathic awareness of our patients can impact on our feelings about inflicting the pain of shocking news for some. The clinic model shows that this communication takes time and has to be delivered in stages like a dance between people, establishing what they know, what they suspect and helping them to put the evidence together with their experience Dooley, J., Bailey, C., and McCabe, R. (2015). While there is no cure for dementia, there is always hope that the decline will not be aggressive and that disease-modifying drugs will be of some use.

There will always be a tension between giving all the news honestly and modifying or delaying it in order to maintain engagement and not inflict unnecessary suffering.

Conclusion

The diminished awareness of the condition of dementia is neither simple nor straightforward. It is often likely to be attributed to loss of brain function but a psychoanalytic model invites us to consider other possibilities, such as active repression and denial of what is too painful to bear. The temptation to collude with this position is understandable when empathic and caring people engage with looking after persons with dementia. We none of us can bear "too much reality" too much of the time. The impact on our own health as carers and professionals needs to be taken into account and factored into any business plan for dementia care services.

Ensuring that people with dementia are helped to understand their own condition allows them a genuine voice in their own future and plans for care.

References

Bailey, C., Dooley, J., and McCabe, R. (2018). 'How do they want to know?' Doctors' perspectives on making and communicating a diagnosis of dementia. *Dementia*, 18(7–8), 3004–3022. https://doi.org/10.1177/1471301218763904

Banerjee, S. (2009). *The National Dementia Strategy UK*. DH. assets.publishing.service. uk/dementia-care/nationalstrategy

Benbow, S., and Kingston, P. (2014). 'Talking about my experiences. . . .' at times disturbing yet positive': Producing narratives with people living with dementia. *Dementia*, 15(5), 1034–1052.

Bollas, C. (1998). *The Shadow of the Object: Psychoanalysis of the Unthought Known*. London: Free Association.

Davenhill, R. (2008). No truce with the furies. *Journal of Social Work Practice*, 147–157. https://doi.org/10.1080/02650539808415143.

Dooley, J., Bailey, C., and McCabe, R. (2015). Communication in healthcare interactions in dementia: A systematic review of observational studies. *International Psychogeriatrics*, 27(8), 1277–1300. http://doi.org/10.1017/S1041610214002890.

Draper, B., Peisah, C., Snowdon, J., and Brodaty, H. (2010). Early dementia diagnosis and the risk of suicide and euthanasia. *Alzheimer's & Dementia*, 6(1), 75–82. https://doi.org/10.1016/j.jalz.2009.04.1229.

Evans, S. (2004). Attachment in old age: Bowlby and others. In S. Evans and J. Garner (eds.) *Talking Over the Years; A Handbook of Dynamic Psychotherapy in Older Adults*. London: Routledge.

Evans, S. (2006). Where is the unconscious in dementia? In R. Doctor and R. Lucas (eds.) *Psychoanalytic Ideas*. London: Karnac Books.

Evans, S. (2008). Beyond forgetfulness: How psychoanalytic ideas can help us to understand the experience of patients with dementia. *Psychoanalytic Psychotherapy*, 22(3).

Evans, S. (2018). Sadism in late life. In A. Sehgal (ed.) *Sadism: Psychoanalytic Developmental Perspectives*, Forensic Psychotherapy. London: Routledge.

Freud, A. (1936). *The Ego and the Mechanisms of Defence*. New York: International Universities Press.

Freud, S. (1901). The psychopathology of everyday life. In *SE*, 6, 1–239.

Freud, S. (1914). Remembering repeating and working through. In *SE*.

Freud, S. (1917). Mourning and melancholia. In *The Standard Edition of the Complete Psychological Works of Sigmund Freud, Volume XIV (1914–1916): On the History of the Psycho-Analytic Movement, Papers on Metapsychology and Other Works*, 237–258

Garner, J. (1997). Dementia: An intimate death. *British Journal of Medical Psycology*, 70(2), 177–184, Pt2. https://doi.org/10.1111/j.2044-8341.1997.tb01897.x.

Garner, J., and Evans, S. (2000). *The Institutional Abuse of Elderly People*. CR 84, College Document. Royal College of Psychiatrists.

Garner, J., and Evans, S. (2018). Psychotherapy and psychiatry of old age. In G. Rands (ed.) *Women's Voices in Psychiatry*. Oxford: Oxford University Press.

Haupt, M. (1997). Emotional lability, intrusiveness and catastrophic reactions. *International Psychogeriatrics*, 8(S3), 409–414. Cambridge University Press. https://doi.org/10.1017/S1041610297003736.

HealthCare for London (HfL) Commissioning Guidelines for Dementia. (2010/11). DH.

Klein, M. (1946). Notes on some Schizoid Mechanisms. *Int. J. Psycho-Anal.*, 27:99–110.

Martindale, B. (1989). Becoming dependent again: The fears of some elderly persons and their younger therapists. *Psychoanalytic Psychotherapy*, 4, 67–75.

MSNAP. (2011). *Royal College of Psychiatrists*. London: MSNAP.

National Confidential Enquiry into Suicide. Personal Communication. (2012). No increase in suicide of older adults following the National Dementia Strategy in which more people given dementia diagnosis.

O'Hanlon, A. McGee, H. Barker, M. Garavan, R. Hickey, A. Conroy, R. et al. (2004). *Health and Social Services for Older People II (HeSSOP II) Changing Profiles from 2000–2004*. Dublin Council on Aging and Older People.

Oliver D. (2015, May 7). Minding our language around care for older people and why it matters. *BMJ Blog*. Available at http://blogs.bmj.com/bmj/2015/05/07/david-oliver-minding-our-language-around-care-for-older-people/.

O'Neill, D., and McGee, H. (2007). Oldest old are not just passive recipients of care. In Letters to the Editor. *British Medical Journal*, 334.

Pinner, G., and Bouman, W.P. (2003). What should we tell patients about dementia? *Advances in Psychiatric Treatment*, 9, 335–341.

Ritchie, C.W., Russ, T., Banerjee, S., Barber, B., Boaden, A., Fox, N.C., Holmes, C., Isaacs, J.D., et al. (2017). The Edinburgh consensus: Preparing for the advent of disease-modifying therapies for Alzheimer's disease. *Alzheimers Research Therapeutics*, 9(85). https://doi.org/10. 1186/s 131950017-0312-4.

Solms, M. (1995). Is the brain more real than the mind? *Psychoanalytic Psychotherapy*, 9(2), 107–120.

Turnbull, O., and Solms, M. (2007). Awareness, desire and false beliefs: Freud in the light of Modern Neuropsychology. *Cortex*, 43(8), 1083–1090.

Watkins, R., Cheston, R., Jones, K., and Gilliard, J. (2006). 'Coming out' with Alzheimer's disease: Changes in awareness during a psychotherapy group for people with dementia. *Ageing & Mental Health*, 10(2), 166–176.

Chapter 6

Dementia and dialogue

Acute hospitals and Liaison psychiatry

Matthew Hagger

A Stranger in a strange land.

Exodus chapter 2, verse 14

Liaison psychiatry

'The success and viability of a social institution are intimately connected with the techniques it uses to contain anxiety' proposed Isobel Menzies concluding her famous study of the nursing service of a general hospital (Menzies, 1960, p. 118). Liaison psychiatry originated in the United States in the 1920s, where physicians and surgeons in general hospitals needed input from mental health professionals to help with their patients. Edward Billings was one of the first people to coin the phrase "Liaison psychiatry" (Thompson and Suddath, 1987).

In the United Kingdom, Liaison Psychiatry has recently undergone significant expansion. Liaison services exist in many UK hospitals, though variability in provision remains(Aitken et al., 2016; Barrett et al., 2015). The reasons for this expansion are complex and wide ranging. For example, it is recognised by policy makers and providers in the healthcare system that a well-funded and functioning Liaison psychiatry team can improve the care for patients, support general hospital staff and save money (Parsonage and Fossey, 2011). There are multiple pressures within the whole health and social care system with acute hospital staff often having little background or expertise in caring for people with mental health difficulties.

Liaison practitioners have educational and ambassadorial roles. They can feed back an expert assessment about an individual patient, challenge stigma (Bolton, 2012) and provide clinical skills teaching for different groups of hospital staff.

Liaison psychiatry teams are usually based in the acute hospitals. They comprise nurses and doctors, though some expanded services include other professions, e.g. occupational therapy and psychology. They may vary in their working practices and capacity depending on funding and working models to include specialists in treating older persons. There has been a recent expansion in specialised services for older people's Liaison in recognition of the prevalence of dementia in acute hospitals (Bourne, 2007; Sampson et al., 2009). Most Liaison teams cover both the emergency department and inpatient wards and respond to both urgent and more routine situations. The vast majority of referrals are made by hospital doctors. It might be that all that is required is advice and/or, as appropriate, providing relevant information concerning the referral. However the vast majority of patients will be seen and if needed further reviewed. Each person referred is discussed by the Liaison team among themselves and at a handover meeting. The person seen may require psychiatric admission or follow up by community mental health services which the Liaison team facilitates. Many people also will not require follow up and the Liaison service communicates about all the people it has seen with the referrer and with the patient's GP. Constant and timely communication is essential.

Psychodynamics in Liaison – *clinical illustration*

> *The Liaison psychiatry team is asked to see JACK, a man in his 70s who is agitated on the ward. Staff describe him as disinhibited and one or two fairly quickly use the word 'nasty' about him such is the depth of feeling he appears to be inducing in others.*

Psychodynamics is primarily about relationships: the thoughts and feelings we have about one another with an emphasis on unconscious processes, ultimately influencing our reactions and behaviour in all situations. Various aspects of Liaison work involve many intrinsic psychodynamic elements, that with skilful handling and supervision can help the patient and the staff looking after them.

Unfortunately, psychodynamics can often be overlooked and it has already been suggested that Liaison Psychiatry has drifted away from its origins in this regard (Jackson, 1990). Liaison work can be complex given the multiple interactions a practitioner can have with their patients, families and other professionals. Teams have to manage various tensions and anxieties, whilst trying to remain focussed on individual patients. Many emotions are being played out in the settings where Liaison services work, for example anxieties about serious illness, life-changing frailty and death. These have their impact on all human feelings although some may be unconscious and cause us to react and behave in ways which are driven by deeper origins than we are necessarily aware of. A calm seemingly "benign" patient with dementia sitting in bed may be experiencing intense emotions themselves and be surrounded by emotional turmoil on the ward.

Historically and indeed up until the present day patients may be referred to Liaison for instances where no clear physical cause can be found for their problems and symptoms. The modern terminology in this area is "Medically unexplained symptoms" and a psychodynamic approach can be helpful also in understanding people presenting in this way. Most people however will also have a clearly established physical condition which the referrer (the treating physical health clinician) believes is affecting their mental health. There are many layers to the interactions that ward staff in the hospital may be having with a patient and their family or significant others. A psychodynamic perspective can help the Liaison worker understand better why a patient has been referred and about what might be going on for the patient at this time in their life.

A Liaison psychiatry professional can bring their own unique perspective to think about the patient in order to aid other staff in their work with that person. The quality of relationships that the Liaison clinician builds up over time with other hospital staff will also affect the milieu: the feel of the environment and the way individual patients (particularly those with dementia) are viewed. Liaison teams may have to bear others' feelings, such as a lot of anxiety, aggression and sadness concerning a patient, whilst helping the ward to process the same experience. The ability to hold the thoughts about various possibilities and uncertainty at the same time is also important. A good example of needing to contain these feelings might occur when a patient cannot return to their own home due to extreme frailty and risk .

Clinical illustration

More difficulties arise when nursing home placement was discussed with him and his family, as his experience of spending times in children's homes when younger is re-activated. He feared that staff wherever he was would behave in a sadistic way. Those who had looked after him felt that he seemed wary of them when they attended to him.

Dementia in the acute hospital

The global prevalence of dementia is projected to increase further over the next decades (Prince et al., 2013) and many people with dementia are admitted to the general hospital, some of them as yet without a dementia diagnosis. A person suffering from dementia can experience spending time in a hospital as difficult and distressing. The somewhat industrialised nature of modern medicine (Illich, 1976) does not always help in this regard where an individuality may be lost amongst pathways and protocols. It is difficult to strike a balance between the demands of individual compassion and that of organisational efficiency (Ballatt and Campling, 2011). Under such circumstances staff have been described as being "irradiated with distress" (Obholzer in Hinshelwood and Skogstad, 2000). In recent years various policy initiatives and approaches have looked to tackle this situation (National Dementia Strategy, 2009) and the work of numerous individuals including the late Tom Kitwood (1997) and other groups have contributed greatly to dementia care. Since 2004 the Butterfly scheme has been adopted in many UK hospitals to improve dementia care and educate and support staff. John's campaign (http://johnscampaign.org.uk) was started by relatives of a dementia sufferer to highlight some of the challenges around dementia care in acute settings.

Working in an environment with little hope for recovery

As the vast majority of those with dementia are older adults, often with extreme physical frailty, those looking after them on an acute ward can be filled with various unwanted or conflicting feelings. The lack of any cure for dementia currently on the horizon and potential resulting therapeutic nihilism surrounding dementia can be potent forces in the milieu. This in itself can affect the person's care sometimes in quite subtle ways. There are also potential threats to a clinician's own "professional narcissism". People who enter medicine do so mainly for altruistic motives but it is also true that making people feel better feels good for us too. When working with older people with dementia, clinicians need to adjust their expectations of a patient's ability to recover and what a "good outcome" might look like. This may involve looking at phase specific problems, e.g. considering Erickson's stages of development through life (Erickson, 1966), and how a patient may become stuck at a certain stage or even regress (Hildebrand, 1982). Putting aside jargon and diagnostic terms one has to look at a patient's feelings of foreboding, dissatisfaction with past achievements and loneliness (Ardern and Garner, 1998). Staff may identify with and experience similar painful feelings to those that the patient is having of hostility, helplessness and frustration. Staff may act these out unthinkingly themselves, sometimes to the patient themselves, sometimes to the relatives or to other colleagues (Davenhill, Balfour and Rustin, 2007). These "acting out" behaviours might include asking for an expert opinion and then ignoring it, identifying strongly with one family member against the others and against the wishes of the actual patient; they often are detrimental to the person or the professionalism of the team. The well-known paper "The ailment" (Main, 1957) described the inevitability of ordinary human feelings amongst care givers. Sutton (2001) highlighted a double jeopardy in dementia of losing one's mind and hence being treated mindlessly.

Clinical illustration continued

Jack is known to have dementia and from initial assessment his overall condition has been worsening over some time. He is particularly agitated when receiving personal care and has lashed out at staff, at times causing injury. The ward charge nurse appears to be at her wit's end as some staff have gone off sick and it is difficult to replace them.

The referral to Liaison psychiatry

A referral of someone with suspected dementia to the Liaison team might read (or sound) something like this: (brevity is common).

Has dementia and has been in hospital for months. Needs placement. Please assess and advise.

Notwithstanding the reality of long stays in hospital it is interesting to observe and speculate about what be going on for this patient and the referring team. With any referral looking at it from a psychodynamic perspective there is much to unpack and decipher. Where has the diagnosis come from (was it inferred on the ward or had Jack been properly assessed by a memory clinic)? Why has this person been referred now (is he medically fit, or have the treating team met insurmountable difficulties when trying to discharge him)? Events that range from the rational to the seemingly incomprehensible can trigger a referral. The reactions the referral produces in the Liaison team can also be linked to the individual patient. Handovers are an opportunity for different team members to ask questions, learn from each other, be challenged and offer opinions. Senior members of the Liaison team often have to consider the dynamics of the individual case and will assess the team's response, seeking to recognise potential strong emotions which may prevent clarity of thought with the case. The senior person also has to provide containment to the team.

Having time and reflective space to think about referrals and consider these aspects can be rare but is really helpful (possibly essential). Thinking rather than unthinking action can provide a brake to incautious, manic activity to do everything one can rather than everything one should (Garner, 2004). Is the patient's distress unbearable to the ward staff? Is something hateful going on? Menzies' words about social defences in nursing staff (1960) are as relevant as ever today. A hospital system which in attempting to reduce responsibility from a junior individual nurse by using hierarchies may risk the professionalism of that individual and their ability to make autonomous and thoughtful decisions. When the Liaison Consultant is asked about medicating the patient to make them stop whatever behaviour is intolerable (whether it is risky or not), there may be another level of disturbance which is tacitly also being requested to relieve in staff themselves. A corollary applies in a dynamic respect here: an individual patient might be tapping into a quite primitive, archaic "state of mind" in a staff member, group or situation.

Clinical illustration

Allen, a man in his 80s, has been admitted with a chest infection. He presents as a loud and boisterous personality on the ward. His family tell one of the ward doctors that his memory has been getting progressively worse over some years and he is repetitive. There is a sense that his family are fearful of him and this may have prevented them going to the GP. They also seem traumatised in some way that is difficult to put a finger on.

Initial assessment

Psychodynamic understanding can be brought into every aspect of the assessment of the individual patient, including the review of the case notes and prior discussion with the ward team. Noticing how one feels and reacts when one first sees the person and during time spent with them may give clues about on-going issues and the anxieties that are affecting them. It is important to listen to what is and isn't being said by staff and families (Garner, 2004). The stress and regressive effects of working in a stressful environment can also lead to one become more defended, e.g. detached and struggling to think about issues like infantilisation (Terry, 1998). Obtaining personal and family history about the person can reveal patterns of relationships that may be repeating themselves in the hospital. This can be challenging when there are cognitive problems present for the individual patient and their informant's (relatives) accounts may be less than objective at times.

Clinical illustration continued

He wants things done quickly as he has always desired in his life. He appears irritable and sometimes shouts at staff. He is very embarrassed about incontinence episodes when his verbal abuse worsens. At times he breaks into outbursts of singing which has a manic quality to it. A referral is made to Liaison psychiatry with a request to move him to a psychiatry ward. The acute ward environment is not felt to be the right place for him according to the staff who feel under pressure to complete their tasks in relation to him. There are differing points of view among his family with some members thinking that he should return home. It emerges during the Liaison team's assessment that he has been being aggressive at home to his wife.

Psychodynamic concepts in Liaison settings: splitting and projection

Splitting and projection are examples of more primitive ego defence mechanisms. Defence mechanisms are largely unconscious psychological manoeuvres thought to develop early in life to deal with both internal and external anxieties. Projection is attributing an unwanted part of oneself, e.g. a thought or feeling onto another. This may take the form of qualities, feelings or wishes which a person is unable to recognise or rejects in oneself. These are then denied as part of the self and located in another person. For those upon whom the projection is made, they may or may not respond strongly. A strong response implies an "projective identification" when the projection has notionally found a "home" and is also located within the other. It is common to feel projective identifications when at work in hospitals. All clinicians are human and feel fear, shame and love all their working day long. A strong feeling may well be due to something being projected into oneself by a person one is looking after. Clinicians may be subject to a whole variety of projections that they will have to process mostly unconsciously whilst having to continue working.

Splitting is about struggling, unconsciously, to manage conflicting parts of oneself. Clinicians looking after a person who is operating this defence, may strongly disagree with each other regarding this patient and the best treatment, thereby reflecting the split.

A person with dementia may be in a more regressed state emotionally will be more likely to be using these two mechanisms, projection and splitting, to cope with their own difficult feelings. Difficult to follow conversation, i.e. confused speech may represent forms of projection. An older person with dementia may experience themselves in a more fragmented way and some aspect of this could be being projected; conveyed by what and how they say something. An example of this occurs in a case observation described in the book *Inside Lives* (Waddell, 1998) where a woman with dementia and her daughter are looking out of the window at a storm. The woman is frightened saying, "take me home please". Her daughter talks quietly with her but then her mother says "but I don't see anyone with guns out there". Her daughter associates this remark to her mother's previous address in Central London during the Second World War. By continuing to talk with her and making links, her daughter provides a containment for these projections. This resurgence of defence mechanisms in dementia may indicate unresolved conflicts or feelings from earlier in the person's lifetime (Waddell, 1998).

These two mechanisms can occur in a range of interactions, from a moment a member of staff shares with the patient on a ward to the interaction of two teams involved in the patients care.

Clinical illustration continued

A member of the Liaison psychiatry team sees Allen and speaks with staff and his family. He seems prickly and domineering with the Liaison clinician. More of his personal history emerges; he came from a large family and grew up in impoverished circumstances. He worked in a steel yard throughout his life and become a foreman who used to order people around. His family and the treating team staff do begin to feel listened to in a containing sense so that a range of views is gathered. A dementia specialist nurse also becomes involved and there is an attempt to use tools such as "My life story" to help him but also to assist the treating team in seeing him differently. They have already engaged with some aspects of his personality and as they start to learn more about him a different dialogue emerges. There is more recognition of what dementia means for him and why he has been so determined to exercise control in such an aggressive way. There is still pressure from some staff and some family members to prescribe tranquillising medication but equally resistance to this from others.

A best interests meeting is held to look at the options around his management on the ward and regarding discharge. This is a chance to discuss the patient in a more rounded sense and look at some of the dynamics that have been occurring, looking at what has and hasn't worked. It can be a chance to acknowledge both the difficult feelings aroused by the patient and also the different pressures, e.g. blockages to certain discharge pathways.

Counter-transference

Blumenfeld (2006) in the context of Liaison psychiatry settings talks about a central role of counter-transference that all care staff have to the patient. There are various definitions of counter-transference with some being narrower in focus.

The feelings that arise within one can be as a result of the patient's treatment of oneself as a healthcare professional and may reflect relationships from earlier in the patient's life.

Empathy with the patient, "tuning in" may include being sensitive to feelings evoked by counter-transference and to make use of them in order to understand the patient better. Holding in mind and reflecting on these feelings in a non-judgemental way towards oneself can be helpful both for those working in Liaison and the staff groups they are working with. Some thoughts and feelings may feel contradictory or unacceptable but can be reflected upon in terms of what might be being communicated when seeing the patient.

Clinical illustration

Janet, a lady in her late 70s, is admitted and treated for various medical problems. She is crying constantly on the ward saying that her husband has just died a few weeks before, but it soon emerges that actually it was some years ago. She is very anxious and often repeating herself. Several staff members have themselves left work in tears and feel overwhelmed looking after her. Other patients whilst sympathetic have complained at times that they cannot sleep. When she is moved to a side room she becomes even more distressed, convinced she is going to die. This leaves the ward staff in a quandary.

Containment

A key factor in dementia care is containment (Davenhill, 2007). It can come from a variety of sources including Liaison teams now acting in a holding manner for those who are working directly with patients on a daily basis – nurses (Williams, 2001). Containment can be an ability to hold uncertainty whilst enabling thinking to go on. A baby or young child needs a containing person who recognises their anxiety and can understand and tolerate it. Helping a child to process their feelings helps them to develop and ultimately to contain their own anxiety (See Chapter 9 on attachment & Affect regulation).

Decisive action can also be containing in certain situations. It can also be about acknowledging the difficulty of a situation and that little can be done that is of help. There may be conflict within staff groups between wishing to care and wishes to get rid of people who feel unbearable (Ardern, Garner & Porter, 1998).

Clinical illustration continued

From informant history it appears she was not talking about her husband's death in the time prior to admission. More history emerges; her husband died in the same hospital and that at the time of his death her cognitive problems were emerging. Family and friends describe some of the difficulties she has had with grieving. There is a sense that admission has re-activated her feelings. Some of the challenges around talking about death in hospitals are evident in this case. It is compounded by dementia, which has been described as a form of dying whilst the person is alive.

Measuring the ability of staff to contain patients and themselves is not straightforward. Staff that feel more contained in their everyday work with all patients will be able to be more mindful and self-reflective. This can enable "presence", i.e. being in touch with the difficult feelings aroused when looking after someone with dementia. Many staff do a very good job of managing the multiple demands made on them, but it is very easy to be pulled out of position and focus, even for a few moments

There are few supervised forums in which one can discuss one's own feelings and thoughts and which can provide a source of reflection and support. The role reversal of relatively young professionals looking after older people with multiple mental health and physical complaints is notable. Working with the patient's family can include helping them to confront loss by giving an accurate prognosis in an honest and kind way. A care giver who can provide a receptive frame of mind, being able to modify and re-communicate things to a patient, can provide a form of containment (Waddell, 1998).

Rustin (1991) talks about how self-knowledge can assist in containing very powerful psychic phenomena. Using one's own mind as a cipher to translate feelings into useful thought may help those with dementia to cope with fear of separation and abandonment by addressing these in moment to moment care interactions. Containment of staff working with the elderly is a key component of a good service Martindale (1989) and staff retention as well as continuity in the team work are essential for this. (Ardern, 1995)

Narcissism

In psychodynamic thinking, narcissism is about struggling to relate to others with all the feelings, e.g. envy, separation and dependence, that this can entail, thinking that one has all the characteristics within oneself to manage. It is important to consider narcissism in patients (and ourselves) and its relationship to ageing (Cohen, 1982). A person may be described as having narcissistic type defences that are exacerbated by ageing. The anxieties induced by dementia may affect these defences giving rise to narcissistic rage (Kohut's, 1972) and a scathing refusal of any help.

"Acting-out"

Acting out refers to a tendency impulsively to speak or act in a way that is related to an underlying anxiety or feeling. This is an unconscious urge and may take the form of aggression and be repetitive in nature. The ability to sit with and think about feelings of hopelessness, disgust, hatred and yet also moments of hope, serenity and humour is very important. People will intrinsically differ in their ability regarding this, but it is true that dementia increases the possibly of acting out behaviour.

On-going review

Liaison clinicians will often have the opportunity further to review patients on the wards. Further review provides more information about the person and to trace an arc of how they are in hospital as well as in their usual lives. Psychodynamic understanding in the initial assessment process and during reviews enables one to see the patient in a more rounded way (Ardern, 1995). Schwartz rounds where the hospital staff gather to look at their own emotional responses to a patient or situation have sometimes focussed on dementia (Wilkinson et al., 2015). Staff who have provided good care often do many of these things implicitly in their work and perhaps Schwartz rounds and similar other initiatives highlight the unconscious processes and how best to deal with them, for patients, between staff and in the wider organisation.

Continuing illustration

It is possible that staff's own personal experiences of death and dementia are reso-nating with Janet's sad reality. However, staff working in a simple, guided way can help her with her grief and again look to help to contain both her and themselves.

Conclusions

Liaison psychiatry teams have an important role in dementia care in acute hospitals. This ranges from the care of an individual patient to interactions with staff teams and beyond in the wider healthcare system. Bringing in a psycho-dynamic perspective can do much to enrich this process in terms of individual understanding of a patient and widening the outlook of all healthcare professionals. Various psychodynamics concepts are helpful in this process; containment particularly so in pressurised environments. Detailed consideration of the individual person with dementia can bring a more humanising aspect to their care and treatment and help individual staff to reflect on their own approach in their work. Work done with staff in the hospital can help to engender a thoughtful and reflective environment and this feeds into a dialogue about dementia care. Various approaches can help in containing clinical staff in their work which places multiple demands on them especially psychologically. There are many pressures which in turn affect the psyche of patients and families and lead to further projection and splitting. Containment for staff, patients and families can be reinforcing and affect outcomes in a positive fashion. Liaison psychiatry with a psychodynamic approach is a powerful movement within dementia care in order to consider the uniqueness of an individual and their relationships with others in helpful and meaningful way.

References

Aitken, P., Bass, C., Lloyd, G., and Mayou, R. (2016). A history of Liaison psychiatry in the UK. *BJPsych Bulletin*, 40(4), 199–203.

Ardern, M. (1995). Psychodynamic aspects of old age Psychiatry. In R. Howard (ed.) *Everything You Need to Know About Old Age Psychiatry*. Petersfield, UK: Wrightson Biomedical Publishing Ltd.

Ardern, M., Garner, J., and Porter, R. (1998). Curious bedfellows: Pschoanalytic understanding and old age Psychiatry. *Psychoanalytic Psychotherapy*, 12(1), 47–56.

Ballat, J., and Campling, P. (2011). *Intelligent Kindness: Reforming the Culture of Health Care*. London: RCPsych Publications.

Barrett, J., Aitken, P., and Lee, W. (2015). *Report of the 2nd Annual Survey of Liaison Psychiatry in England*. https://www.crisiscareconcordat.org.uk/wp-content/uploads/2015/10/2a-Report-of-the-2nd-Annual-Survey-of-Liaison-Psychiatry-in-England-20-.pdf

Blumenfeld, M. (2006). The place of psychodynamic psychiatry in consultation-liaison psychiatry with special emphasis on countertransference. *Journal of the American Academy of Psychoanalysis & Dynamic Psychiatry*, 34, 83–92.

Bolton, J. (2012). 'We've got another one for you!' Liaison psychiatry's experience of stigma towards patients with mental illness and mental health professionals. *The Psychiatrist*, 36(12).

Bourne, J. (2007 [2012]). *Improving Services and Support for People with Dementia: National Audit Office*. London: The Butterfly Scheme.

Cohen, N.A. (1982). On loneliness and the ageing process. *The International Journal of Psychoanalysis*, 63(Pt2), 149–155.

Davenhill, R. (2007). No trace with the furies: Issues of containment in the provision of care for people with dementia and those who care for them. In R. Davenhill (ed.) *Looking Into Later Life: A Psychoanalytic Approach to Depression and Dementia in Old Age*. London: Karnac.

Davenhill, R., Balfour, A., and Rustin, M. (2007). Pschodynamic observation and old age. In R. Davenhill (ed.) *Looking Into Later Life: A Psychoanalytic Approach to Depression and Dementia in Old Age*. London: Karnac, 129–144.

Erickson, E.H. (1966). Eight ages of man. *International Journal of Psychiatry*, II, 281–300.

Garner, J. (2004). Dementia. In S. Evans and J. Garner (eds.) *Talking Over the Years*. Hove: Brunner-Routledge.

Hildebrand, H.P. (1982). Psychotherapy with older patients. *British Journal of Medical Psychology*, 55, 19–28.

Illich, I. (1976). *Limits to Medicine: Medical Nemesis – The Expropriation of Health*. London: Marion Boyars.

Jackson, M. (1990). Psychosomatic symptoms: Psychodynamic treatment of the underlying personality disorder. *International Review of Psycho-Analysis*, 17, 388–390.

Johns Campaign: https://johnscampaign.org.uk/#/

Kitwood, T. (1997). *Dementia Reconsidered: The Person Comes First* (Rethinking Ageing). Milton Keynes: Open University Press.

Kohut, H. (1972). Thoughts on narcissism and narcissistic rage. *The Psychoanalytic Study of the Child*, 27, 360–400.

Living Well with Dementia: A National Dementia Strategy. (2009). London: Department of Health.

Main, T.F. (1957 [1989]). The ailment. In J. Johns (ed.) *The Ailment and Other Psychoanalytic Essays*. London: Free Association Books.

Martindale, B.V. (1989). Becoming dependent again: The fears of some elderly patients and their younger therapists. *Psychoanalytic Psychotherapy*, 4(1), 67–75.

Menzies, I.E.P. (1960). A case-study in the functioning of social systems as a defence against anxiety: A report on a study of the nursing service of a general hospital. *Human Relations*, 13(2), 95–121. http://doi.org/10.1177/001872676001300201.

Obholzer, A. (2000). In R.D. Hinshelwood and W. Skogstad (eds.) *Observing Organisations: Anxiety, Defence and Culture in Health Care*. London: Routledge.

Parsonage, M., and Fossey, M. (2011). *The Economic Evaluation of a Liaison Psychiatry Service*. London: Centre for Mental Health.

Prince, M., Bryce, R., Albinese, E., Wimo, A., Ribiero, W., and Fern, C.P. (2013, January). The global prevalence of dementia: A systematic review and metaanalysis. *Alzheimers Dementia*, 9(1), 63–75. e2.

Rustin, M.E., and Trowell, J. (1991). Developing the internal observer in professionals in training. *Infant Mental Health Journal*, 12(3), 233–245.

Sampson, E.L., Blanchard, M.R., Jones, L., Tookman, A., and King, M. (2009). Dementia in the acute hospital: Prospective cohort study of prevalence and mortality. *British Journal of Psychiatry*, 195, 61–66.

Sutton, L. (2001). When late life brings a diagnosis of Alzheimers disease and early life bought trauma. A cognitive-analytic understanding of loss of mind. Unpublished paper.

Terry, P. (1998). Who will care for older people? A case study of working with destructiveness and despair in long term care. *Journal of Social Work Practice*, 12(2), 209–216.

Thompson, T.L., and Suddath, R.L. (1987, March). Edward G. Billings, M.D.: Pioneer of consultation-liaison psychiatry. *Psychosomatics*, 28(3), 153–156.

Waddell, M. (1998). The last years. In *Inside Lives: Psychoanalysis and the Growth of the Personality*, Tavistock Clinical Series. London: Duckworth.

Wilkinson, P., Caudle, H., Nargis, F., and Hagger, M. (2015, June 1). Supporting compassionate care: Lessons from introducing Schwartz Rounds into a district general hospital. *Future Hospital Journal*, 2(Suppl 2), s13.

Williams, A. (2001). A literature review on the concept of intimacy in nursing. *Journal of Advanced Nursing*, 33(5), 660–667.

Chapter 7

Psychodynamic interventions in dementia

The Australian and New Zealand experience

Neil Jeyasingam

> *She listened in a way that made slow-witted people have flashes of inspiration.*
> *It wasn't that she actually said anything or asked questions that put such ideas*
> *into their heads. She simply sat there and listened with the utmost attention and*
> *sympathy, fixing them with her big, dark eyes, and they suddenly became aware*
> *of ideas whose existence they had never suspected. . . . And if someone felt that*
> *his life had been an utter failure, and that he himself was only one among mil-*
> *lions of wholly unimportant people who could be replaced as easily as broken*
> *windowpanes, he would go and pour out his heart to Momo. And, even as he*
> *spoke, he would come to realize by some mysterious means that he was abso-*
> *lutely wrong: that there was only one person like himself in the whole world,*
> *and that, consequently, he mattered to the world in his own particular way.*
>
>

Momo, Michael Ende (1985:11)[1]

Perspectives in psychodynamic theory in Australia and New Zealand are primarily dominated by the Conversational Model, developed by Robert Hobson and Russell Meares. Intended as an interpersonal modality for younger adults presenting with personality disordered features, it has had little application in older adults, and for that reason it is rarely used in cognitively impaired individuals, let alone in dementia settings. Beyond this modality, psychodynamic interventions are in their infancy in many regions.

However, there is considerable heterogeneity in old age mental health services across the nations, owing to the organic way in which services were formalised from existing practices, rather than centrally planned according to any heuristic. The Faculty of the Psychiatry of Old Age was only established within the Royal Australian and New Zealand College of Psychiatrists in January 1999. Some public services were only designated as Specialist Mental Health Services for Older Persons as recently as 2005. Psychogeriatrics as a whole shows enormous variability within the country on multiple levels – regarding which part of government is responsible for service provision, and whether dementia is regarded as a mental illness. As an example, in 1997–98 per capita expenditure on psychogeriatric services varied from A\$76.21 to \$174.66 in Western Australia. (Draper et al., 2005)

This inconsistency in service delivery naturally leads to significantly inadequate services in certain areas, however it also leads to surprisingly creative interventions in some others, with pockets of innovative interventions for older persons with cognitive impairment that have psychodynamic underpinnings for their rationale. This chapter will outline in detail three examples of these interventions for the reader to consider. It is suggested that, when systematic evidence is lacking, the question of how to design an old age service that effectively uses psychodynamic theory in a largely critical broader administrative culture is perhaps best informed by serendipity.

A psychodynamically informed behaviour advisory service

Behavioural and Psychological Symptoms of Dementia (BPSD) are a common concern for people with dementia, and tends to be the domain of old age psychiatry because of its history of managing mood disorders, psychotic symptoms, and engaging with and trying to understand distress. Behavioural advisory services for dementia are a relatively new phenomenon in Australia, with fragmented interventions in different areas in the setting of trying to operationalise their administration and scope of practice (Brodaty, Draper and Low, 2003). Following recognition of the value of services operating by a consultation-liaison model (as opposed to the relying solely on the expertise of inpatient staff in specialised units), this was reflected in policy directions in acute and mental health sectors in Australia (Brodaty and Cumming, 2010). Residential care facilities now provide care to people with increasingly complex medical conditions and dementia-related behavioural disorders who would have previously been cared for in the medical or psychiatric hospitals (Brodaty and Cumming, 2010) This has been in conjunction with an increased emphasis on patient-centred care (Kitwood, 1997), which is a humanistic appraisal of a patient with dementia in terms of understanding the person, rather than merely an agglomeration of behaviours.

Within this framework, the Dementia Behaviour Management Advisory Service of New South Wales (DBMAS) deserves special mention as one of the few advisory services that relies on the clinical expertise of its clinical director, a psychodynamic psychotherapist.

Referrals to the DBMAS service come from people living with dementia (whilst patients are able to self refer, this rarely occurs directly but usually following transfers from the nation's central Mental Health AccessLine following decisions made by triage clinicians), the family carers of people living with dementia, staff and volunteers working with people with dementia (such as community and residential aged care staff, general practitioners, staff of mental health services for older persons, and hospital staff) (DBMAS.org.au, 2017). Initial assessments are completed by DBMAS clinicians, who consist of registered nurses, registered mental health nurses, occupational therapists, physiotherapists, social workers, medical specialists, psychogeriatricians and geriatricians, neuropsychologists, clinical psychologists, speech pathologists, dieticians, and nurse practitioners. If it is felt that the patient requires a medical assessment, this is provided by Professor Stevenson, who was trained under the Conversational Model with Russell Meares. An expert in older adult personality disorders (Stevenson, Brodaty, Boyce and Byth Wilson, 2012) and extensively published on psychodynamic psychotherapy, this service provides unique insights into patient functioning. Starting as a smaller local advisory service, it has expanded to receive funding for state-wide behaviour assessments following the success of its interventions as of 2016. Formative evaluations of outcomes are not yet available at time of writing.

Within this framework, an anonymised case illustration will serve as an example of the practice and the output of this service:

> *I note that Mr X's loss of his carer's role is likely leading to his repeated intrusions to other residents of the facility, particularly his predilection towards entering the rooms of other female residents, which does not appear to be a predatory behaviour but often related to hearing calls from them and an effort to be supportive. His greatly deteriorated language capacity makes it difficult for him to make his ideas heard by others, but I also suspect his practice of hoarding food in his room (to the point of its spoiling) probably relates to his traumatic experiences in his home country's civil war. Opportunities to reorient as well as to introduce familiar events have not been successful, as they have rather rekindled his early traumatic experiences.*

This case vignette demonstrates the effectiveness of the service – in an effort to understand this gentleman's behaviour in the context of his premorbid (and current) personality, a 'difficult' person becomes a caring person who attempts to help others. His food hoarding suggests years of earlier famine and hunger and misdirected attempts to avoid ever experiencing such horror again. The very act of reframing this man's narrative may assist the staff in tolerating his behaviour better, and finding new ways to help him integrate with the present.

It is important to note that the framework of this service is essential in understanding its progress. Ownership of the DBMAS Service comes from Hammond-Care, a private organisation registered as a Christian Charity. (hammondcare.com.au, 2017), this led to a novel intervention in the setting of failure of the institution-first approach, which eventually led to a policy shift funding successful private interventions that had a person-centred, broad-based consultation-liaison philosophy.

However, there are limitations. Only psychodynamic assessments, if appropriate, are made, but there is no capacity for psychodynamic psychotherapy, nor any other direct intervention (such as art or music therapy), as the service is consultative only and makes recommendations utilising target organisation's own resources. Whilst providing this interpretations of patient behaviour is provided to the staff as a whole, it relies on the target organisation's internal communication strategies to see that these ideas spread and are used by the appropriate clinicians.

In addition, these assessments are made only following a second-tier request for a medical assessment, which is in itself highly limited due to the competing demands on the director's time.

The capacity for dynamic interpretations is largely limited towards the skill of its assessors – principally, its clinical director. However, the flow-on effect through the rest of the service is a validation of the person-centred approach, encouraging an interest in the patient's internal world amongst all staff are involved in their care.

An old age outpatient psychotherapy service

Following an interest in psychodynamic psychotherapy and an awareness of a relative dearth of available services for older people, Australia's first psychotherapy service specifically for older persons was set up in 2002 (Payman, 2010).

The St George's Hospital Aged Psychiatry Service was established in 1995 at the hospital campus in Kew, Melbourne. The move to St Georges followed the closure of Mont Park as part of the process of deinstitutionalisation across the state and mainstreaming of psychiatric services.

In April 2002, an outpatient psychotherapy clinic commenced at Normanby House. Its purpose was to provide psychotherapy assessment and treatment for patients over 65 from the St Georges catchment area. The clinic ran according to a shared public-private model, in which public patients incur no cost for treatment and the psychotherapist is remunerated by the government's Medicare rebate for specific item numbers. Therapies offered were in one or more of five different therapies: psychodynamic psychotherapy, CBT, grief counselling and therapy, supportive psychotherapy, and social skills training, with recognised limitations in the lack of reminiscence therapy or interpersonal therapy.

Patients were not screened for cognitive function prior to receiving therapy, and in the assessment of the first 51 patients' studies, one patient was identified as having dementia, and regrettably was found inappropriate for therapy due to the aforementioned cognitive deficits. In addition, of the eight patients who were deemed suitable for psychodynamic psychotherapy, only three had over 40 sessions of therapy. The other six patients received between 3 and 11 sessions. Nobody over the age of 85 received psychodynamic psychotherapy. In direct consultation with the unit's director, it interestingly arose from a conflict between the unit's director (and principle therapist) and his own supervisor, as there was reticence from the latter for the oldest old to undertake psychoanalysis. As for the five patients who did not receive more than 40 sessions, these were patients who dropped out of therapy, with transport difficulties cited as the primary obstacle.

Although not providing interventions for dementia, the experience of this clinic (at time of its publication, the only such clinic in the world) provided a useful roadmap for interventions in future. In direct communication with its director, the lack of screening for cognitive deficits appears to have been a deliberate intervention, as it determined successful interventions based on progress through therapy, not in terms of assuming invalidation based on arbitrary benchmarks.

In an unusual fashion, this may have led to several individuals with cognitive impairment receiving psychotherapy that they may not otherwise have received. This traditional bar could arguably be seen as a bias or prejudice against cognitive impairment.

The study also identified benefits with an eclectic approach, combining multiple models of psychotherapy. It notably identified that long-term therapies had very limited benefit (at least within the limitations of this study, and one is reminded of the conflicted perspectives between the unit's director and his psychotherapy supervisor), which prompts an exploration of brief psychodynamic models of therapy, which are (at time of writing) enjoying a renaissance in several organisations around the world. (Mantosh, Priyanthy and Lynn, 2008).

The Normanby service is an extremely limited service, however it is also the first of its kind and provides a novel – and expandable – model for delivery of psychotherapeutic services to a wider subset of the population. Its value as a pioneer service cannot be underestimated.

An old age multidisciplinary service

The Faculty of Old Age Psychiatry in Australia was only established in January 1999, and New South Wales' Specialist Mental Health Services for Older Persons was consolidated relatively recently (from 2005) as a means of identifying existing older persons' support services and unifying them into a strategic plan across the state. The Hornsby Ku-Ring-Gai service, HKSMHSOPs, despite preceding this formal plan, was created with a significant degree of staffing and coordination. Its core, a community-based multidisciplinary team covering a catchment area of approximately 205,000, comprises a senior triage nurse and several allied health clinicians (comprising occupational therapists, social workers, psychologists, and registered nurses), operating according to an assertive case management model. There is also a limited inpatient facility onsite, with admissions possible to the adult mental health inpatient unit, with a dedicated social worker, registrar, and consultant psychogeriatrician, who also supervises the community team.

The consultant psychogeriatrician is also a founding member of the Faculty of Psychotherapy with the Royal Australian and New Zealand College of Psychiatrists, with a specific interest in psychodynamic psychotherapy, as adapted for older adults. He also operates as a psychotherapy supervisor in private and public practice.

The service receives referrals for older persons in their own homes, in residential facilities, and from the hospital's emergency department, short stay psychiatric unit, and medical and surgical wards. The service's overarching organisation, Hornsby's Mental Health Service, has approximately 15–20 registrars at any one time. These training psychiatrists, as part of college accreditation, are required to complete a long term psychotherapy case with appropriate supervision.

Within this setting, therefore, there are several referrals of patients with varying levels of cognitive impairment that can then be connected to psychotherapeutic interventions and assessments on an as required basis. The service receives in excess of 700 referrals per year. Of these, about ten are assessed as having a potential benefit from psychodynamic psychotherapy, and about five proceed to be accepted for the same. It is possible that these numbers would increase if there were more clinicians available for purposes of psychodynamic assessments.

Given that the registrars are required to provide these interventions as a part of their training, this leads to a reasonable pool of therapists. The consultant psychogeriatrician provides brief psychodynamic interventions, but also supervises registrars in long term psychotherapy. A brief case vignette illustrates the kinds of patients seen:

72 year old Mrs Y had had considerable interpersonal dysfunction well before admission to a nursing home. She had a moderate cognitive impairment (of vascular aetiology) leading to a Mini Mental State Examination of 22/30, but with reasonably intact short term memory. It is notable that this is not an insurmountable degree of impairment in most circumstances, however her interpersonal dysfunction was a very likely contributor to – if not the primary reason for – her transfer to supported residence.

She was a voluntary resident at a nursing home that was locked due to a mixed population of residents, including severe dementia. She was referred due to making suicidal threats and absconding (leaving without notifying staff) from the facility on three separate occasions, being found wandering (but more accurately, purposefully escaping from a restrictive environment) along the road outside the property. She was angry and refusing to engage with any staff member, and often kept to herself in a dining hall that had to be evacuated from any other residents. She had two daughters, estranged from one due to disapproving of her daughter's sexuality, and a very poor relationship with the second, citing her being in a nursing home proof of being abandoned – which, arguably, may not have been incorrect. She was assessed and noted to have a reactive affect and longstanding interpersonal difficulties, and was introduced to a junior registrar with a view to an assessment regarding appropriateness for long-term psychotherapy. The registrar would come to visit her in her nursing home, and sessions often took place in her own room. The registrar noted a reasonable attachment during the assessment sessions, and admission of very poor maternal attachment to her children, with an awareness of a difficulty connecting with other people throughout her life, and anger at the perception of cognitive impairment. Following this, and with assessment by the consultant psychogeriatrician, she was deemed to have capacity to agree to a long-term intervention, with risks and potential benefits explained to her.

The sessions were marked with considerable resistance, with the patient never outright refusing to see the (female) registrar, but often citing multiple excuses – such as frequently needing to go to the bathroom during time allocated to sessions. This resistance was not present during initial assessment, but occurred a few sessions into therapy, despite an initial contractual and full agreement to have therapy. Therapy occurred in the patient's room due to the patient's preference. There was limited insight, with denying any personal difficulties, and changes in the frame to have the patient seen in a separate, neutral room (despite patient preference) rather than her own room was associated with improved engagement. Suicidal ideation considerably reduced, and the sessions moved from ventilation of anger directed at her children through to anger directed at the patient's mother. There were descriptions of the patient's own mother being cold and unfeeling – with notably similar language used previously to describe her children.

In the last ten sessions, the staff in the nursing facility noted a prodigious improvement in the patient's functioning, from initially refusing to engage with any person through to knowing every resident and staff members' name. There was no more suicidal ideation, and whilst the patient remained 'grumpy' and requiring episodes of privacy, there were no more behavioural concerns. Termination was successfully negotiated, and ongoing arms-length Liaison with the facility verified that the improved behaviour was sustained for a year after termination.

One could see this patient as being initially wilful and unlikeable, probably due to failure of attachment as an infant and growing up with a feeling of being unloveable – which was brought into the room with her – but also demanding. This poor relationship with her daughters likely led to her being transferred to a facility, together with her difficulty engaging with any support due to frequent suicidality. This puts in a new light her 'delinquent' behaviour of absconding from the facility – a childlike behaviour perhaps because she feels once more like a child, disenfranchised and thrown back into a familiar scenario.

One could question the significance of her room – required by the patient initially as the location for therapy, she started to retreat soon into therapy by leaving to her bathroom, which became her new 'safe space'. The physical difficulty with moving from the new therapy room back to the bathroom reduce the ease of this defence, and was marked with a major improvement in the course of therapy.

The improvement in her interactions with staff did not arise from breaching her confidentiality, or disclosing the detail of her therapy – documentation in staff notes comprised only issues of risk and issues requiring immediate communication. This improvement was notably patient-led, with staff finding gradually that the patient was starting to talk to other residents first, and then eventually to every person in the building.

A personal experience

Early in my training, and shortly after being exposed to psychodynamic psychotherapy, I was working in an older adult inpatient unit that had a small community role. Under the hospital's surveillance was a nursing home facility that had a regular visiting psychogeriatric clinic. It was my role as registrar to review patients at the nursing home, which was purpose built to accommodate patients with a high mental health comorbidity. One of these patients was a 74-year-old woman with moderate Alzheimer's, transferred to the nursing home due to profound social isolation as well as behavioural concerns. She was brought to our attention due to having considerable agitation, with violent fluctuations in mood, verbal agitation, and attacking staff when they attempted to attend to her personal needs. She had very limited mobility and was dependent on a walker, yet angrily refused showers, preferring to yell in her room. Her Mini Mental State Examination score was under 14, and she had profound short-term memory loss, as well as appeared to be exhibiting some tangentiality.

There was a trial of antipsychotic therapy, but this was curtailed due to her refusal to accept medication. She was well in other respects and fortunately did not need treatment for chronic physical illnesses.

Following discussion with her general practitioner and what was left of family willing to speak with us, much of her earlier history became filled in. She had suffered repeated sexual abuse as a young child, with systematic abuse occurring for at least three years throughout her adolescence. It was in late adolescence that severe emotional disturbances manifested, with angry outbursts and self-harm attempts. There was also impulsivity, with several brief and catastrophic relationships. However, in adulthood a marked change occurred when she fled her traumatic life to become a nun. Within the confines of the convent, she was relatively stable, but apparently remained prickly and difficult to engage, with minimal meaningful relationships. It was about three years ago when memory changes first were noticed with her, and she never accepted a diagnosis of dementia, up to and including admission to her nursing home.

I had noted a likely premorbid borderline personality disorder, and interesting longstanding attachment disruption. At that stage of training I spoke to my supervisor regarding trialling a brief psychodynamic intervention for this woman, given her considerable management difficulties. Finding the concept unusual, I was nevertheless permitted to proceed with seeing this patient for therapy, as well as with consent provided by her family. I sought and had external psychoanalytic supervision for the process, as my training supervisor (a psychogeriatrician) had little experience of psychotherapy in older adults.

I met with the patient to discuss her experiences, using an open and flexible frame of meeting in public sections of the nursing home (as she refused to be redirected), but nevertheless giving her the option to move to where she wished, as well as to discuss whatever she wished. She described feeling angry at all staff, which I reflected back to her, and offered opportunities to discuss her past – which she declined. There was marked poverty of thought, and considerable emotional material on a superficial, shifting basis. Sessions lasted barely half an hour, and after three sessions the task seemed too difficult, perhaps for us both, as she had no apparent recollection of my previous engagements or our previous sessions.

There was no opportunity to build on previous session materials, and all that could be done was reflect on her current emotions and how they had been long-standing. We terminated after just four sessions.

However, a few weeks after terminating therapy, staff came to me in consider-able gratitude, finding that her behaviour in the nursing home had been consid-erably better. Despite no changes in medication, she was no longer abusive or aggressive to staff, and they had found a marked change in her pattern of engage-ment. She was still rude and dismissive, but she was now considerably calmer, and on occasion even thanking staff for their help. This remarkable change per-sisted for at least two months after the therapy occurred, with no other identifiable contributor to this change.

I reflected this back to my training supervisor, but was soon to discover that the educational experience was not over. Soon after this, I was brought up in front of the area's director of training, as well as my training supervisor, for a disciplinary meeting. Apparently the issue of contention was that I had failed to recognise that the practice of psychodynamic psychotherapy was 'worthless' for patients with cognitive impairment, and that I had been permitted to start see-ing this patient in order to realise this for myself. In addition, the fact that I had persisted for four sessions showed a gross lack of insight into appropriate patient selection and therapeutic process, and I must have misrepresented my practice to my psychoanalytic supervisor in order for them to allow me to continue as long as I did.

Fortunately, there were minimal professional repercussions, but the experience speaks volumes about the use of psychotherapy. There is considerable fear with the use of certain therapeutic techniques, despite the use of appropriate consent processes, objective goals of therapy, and appropriate supervision for clinical practice. This conservative approach is not without merit, as older people with dementia are a vulnerable population, and psychodynamic interventions can inflict considerable pain. However there are significant potential benefits. I note for example that my experience has been mirrored by others (Burns, 2005), with finding significant carer-reported improvements in patient functioning despite no apparent gains in insight. The essential issue that stands, however, is the need to provide interventions that are of benefit to the patient, particularly in settings where there is no alternative.

It is also worth speculating as to why my clinical supervisor and director of training had such a severe reaction to the episode. These were senior, well-respected clinicians with extensive experience in the care of the elderly, and I still respect their considerable accomplishments. Perhaps the unwillingness or discomfort with thinking about people with dementia comes from a hope that there is no further thought or desire present in a person with dementia. The reader will excuse my insolence for suggesting a perhaps more pragmatic reason – I'm reminded that Freud argued against the use of psychotherapy for any patient over the age of 50, when he himself was aged 49.

Discussion

There are multiple opportunities suggested by the aforementioned descriptions. I suggest that a connecting factor is the presence of a lead medical clinician who has specialist level training in both old age psychiatry and psychodynamic psychotherapy. Older adults have major difficulties in access of therapies and mobility, as well as a therapeutic community that is largely unaware of the indications for psychotherapy.

An outpatient service has clear benefits for clinician interaction, ease of administration, and staffing. There are also considerable opportunities for peer review and dissemination of ideas, particularly in eclectic settings with multiple therapists seeing the same patient for different reasons. This leads well into research opportunities. However, it also greatly limits potential access for less mobile patients, and is highly dependent on acquiring referrals from a community that may not understand their indications.

Meanwhile, a community service with a wider range of referral criteria increases the likelihood of patients presenting that are indicated for therapeutic interventions. However, even with clinicians who are experienced in assessment of appropriateness for psychotherapy, a very small proportion of patients will be indicated for therapy. In addition, there needs to be a mechanism for where the therapy will practically happen – together with accommodation of the setting components that will affect therapy. There is also the risk of marginalisation of therapeutic skill, with an expectation of only certain individuals within the service having an obligation to think 'dynamically'.

The reader is thus encouraged to consider therapeutic interventions for the elderly not only in terms of the evidence and philosophy for their interventions, but also in terms of the realities of service design and provision amongst overarching government policy. To do so is to create an intervention that can potentially validate individuals to a level never previously envisioned, as well as create a stable self-maturing enterprise with benefits for patients as well as therapists.

Note

1 Original English language translation copyright Burke Books Publishing Company Limited 1974.
Published as The Grey Gentlemen, Copyright K. Thienemanns Verlag. Stuttgart. 1973.
Reproduced by permission of AVA international GmbH · Autoren- und Verlagsagentur · Hohenzollernstr. 38 Rgb · D-80801 München.

References

Brodaty, H., and Cumming, A. (2010, September). Dementia services in Australia. *International Journal of Geriatric Psychiatry*, 25(9), 887–995.

Brodaty, H., Draper, B., and Low, L. (2003). Behavioural and psychological symptoms of dementia: A seven-tiered model of service delivery. *Medical Journal of Australia*, 178(5), 231–234.

Burns, L. (2005, August). Brief psychotherapy in Alzheimer's disease: Randomised controlled trial. *British Journal of Psychiatry*, 187, 143–147.

DBMAS.ORG.AU. (2017). *DBMAS website* (online). Available at dbmas.org.au [accessed 7 March 2017].

Draper, B., Melding, P.S., and Brodaty, H. (2005). Psychogeriatric services: Current trends in Australia and New Zealand. In B. Draper, P. Melding, and H. Brodaty (eds.) *Psychogeriatric Service Delivery and International Perspective*, 1st ed. Oxford: Oxford University Press.

Ende, M. (1985). *Momo*. Illustrated ed. New York: Doubleday, p. 11.

HAMMONDCARE.COM.AU. (2017). *Hammondcare official website*. Available at hammondcare.com.au [accessed 7 March 2017].

Kitwood, T.M. (1997). *Dementia Reconsidered: The Person Comes First*. Buckingham: Open University Press.

Mantosh, D., Priyanthy, W., and Lynn, S. (2008). Techniques of brief psychodynamic psychotherapy. In *Textbook of Psychotherapeutic Treatments*. VA, United States: American Psychiatric Publishing.

Payman, V. (2010). An outpatient psychotherapy clinic for the elderly: Rationale, establishment and characteristics. *Asia-Pacific Psychiatry*, 2(4), 191–200.

Stevenson, J., Brodaty, H., Boyce, P., and Byth Wilson, K. (2012). Does age moderate the effect of personality disorder on coping style in psychiatric inpatients? *Journal of Psychiatric Practice*, 18(3), 187–198.

Chapter 8

Art therapy with people with dementia

The present and the past

Angela Byers

I will work out the divinity that is busy within my mind/and tend the means that are mine.

Pindar (c. 530 BC)[1]

Introduction

The epigraph describes the aesthetic sense which remains in dementia. In this chapter I will describe the practice of art therapy with people with dementia by portraying it from three different viewpoints: the first viewpoint is my own, a description of an art therapy session taken straight from the notes which I wrote as soon as possible after the session;[2] the second viewpoint comprises themes from the literature about art therapy and working with people with dementia; the third viewpoint is directly from clients in the form of comments given by two people with dementia who are currently having art therapy.[3]

What I have written is the result of studying the texts, listening to patients and extracting what I perceive as the main themes. Then, in comparing the themes, I have created a picture which suggests a 'three-dimensional' view of art therapy.

View from a session

I begin with an account of an art therapy session with a man with mild dementia, which illustrates one person's way of getting involved in the process of art therapy. It describes elements about the effects of using art, about the relationship between patient and therapist, and about how the patient's dementia can affect the process.

I created this account not only from my notes, which included some of my immediate reflections, but also my thoughts on re-reading them three years later.

Mr A was 78 and had been referred to me after a stay in hospital, following a breakdown in his relationship with his wife who was simultaneously receiving counselling. This was his eighth session in one-to-one art therapy with me.

I had organised his transport to art therapy because we had agreed that he would not be able to negotiate public transport and arrive on time.

On this day we entered the room and he hesitated, asking me where I was going to sit. I said 'probably there', pointing to a chair and he put his coat on the other one. I answered straightforwardly to enable him to feel at ease at this point of the session.

He told me he had been to an exercise class. He didn't think he was doing well but the 'man' had said he was. I thought about previous sessions when he had said he was not doing well and we had established that he was lacking in confidence, how he had been bullied by his father and brothers, never learning to read and write.

He then said, 'I never know what is going to happen, I am too ill to learn new things.' I asked, 'Why?' He said, 'Well I'm eighty' and then he hesitated and said, 'And so I will go until I'm dead'. I nodded so as not to interrupt the effect of this powerful statement.

Then he said, 'What are we doing today?' It was strange for me because I thought that by now he knew what he was doing, he recognised the room and he did recognise a lot; but there again he might not, I might have been assuming that he did; was this organic, a lapse of memory? Or his personality, being cautious? Or a bit of both?

I tried unsuccessfully to encourage him to decide and then said 'Well, there's me to talk to, the art materials to use'. He still asked me what I wanted him to do, so I asked if he would be able to use the art materials. I gave him choices, showing him the different materials and added 'Here's your folder with the drawings you did before'.

He was interested in the clay, which he had never used with me before. It seemed that he was attracted by this tactile, real stuff, moving from mind to body. He asked if he could see it.

He poked the clay and asked, 'It's to make a model?' He was still being cautious: after all when he was a child he was constantly told he'd got things wrong. I said 'yes'. He warned, 'I'll make a mess'. I replied, 'I can wipe it clean'. He said 'That'll take you extra time.' I said that that was alright.

He said 'I don't know what I could do', 'What could I make?' However by this time he had actually taken out a piece and made a sausage shape; the clay had invited him to touch it and work with it.

I said 'have a look at it; you see what you think it looks like'. By now he had taken the lead, albeit unconsciously, and I sensed that I could go from there; I could be direct to encourage his process, one thing leading to another.

He did look at it and then he attached four legs and turned it round so it stood on its legs. He did this silently and so I was quiet.

I tried not to interrupt the actual image-making process, because this was a special time when he was with himself. He would be aware of me watching, he was not completely alone; but I expected that he would be having a sort of conversation with himself, which would be interwoven with his manipulating the materials and with the creative process, in which one thing leads to another.

I saw that he modelled what I thought were some scales on the model's back and a big mouth, like a fish, and two dents for eyes (see Figure 8.1).

As he worked Mr A said his brain wasn't working and I asked 'in what way?' He just repeated it, so I asked if he couldn't concentrate and he said 'yes'.

After a while he said it was no good.

He said it was supposed to be a mouse and I said I'd thought it was a lizard, but that 'both run quickly' and I added 'I like the shape, I think it flows'.

He smiled. He said 'like a child'.

I asked him, does it remind him of school? He replied 'school'.

He told me how his father had undermined his attempts to learn.

He smiled and then he said, 'But now I'm grown up and I'm here'. I said, 'You got away from your Dad'. He said, 'Yes'. I said 'But he's still in here isn't he?' I pointed at my head and he said, 'Yes'.

We talked about the model. I asked what he associated with the mouse. He said, 'They're destructive'. I said I thought it looked as though it was watching for when it could run.

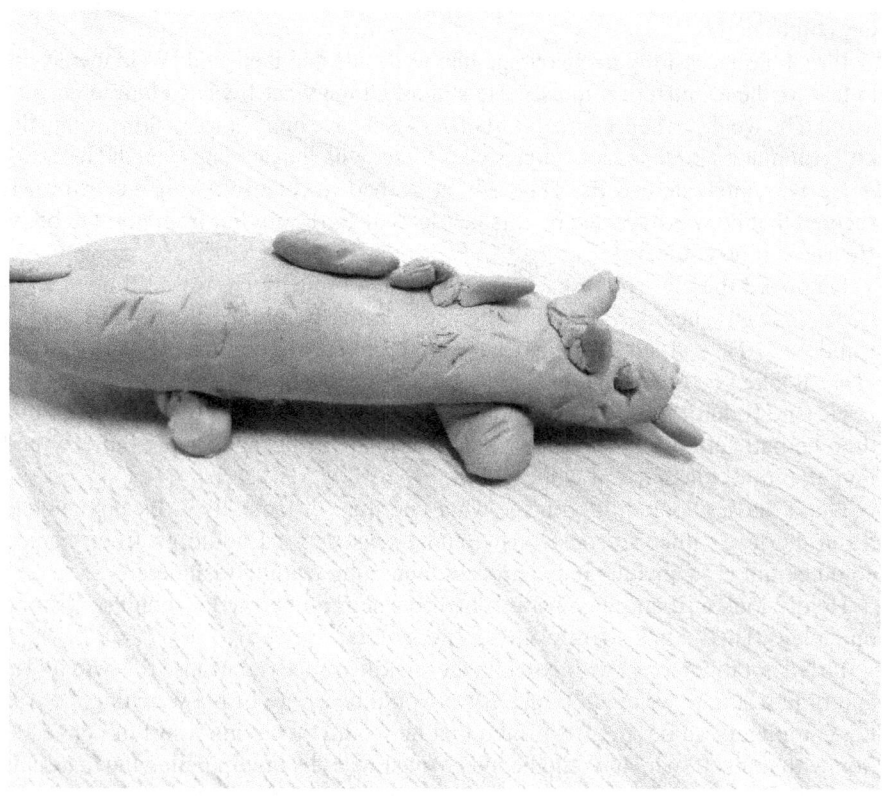

Figure 8.1 Mr A's Model

Perhaps he was afraid that I might see something destructive in him and I was afraid that I might frighten him and then he would run away.

He said he would do more and I warned him that I was going to check the time: the process of making an image is affected by the knowledge of when the session will end. So I would count down for people with dementia, letting the patient know we had fifteen, ten, then five minutes before I ended the session.

He said his brain wouldn't let him be creative. I said, 'but this is creative'. I said, 'Perhaps your brain forgets what you were doing'. He seemed to agree.

He then worked until it was time to finish.

I asked if the front coils were teeth and he said he had given it whiskers. This now makes me think about his sensitivity, he was constantly feeling (as with whiskers) to see if he was doing the right thing.

He said the bits on the back showed the hair standing on its end when you put your hand on its back. I thought of fear, or aggression, I imagined the moment of deciding whether to flee or fight.

Summary

The description illustrates Mr A's measured involvement in the process of art therapy during one of his sessions. Initially he was hesitant, but moved gradually to choosing and using a material, first in an unconscious way, then with a more conscious engagement. Both of us could associate to the model he was making, and make links to his long-term memories and their effects.

It illustrates my dilemma over his hesitations, being unsure whether they were due to dementia or childhood events; also the changes in my approach as Mr A became engaged in his model.

In some ways this process was no different to the process in a session with someone who does not have dementia. But other dimensions were added by my involvement in practical issues such as his transport arrangements, my giving simple choices and my not being sure whether some of his actions were due to dementia or lack of confidence, or both.

By arranging his transport, I made sure that he could get to the session and then go back home again; by adapting my interventions, I enabled his involvement; yet it was the creation of his model which enabled us to converse, using our associations to it.

This is an illustration of an art therapy session with someone with dementia.

In order to discover how other art therapists have approached this work, I will now describe the main themes which I found in the literature.

A view from the literature

Art therapists have been writing about their work with people with dementia since the early 1970s: most of their papers were published in English in the USA and the UK. For the purpose of this present chapter, I have collated the most reported themes from this literature, as well as from a few other significant papers, in order to present the art therapists' point of view.

Most of the published literature centers upon case study material, including detailed observations out of which the authors discuss and theorise the practice of art therapy undertaken with this client group. There are also seven papers which describe research studies (Knapp, 1994; Wood, 2002; Rusted et al., 2006; Kim et al., 2009; Mihailidis et al., 2010; Kim et al., 2012; Kim et al., 2013). However these studies differ from each other in purpose, methodology and rigour, so it is not possible to generalise research priorities or outcome from them.

I have presumed that the most reported themes from all of the literature I surveyed demonstrate some consensus of expert opinion. Although the details which I will discuss refer to papers which have been published more recently, the themes have almost entirely been drawn from the survey as a whole, except the last one which involves developments in neuroscience. The first of these themes is that art therapy facilitates communication, for example through self-expression (Baines, 2011) and the use of metaphors. Metaphors provide another 'channel for communication' (Urbas, 2009), often of feelings (Kamar, 1997) and are described by Cossio (2002) as 'utterly personal' and 'sometimes secret and unintelligible even for the person who makes them' (47). This visual form of communication is particularly significant for people with dementia, even if it must be sensed rather than interpreted.

Communication becomes more complex in art therapy groups. Stephenson (2016) shows how group members can influence each other's art making process, consciously or unconsciously; Golebiowski (2015) says that 'a single image made by one person can resonate with all group members, uniting and moving them to a deeper level of understanding and commitment to each other' (223); Ashby (2015) adds that the 'social dynamics of the group' are 'an important source of support and benefit' (208).

Indeed Rusted et al. (2006) report 'improved sociability' in the results of their randomised controlled trial of art therapy groups, adding that the group members in the trial showed positive changes in mood also.

Rusted et al. were studying art therapy groups, not art groups. So what makes art therapy different from other ways of working with art? Most of the papers state that the processes in a session and of making artworks are more significant than are the finished images, whilst Tyler (2002) adds that a patient's process develops from session to session over time.

The word 'process' can become bland with overuse, so it is encouraging to find details of what it involves. For example, many authors describe how a person with dementia is engaged or concentrating more than usual whilst using the art materials. The process of making an image 'involves constant decision making' (Ashby, 2015) and can provide a sense of autonomy (Norris and Bush, 2015) and control (Harlan, 1993; Urbas, 2009), feelings which are frequently undermined by the symptoms of dementia as well as the responses of other people.

During this process thoughts and feelings 'emerge' from spontaneous activity (Golebiowski, 2015) and can be expanded whilst images are being created (Falk,

2002; Baines, 2011). This involvement often leads to people with poor short-term memory remembering an image made previously, or remembering the art therapy room or objects within it (Falk, 2002; Waller, 2002).

Baines (2011) says that the creative aspect of the process makes art therapy 'meaningful' and Urbas (2009) says that it is significant because it involves the 'self'.

Creativity is another theme which is frequently discussed. Some describe it as an artistic struggle (Shore, 1997), conflictual but liberating (Shore, 1997; Cossio, 2002) and giving 'intense consolation' (Cossio, 2002, p. 47), through which 'mood is elevated, and the individual is able to experience a sense of personal identity' (Norris and Bush, 2015, p. 3). In structuring a session, most authors recommend a directive approach, in which instructions or a theme are given, whilst several, mainly British, authors work non-directively and follow their patients' leads, thus working in a more traditionally psychoanalytic way: listening and creating an environment which 'holds' the patient (Winnicott, 1965), enabling them to communicate and paying attention to transference and countertransference. This involves consistency in time and place (Falk, 2002; Tyler, 2002) and 'professional and psychodynamic boundaries' (Golebiowski, 2015, p. 226).

The therapeutic relationship changes according to the severity of a patient's dementia. In the case of mild dementia, it is possible to converse with words and therefore to work more overtly from a psychoanalytic viewpoint. In the late stages conversation will be difficult or impossible and psychoanalytic work focusses more on countertransference, as an indication for the therapist about their own difficulties with engaging (Harlan, 1990; Byers, 1998) and as a tool for understanding the patient (Berardi, 1997; Shore, 1997; Byers, 1998).

Such attentiveness is valuable because, as Kitwood (1997) has brought to our awareness, there are 'many processes that work towards the undermining of people who have dementia' (45), and Cohen (2006) observes that attitudes towards people with dementia tend to be problem-focussed. So Jensen (1997) says we should look for 'remaining strengths' in order to acknowledge their senses of self, whilst Levine-Madori (2012), Urbas (2009) and Baines (2011) promote positive reinforcement in the approach to art therapy which they describe. Yet I suggest that there is a danger of not acknowledging difficult and depressed feelings; thinking psychoanalytically we want to know the whole person, the strengths and the feelings, positive and negative. So it is that Harlan (1993) says 'Clients may feel that their remaining capacities for judgement and discrimination are being recognised when their own negative appraisals of the art work are acknowledged' (104).

Aside from the therapeutic relationship, some art therapists have focussed on the use of art making and images to diagnose dementia (Knapp, 1994) or a person's stage of dementia (Wald, 1984; Kim et al., 2012). These studies use quantitative methods which narrow the focus, overlooking the interpersonal quality of art therapy.

However, the link between the brain and image making has often been of interest. Back in 1979 Edwards referenced research which demonstrated that the two sides of the brain control different types of mental activity. Baines (2011), Ashby (2015), and Norris and Bush (2015) all say that art making uses the whole brain, right and left side, suggesting but not demonstrating that this is helpful for dementia.

Some art therapists have been influenced by recent developments in neuroscience. Galbraith et al. (2008) and Levine-Madori (2012) have devised programmes to stimulate people who have mild cognitive impairment and early-stage Alzheimer's Disease, using art therapy as a component. Both publications include reference to experimental research into brain plasticity which demonstrates that 'the brain can make new cells when stimulated by visual, auditory, sensory, verbal, or kinaesthetic stimuli' ((Diamond, 2000, in Levine-Madori, 2012, p. 87) and longitudinal studies which demonstrate that people are less likely to develop dementia if they have had 'an active intellectual life' (Levine-Madori, 2012, p. 89). The programmes they describe are intended to delay the symptoms; but I suggest that they have not yet produced enough convincing evidence. Indeed Mirabella (2015), who has contributed to many publications which describe experimental research into brain plasticity, points out that such changes in the brain 'take time to become established, especially in nonhealthy brains' (197); he suggests that the interventions used by most arts therapies do not continue for long enough. However, he says art therapy for people with dementia can enhance 'self-confidence', 'improving interpersonal functioning' (197), which is necessary to improve 'the personal and social lives of patients and caregivers' (198): surely a valuable contribution.

Jensen (1997) makes a pertinent point when she says that some are not motivated to have art therapy; Waller (2002) says that low motivation is exacerbated when there is a lack of managerial support for art therapy groups. Queen-Daugherty (2001) suggests that the words 'art' and 'therapy' can put people off, and she waits 'for the group to become familiar with the space and engaged in dialogue before introducing the art materials' (28).

Yet the BAAT approved guidelines (Art Therapy & Outlook on Later Life (ATOLL) BAAT Special Interest Group, 2015) suggest 'The art therapist must pay close attention to the patient's willingness to engage in the art therapy process and to ensure that the rights of the patient are maintained at all times' (7), although, 'Offering a place to come and talk or watch can take some of the pressure out of attending, reducing expectation and fear of "failing"' (11).

Art therapy may seem foreign to those who have never been involved in art or therapy, whilst dementia and other people's responses to it can undermine a person's confidence and create apathy. Yet some may encourage people to attend over enthusiastically. The guidelines (2015) acknowledge this dilemma.

Summary

I have distilled several themes from the literature about art therapy with people with dementia; most of these are enduring, reappearing frequently in the papers, although they are not substantiated by a body of research which is reliable enough to be used as evidence.

There have been subtle changes in the literature over time which run parallel to changes in attitudes towards people with dementia. Recently? there has also been a more radical shift towards linking attributes of art therapy to changes in the brain, with a debated claim that art therapy could be a form of treatment for early stage dementia (Galbraith et al., 2008; Mirabella, 2015).

Nevertheless the enduring qualities have relevance: the process of using art materials in a therapeutic setting is seen as more beneficial than the quality of the finished image; art therapy is an agent for expression and fuller communication and, being a creative activity it is meaningful; finally art therapy can be a group activity which is inclusive and generates improved social interaction.

Views from patient/participants

The views of patients are important, if not essential, in any description or research about the experiences of people with dementia (Knauss and Moyer, 2006). However, their views are typically missing in the literature. There are many ethical considerations which may lead to such omissions, concerning the vulnerability of people with dementia and their potential susceptibility to misunderstanding or persuasion. With these considerations in mind, I have been able to gain the consent of two individuals to participate in short interviews. Both were receiving art therapy with separate therapists other than myself. Participant A was having individual sessions and participant B was part of an open art therapy group; I talked with them outside of these sessions.

Because there were only two of them, their views obviously cannot be considered as representative of the recipients of art therapy as a whole; yet they do add a third view to this chapter, thus serving to broaden its perspective.

The interviews were unstructured, although on occasion, in order to get to a point more quickly, I found myself asking direct questions; this was to remind them that I wanted to hear about their opinions of art therapy before they forgot their sessions.

Both participants showed that they had positive feelings towards their therapist or co-therapist. Participant A said he accepted the therapist because he was easy with him and he could be easy with the therapist, participant B said that she very much liked the co-therapist, having forgotten the therapist whom she had not seen so recently. Participant A said that he appreciated that he was not told when and what to draw, supporting this statement with long-term memories of being under pressure to produce drawings for others.

Participant B described the art making as a time to 'create', to 'create' being better than to 'destroy'. She described the conversation in the group as a time when you 'learn, for everybody, not just for yourself'.

I asked about the quality of the art materials and was told that they need to be 'strong'. One of the rooms where art therapy took place was appreciated as bright and airy, making it an environment where participant B could talk about personal matters.

Drawing these themes together, I conclude that these two participants value a calm and/or friendly approach which allows some autonomy when needed over choices about what to do and when to do it.

I also conclude that the quality of the art materials is significant for some and that the environment influences a person's wish to talk about personal matters.

Art therapy was valued as enabling autonomy and creativity, and art therapy groups as a time for learning together.

Conclusion

In this chapter I have presented the practice of art therapy from three different viewpoints: a vignette of a session, the combined views of art therapists in the published literature, and the responses of two patient/participants to short interviews with myself, as author of this chapter. The three views correspond with each other but are expressed differently. I will illustrate this point with some examples.

All of the literature emphasises that the processes in art therapy are more significant than the finished objects; the vignette expands on this, illustrating the way in which the final image is a culmination of processes.

Although the participants do not discuss such processes, one of them remembers being able to 'create' rather than 'destroy'. Many of the papers refer to 'creativity', some observing it as challenging, involving the self and adding meaning to their patients' experience of art therapy. In the vignette, I observed Mr A's apparently unwitting creativity with the clay.

Communication is another feature. The vignette describes how it evolves through action, words, the use of clay, and the metaphors embodied in the clay. For one of the participants, the word 'learn' expresses something of this.

When she says learning is 'for everybody, not just for yourself', she is talking about her experience in the art therapy group and this corresponds with descriptions, in the literature, of art therapy groups as inclusive and generating social interaction.

But in individual sessions there is more emphasis on the relationship between therapist and patient. One of the participants simply describes this relationship as 'easy' both ways, whereas the vignette goes into detail by showing some shifts in the relationship.

Altogether there is an interweaving of the different views of art therapy, showing this therapy as a phenomenon which shifts but also has enduring qualities. We see that art therapy has much to offer even though it is not yet an evidence-based intervention.

I could not have spoken to people with dementia without the help of the arts therapists and other professionals, who went out of their way to make it possible. I am very grateful to them and also to the participants themselves, who were generous with their time and their opinions.

Notes

1 Republished with permission of University of Chicago Press, from 'The Odes of Pindar', translated by Richmond Lattimore (1st edition, year of copyright 2018); permission conveyed through Copyright Clearance Center, Inc.
2 Mr A has given permission to use parts of his therapy for publication.
3 The two clients have given permission for their comments to be included in a chapter for publication.

References

Art Therapy & Outlooks on Later Life (ATOLL) BAAT Special Interest Group. (2015). *BAAT Approved Guidelines on Art Therapy with Mild to Moderate Dementia*. Available at www.baat.org.

Ashby, E. (2015). Reframing and reconnecting: An art therapy group for people with dementia. In S. Weston and M. Liebmann (eds.) *Art Therapy With Neurological Conditions*. London and Philadelphia: Jessica Kingsley Publishers.

Baines, P. (2011). Art therapy and dementia care. In H. Lee and T. Adams (eds.) *Creative Approaches in Dementia Care*. London: Palgrave Macmillan.

Berardi, L. (1997). Art therapy with Alzheimer's patients: Struggling in a new reality. *Pratt Institute Creative Arts Therapy Review*, 18, 23–32.

Byers, A. (1998). Candles slowly burning. In S. Skaife and V. Huet (eds.) *Art Psychotherapy Groups*. London and New York: Routledge.

Cohen, G. (2006). Research on creativity and aging: The positive impact of the arts on health and illness. *Generations: Journal of the American Society on Aging*, 30(1), 7–15.

Cossio, A. (2002). Art therapy in the treatment of chronic invalidating conditions: From Parkinson's disease to Alzheimer's. In D. Waller (ed.) *Arts Therapies and Progressive Illness: Nameless Dread*. East Sussex and New York: Brunner Routledge.

Diamond, K. (2000). *Older Brains and New Connections*. San Luis Obispo, CA. Available at http://davidsonfilms.com.

Edwards, B. (1979). *Drawing on the Right Side of the Brain*. Los Angeles: J. P. Tarcher Inc.

Falk, B. (2002). A narrow sense of space: An art therapy group with young Alzheimer's sufferers. In D. Waller (ed.) *Arts Therapies and Progressive Illness: Nameless Dread*. East Sussex and New York: Brunner Routledge.

Galbraith, A., Subrin, R., and Ross, D. (2008). Alzheimer's disease: Art, creativity and the brain. In N. Hass-Cohen and R. Carr (eds.) *Art Therapy and Clinical Neuroscience*. London and Philadelphia: Jessica Kingsley Publishers.

Golebiowski, M. (2015). 'My coat or yours?' Generating peer support and interpersonal relationships through art therapy for minority ethnic people experiencing early onset dementia living at home. In S. Weston and M. Liebmann (eds.) *Art Therapy With Neurological Conditions*. London and Philadelphia: Jessica Kingsley Publishers.

Harlan, J. (1990). Beyond the patient to the person: Promoting aspects of autonomous functioning in individuals with mild to moderate dementia. *Art Therapy: Journal of the American Art Therapy Association*, 4(28), 99–105.

Harlan, J. (1993). The therapeutic value of art for persons with Alzheimer's disease and related disorders. *Loss, Grief and Care*, 6(4), 99–106.

Jensen, S. (1997). Multiple pathways to self: A multisensory experience. *Art Therapy: Journal of the American Art Therapy Association*, 14(3), 178–188.

Kamar, O. (1997). Light and death: Art therapy with a patient with Alzheimer's disease. *Art Therapy: Journal of the American Art Therapy Association*, 35(4), 118–123.

Kim, S., Betts, D., Kim, H.-M., and Kang, H.-S. (2009). Statistical models to estimate level of psychological disorder based on a computer rating system: An application to dementia using structured mandala drawings. *The Arts in Psychotherapy*, 36(4), 214–221.

Kim, S., Kang, H., Chung, S., and Hong, E. (2012). A statistical approach to comparing the effectiveness of several art therapy tools in estimating the level of a psychological state. *The Arts in Psychotherapy*, 39(5), 397–403.

Kim, S., Kim, J., and Hong, E. (2013). A computer system for the face stimulus assessment with application to the analysis of dementia. *The Arts in Psychotherapy*, 40(2), 245–249.

Kitwood, T. (1997). *Dementia Reconsidered: The Person Comes First*. Berkshire and New York: Open University Press.

Knapp, N. (1994). Research with diagnostic drawings for normal and Alzheimer's subjects. *Art Therapy: Journal of the American Art Therapy Association*, 11(2), 131–138.

Knauss, J., and Moyer, D. (2006). The role of advocacy in our adventure with Alzheimer's. *Dementia*, 5(1), 67–72.

Lattimore, R. (1947). *The Odes of Pindar*. Chicago: University of Chicago.

Levine-Madori, L. (2012). *Transcending Dementia Through the TTAP Method*. Baltimore: Health Professions Press.

Mihailidis, A., Blunsden, S., Boger, J., Richards, B., Zutis, K., Young, L., and Hoey, J. (2010). Towards the development of a technology for art therapy and dementia: Definition of needs and design constraints. *Art Therapy: Journal of the American Art Therapy Association*, 37(4), 293–300.

Mirabella, G. (2015). Is art therapy a reliable tool for rehabilitating people suffering from brain/mental diseases? *The Journal of Alternative and Complementary Medicine: Research on Paradigm, Practice and Policy*, 21(4), 196–199.

Norris, K., and Bush, J. (2015). *Creative Connections in Dementia Care: Engaging Activities to Enhance Communication*. Baltimore: Health Professions Press, Inc.

Queen-Daugherty, H. (2001). From the heart into art: Person-centred art therapy. In A. Innes and Karen Hatfield (eds.) *Healing Arts Therapies and Person-centred Dementia Care*. London and Philadelphia: Jessica Kingsley Publishers.

Rusted, J., Sheppard, L., and Waller, D. (2006). A multi-centre randomised control group trial on the use of art therapy for older people with dementia. *Group Analysis*, 39(4), 517–536.

Shore, A. (1997). Promoting wisdom: The role of art therapy in geriatric settings. *Art Therapy: Journal of the American Art Therapy Association*, 14(3), 172–177.

Stephenson, R. (2016). Color my words: How art therapy creates new pathways of communication. In L. Carozza (ed.) *Communication and Aging: Creative Approaches to Improving the Quality of Life*. San Diego: Plural Publishing Inc.

Tyler, J. (2002). Art therapy with older adults clinically diagnosed as having Alzheimer's disease and dementia. In D. Waller (ed.) *Arts Therapies and Progressive Illness: Nameless Dread*. East Sussex and New York: Brunner Routledge.

Urbas, S. (2009). Art therapy: Getting in touch with the inner self and outside world. In E. Moniz-Cook and J. Manthorpe (eds.) *Early Psychosocial Interventions in Dementia: Evidence-Based Practice*. London and Philadelphia: Jessica Kingsley Publishers.

Wald, J. (1984). The graphic representation of regression in an Alzheimer's disease patient. *Art Therapy: The American Journal of Art Therapy*, 11(3), 165–175.

Waller, D. (2002). Evaluating the use of art therapy for older people with dementia: A control group study. In D. Waller (ed.) *Arts Therapies and Progressive Illness: Nameless Dread*. East Sussex and New York: Brunner Routledge.

Winnicott, D.W. (1965). *The Maturational Processes and the Facilitating Environment*. Reprint, London: H. Karnac (books) Ltd, 1990.

Wood, M. (2002). Researching art therapy with people suffering from AIDS related dementia. *The Arts in Psychotherapy*, 29(4), 207–219.

Chapter 9

Attachment in confusional states and in dementia

Theory into practice

Sandra Evans

I fear not death, but am concern'd that I
Should here by shipwreck in this manner die
Happy's the man whom favourite ills invade
Whose body in its Nature earth is laid

(Ovid Elegy II)

Introduction

Attachment theory stands alone but is also the basic part of a model in the burgeoning discipline that is neuro-psychoanalysis. This chapter examines research in attachment and in neurology, including recent developments that further our understanding of people with dementia and their carers. Neuro-psychoanalysis promises much as the bridge between the "object relations" psychoanalytic work of the mid part of the 20th century and the modern neurobiology of empathy and relationship-building, as highlighted by Shore and others. Much has happened since Bowlby expanded on the discoveries of ethologists like Konrad Lorenz and his "Imprinting Studies". Mary Main developed the Adult Attachment Interview and Mary Ainsworth took the work further in the "Strange Situation" studies, which examined the quality and strength of attachment styles of children to their mothers (2015).

We know now that attachment styles are robust throughout life, on into old age including dementia (Bowlby, 1969; Meisen, 1993). We know of specific dementias and neuro-degenerative disorders which can attack the very parts of the brain which hold the emotional responses that glue relationships together and afford the capacity for empathy. For example, those that involve the frontal lobe will diminish these responses and awareness, particularly fronto-temporal dementia (FtD).

Equally and by contrast, the reflected response to those with FtD may be very hard to sustain when that person shows no affection or warmth. The discovery that the hormone oxytocin (which is released naturally via the hypothalamic-pituitary axis shortly after parturition and which is involved in milk let down) encourages bonding between mother and infant after birth and, when given parenterally in a spray, can temporarily increase empathy in FtD, is exciting. In terms of elucidating further neurobiological links with attachment theory it is genuinely fascinating; but here is a use which may also be of some practical help in the realm of dementia care (Finger et al., 2015).

This research is building evidence for the continuation of human feeling, at whatever level of consciousness in people; even those with very advanced dementia and insists that we always think of their lived experience in all situations of care. Of course, this insistence on valuing continued empathic responses to the suffering of people with dementia, will bring additional emotional demands on those caring for them. Sharing in the anxieties, bewilderment and grief of a person with dementia is the essence of our humanity. It can however be a painful experience and hard to bear at times. This should mean that ongoing support for carers *ought to be* built in to any civilized system of care. It remains a moot point, though, who may do this work and how will this be paid for (Evans, 2015)

The history of attachment and its impact in medical arenas: images from the Robertson film

In the late 1950s John Bowlby's collaborative work with the Robertsons revolutionized the way in which small children were treated as hospital inpatients, particularly in family visiting, which previously had been restricted (Robertson and Roberston, 1967). The images of a little girl being admitted to hospital and being processed by a system which took little interest in her fear at being alone with strangers, her pain at injections or her illness and her pining at being separated from her parents were sobering indeed. This film and its message eventually did much to reduce the trauma of separation caused by hospitalization and helped alleviate children's fears. It also did much for the parents who must have suffered anguish and guilt at leaving their sick infants.

Bowlby demonstrated the importance of consistent loving attachments in the early life of the child and the adverse effect of separation through distance, both geographical and emotional. He was clear that a critical period of emotional and intellectual development casts a long shadow upon each individual's later adult life and that adverse experiences impacted on the ability to have fully satisfying relationships. This assertion was later supported by sociological research (Brown and Harris, 1978), who highlighted the mitigating effect of a confiding relationship on the mood disorders of women in Camberwell (a borough in South East London known for its high levels of social deprivation and poor social housing) who had lost their own mothers before they had reached the age of 11.

More than 60 years on, we are concerned now with the emotional lives of older people, particularly those with dementia, in ways which were unimaginable when Bowlby and Robertson likened the sad images of the tearful two year old in the hospital to that of a depressive illness. Gone (mostly) are the vast Nightingale wards from most hospitals and the enormous sitting rooms in residential care homes, where old people were often rendered incapable of communicating with their neighbour by dint of ignorant poor positioning of chairs: jamming chairs parallel to each other making it difficult to see one's immediate neighbours in order to maximize use of space. People were rarely physically in a position to face each other for an exchange of greeting or a conversation. Consideration of older peoples' psychological and social well-being have been championed by the likes of Tom Kitwood and the Dutch researcher Bere Miesen, who have been only part of a growing interest in psychoanalytic theory and how it might pertain to older people.

More recently, the emergence of neuro-psychoanalysis involving the work of researchers such as Mark Solms (1995) has also fired the interests of old age psychiatrists and psychologists. Perhaps because the ageing brain and its vicissitudes complimented a purely biological viewpoint in examining mental disorders associated with old age, only a few old age psychiatrists ever trained as psychotherapists. For those that did, their efforts were often viewed as redundant or optimistic in the extreme. "Curious Bedfellows" (Ardern et al., 1998) was a phrase apposite to considerations of this kind. There is still more improvement necessary; "Improving Access to Psychological Therapies" (IAPT), for example which delivers psychotherapy to older people as well as younger patients is still struggling to see even 7% overall of the people over the age of 65 referred to the services (IAPT, 2014). IAPT is funded to offer psychological support to *carers* of people with dementia (Burns, 2017), but currently any request for psychological support for those with a diagnosis of dementia – no matter how early on in the disease process and irrespective of their ability to make use of any therapy, is strictly the domain of the specialist services in dementia care. Resources are very limited. What must be combatted however is an automatic assumption that people with dementia will not be able to make use of a psychological approach. The relational approach of attachment theory (Schore, 2001, 2014) is of particular interest to those friends and family of people with dementia; clinicians too rely on their ongoing rapport with their patients to manage the adversity of continuing illness and decline. The brains of social beings have developed in a way to protect from too much stimulation from fear by a process of affect regulation and this will continue to some degree during the dementia process.

The limitations of a purely neuro-psychiatric perspective

This delineation of those in hospital care with and without dementia may have greater repercussions on older people's services and access to treatment than previously imagined. Thinking in a purely biological framework threatens to reduce thinking about people's attachment needs, which in turn increases people's risk of developing anxiety or depression within that service system. For example, because older people are more likely to suffer from physical health problems which may impact on their ability to think and remember, they may be *assumed* to have dementia, even when they do not. Modifiable confusion and reversible causes of memory problems are very common.

Older people are also at increased risk of stroke disease or suffer age-related changes to their brains. Therefore even when very modest recall difficulties are detected, many therapists refer their patients immediately to older people's services. It is most likely that this occurs out of concern for the patient, but it is possibly also linked to fears of damaging that person or missing something vital (Evans, 2008). The trend overall has been, however, to treat the psychological and emotional difficulties of older people merely as though it were some aspect of a brain disorder – distinct from the person. Of course some late life depression is been linked to prodromal dementia; these a*re associations*, but the story doesn't *end* there. There exist other explanatory relationships which are not so one-directional but which do not absolve the observer from the responsibility of addressing it beyond prescribing medication (Evans, 2004). We must not fail to think about people who cannot think easily for themselves.

A neuropsychiatric mental state examination or brain imaging will perhaps reveal where the brain lesions might be but probably will not be useful in considering treatment strategies for BPSD, over and above the decision to prescribe a cholinesterase inhibitor (anti-dementia drug) or a sedative. Attachment theory, by contrast, exemplifies the continuing convergence of psychoanalytic thought and neuropsychiatric research (Gabbard, 2000), potentially leading to treatment and management strategies having potential influence on brain functioning. It can explain in part at least *why* people behave in particular ways and can decode some obscure communications by considering emotional and interpersonal aspects.

We know for example that areas of the orbito-prefrontal cortex are highly relevant during early development of the brain with respect to attachment, affect regulation and theory of mind (Coan, 2016). Dementia, being a number of heterogeneous disorders, all of which attack the brain including the orbito-frontal cortex and other brain regions in many different combinations of ways will present in equally rich and varied ways. No two people dement in the same way. The very originality of personal history and characteristics (including attachment style) have their singular effect on the failing mind; however certain principles pertain. For example, Alzheimer's Disease tends to present first with some loss of awareness of there being a problem, some temporal confusion and short-term memory loss. The impact of the changes may not be so clear to the person affected, but their relationships will remain important and to the fore. The person with a fronto-temporal dementia may struggle with empathic responses but will still crave physical contact and will still need to be treated with kindness and respect. They will still value the relationships built up over a lifetime. This is why Bowlby's work on attachment, separation and loss continues to be highly relevant to old age psychiatry and the understanding of the patient experience.

Case illustration

A woman with a young onset dementia of Alzheimer's type with frontal lobe prominence is seen in the memory clinic for a follow up appointment. Her verbal communications have diminished to single-word answers and she demonstrates emotional lability consistent with a frontal lobe syndrome. In response to statements from the clinician with whom she is familiar, she wraps her arms around their shoulders and kisses them on the cheek. This happens several times in less than a half hour. The counter transference experienced is one of a caregiver responding to a vulnerable person.

This disinhibited behaviour could be construed as BPSD-behavioural and psychiatric symptoms of dementia (or inappropriate behaviour in the consulting room). It is as a direct result of brain damage after all. It is also a demonstration of the empathic, non-verbal communication of the right brain, when words are no longer so meaningful, although facial expression and the tone of the voice is being responded to (Schore, 2001). In addition it is an expression of a woman's feelings, an aspect of her personality, released and enhanced but not, according to her family, fundamentally changed.

Discussion

In what way is attachment theory useful in this situation? Fundamentally what is helpful is the reminder that this is a *normal* human response in a stressful situation. We are aware that the woman has a dementia, but we can relate to her feelings and respond to them appropriately. She is unable to articulate verbally that she is distressed and in need of comfort. We could think of this as BPSD and distance ourselves from the communication, but this would not serve her well nor help her family (*who might otherwise be embarrassed*) to understand and manage the emotional demands of her illness, when *they* could still be supported to hold her feelings in mind.

If we should multiply that scenario several thousand times across every acute hospital ward, care home or home care situation and we can see just how the influence of attachment theory does and will benefit the lives of many. Adopting a psycho-educational approach to disseminate this knowledge, helping people gain the skills and confidence to practice this approach, could change the way people are cared for yet further than the improvements already made in the last century. To some extent this has started already with Health Education England adopting a range of interventions to teach NHS staff, particularly in "patient-centred care" (Kitwood, 1997; Brooker, 2007) and communication skills (HEE, 2015). It is quite clear however that there is a continued lack of this fundamentally simple approach across the country and many areas of the NHS are performing poorly (personal communications from fellow clinicians).

Caring for the carers

As a further example, a person with dementia may require more time and empathic interest shown in order to understand their daily domestic and personal needs. Unfortunately, task-based care and low staffing levels (Francis, 2012) in care settings with older adults are still commonplace.

This "detachment" of task from "care", which may allow routine pieces of work to be performed efficiently, will be at the cost of being able to observe and respond to need. The catalogues of neglectful practices in NHS and care home settings, as well as those in peoples' own homes, is caused largely by this de-coupling of task-based care and attention (Garner and Evans, 2000, 2004). The media often focusses on the so-called cruel carers; but more carers are in fact giving much more than they are paid to do.

Vega-Roberts writing in Obholzer and Robert's 1994 *The unconscious at work* describes the tendency of staff teams to focus attention on physical tasks with a clear completion time, to the extent that quality of interaction may be forgotten altogether. Feelings of anxiety, fear or even disgust may be stirred up in the caregivers. Fears may be about our own fate as we become older and undoubtedly fears contaminated by feelings about older people in our own attached lives, grandparents and parents, as described by Brian Martindale in 1989.

The demand to give empathic care may be overwhelming for some and needs to be supported through institutional systems that allow caregivers to recover. Family caregivers need ongoing support; a fact recognized by the Alzheimer's Society, which has self-help blogs, carers' forums and local networks to provide carers' groups and other support. We know from research in this area that high levels of attachment avoidance can be negatively associated with adult children's intentions to take care of parents in future (Karantzas et al., 2010) and positively associated to the institutionalization of family members with dementia (Markiewicz et al., 1997) and that anxiously preoccupied carers over compensate, often caring beyond the needs of the family member (Meisen & Jones, 2006). By contrast securely attached family carers found the losses brought about through dementia easier to accept (Ingebretsen and Solem, 1998), and care easier to give.

Professional caregivers may not however give much thought to their own emotional makeup; money does not provide motivation for this demanding work that needs singular qualities in a person to do it well: qualities that are rarely adequately rewarded financially and yet the recruitment to such services are haphazard at best. Attachment theory gives us precedence to argue for a more systematic recruitment and career structure with progression for professional carers. Rather than tendering bids for service-provision from "for-profit" organizations, local authorities could devise a more robust scheme for providing quality care which would reduce the perennial recruitment and retention difficulties. Ultimately ensuring that "care" falls under the same publicly funded system as health will reduce the risk of the most vulnerable people suffering neglect.

Caregivers, both professional and family, often can be called upon to provide a symbolic attachment figure to someone with dementia, as discussed by Meisen and Jones (2014). Using a modified strange situation, he demonstrated the "Parental Fixation" of people in advanced states of dementia who demonstrate more overt attachment behaviours such as calling out or clinging. The tolerability of these highly charged and difficult-to-contain behaviours is limited and, in the author's experience, people exhibiting this degree of anguish are only ever cared for in NHS continuing care wards. Agnosias or misidentification syndromes may make the revisiting of these primal attachment behaviours quite distressing to family members, particularly when they are highly emotionally charged. One's patient or own parent calling out for a mother long dead can be heartbreaking to witness. Containing those affects and regulating them is what good quality carers do (Bateman and Fonagy, 2010). Such work derived from understanding affect regulation led to mentalization being devised to assist people with emotional instability. It is in fact mirroring the kind of responsiveness seen in mothers and small infants, applying the support of a functioning second brain (and mind) (Strathearn et al., 2009). Here one might suggest that helping professional carers to be aware of their own good practice by providing a psycho-dynamically informed supervision and further teaching may ensure that they continue to provide high quality care. Poorer practice might also be reduced as a result.

Clinical illustration

Agnes had only recently arrived at a care home having been placed by the Local Authority. She was very hard to manage and almost impossible to engage. She used monosyllabic language only. Her only living relative was not contactable and the care home placement soon broke down, mainly because of her constant cries for help.

In an NHS nursing home for people with severe dementia equipped with a better staffing ratio and trained nurses, her calls for help were soon established to be demands never to be left alone. She was managed without the use of medication and settled into a kind of existence. The nursing staff needed regular support from the senior doctors and senior nurses; mainly just confirming that they were doing a good job. This was not a hugely sophisticated strategy, merely a systemic understanding of the need to support and contain those nurses who were empathically tuned in to Agnes and who were responding to her needs. The nurses were taking in Agnes's distress and processing it in their own minds, giving back to her the metabolized products of their own, containing minds. This is an active process requiring real work by the nursing staff. It contrasts strikingly to media reports of nurses and carers shouting at patients, smacking them or taunting them, highlighting what can be achieved by caring institutions following simple guidelines and spending appropriately on care (Garner and Evans, 2000).

Mood disorders in dementia: depression after loss

Anxiety is the most common mental disorder (Evans and Katona, 1991), and is extremely common in older people. Anxiety is often closely linked with depression in older patients and is often difficult to separate from low mood, so that a "pure anxiety disorder" is uncommon. Late onset depression tends to be associated with loss: including loss upon loss, often defined as the "après coup" or the after strike where a later loss puts one in touch with an earlier loss or trauma which was buried deep in the psyche. The subsequent loss is consequently experienced particularly strongly (Freud, 1895; Perelberg, 2006) as it holds all the pent-up grief of previously unacknowledged pain. We might see such a phenomenon in our ageing patients whose only experience of loss or separation was during the World War II evacuations when small children in the UK, usually in big strategic towns such as London, were sent away from family for their own protection. The East End of London bombings were particularly a cause of inner city children ending up in farms in Norfolk for example, living among strangers. A man with advancing dementia who would not let his elderly sister out of his sight began to talk repeatedly about being billeted with his sister when they had been sent far from their mother. This second loss of the dementia was putting him in touch with how devastating it was to have his family torn apart in that way. Anxiously attached children would have suffered all the more, which may explain to some extent the differences in response to childhood wartime evacuation from one person the other.

Loss aside, a particularly treatment-resistant depression may be heralding dementia. There are often brain-imaging clues such as an exceptional burden of subcortical, periventricular infarcts (areas of brain cell death), which indicate that early dementia might be part of the diagnosis. The more interesting question is this: what pathways are these lesions disrupting to give rise to this alteration in mood, particularly in people who have never know depression in their lives? (Evans 2006).

Ageing commonly but not inevitably brings with it a series of exceptional stresses and losses as physical health declines, mental processing changes and older generations die, followed by the death of one's contemporaries (Murphy, 1982). Murphy identified the effects of different life events that can trigger depression in later life from the ones more likely to do so in younger people's mood disorder (such as the death of the neighbour's cat). Both Murphy's and Brown and Harris's cohorts however had similar protective factors – particularly the presence of a confiding relationship, and the hint (Lowenthal, 1965) that the ability to have relationships – even in the historic past – is a protective factor against depression. Here was a suggestion that attachment style was pertinent even in mood disorders in late life (Andersson & Stevens, 1993), and that the (Evans, 1998) avoidant, anxiously attached or dismissive person was less able to summon the emotional resilience to weather those losses (Ingebretsen and Solem, 1998). Balfour's Chapter 10 in this book details a more in-depth analysis of couple relationships in dementia and further empirical evidence that this is indeed the case.

The psychoanalytic concept of delayed reaction, or *Nachträglichkeit*, was put forward by Freud from 1895 in his early work *A Project for a Scientific Psychology*. A memory is repressed which becomes a trauma later when a similar, memorable and consciously appreciated trauma occurs. The theory of deferred action was developed by Freud in the *Studies on Hysteria* (1895 and 1896).

Case illustration – Barbara

Barbara is in her eighties and in a state of mild to moderate cognitive impairment when she loses her husband. She starts to attend her GP surgery repeatedly asking for sleeping tablets and although she is not suicidal, she is clearly depressed in the context of bereavement. She is also forgetting to eat and neglecting herself. She is very distressed. Her sleep is very poor.

Her GP has time and the skilful approach to find out a bit more about her. She lost her own father in World War II when she was very young and Barbara's mother went into a "decline". Barbara herself was evacuated from London during the blitz and missed her mother terribly, not making friends easily and being a rather quiet child. She married young and sadly lost her first child due to a stillbirth. She became depressed following the birth of her second child and needed inpatient treatment. She did not conceive further children. She suffered a further depressive episode when she discovered her husband was having an affair; on this occasion she received outpatient treatment only.

Her son reports that she phones him night and day in an anxious state and sometimes mistakes him for his late father. She seems to need the reassuring sound of his voice.

Discussion

In Barbara's case we can hypothesize that her father's death precipitated her mother's depression and probable emotional withdrawal. Little Barbara was likely to have experienced an insecure attachment of anxious or ambivalent type. The repeated patterns of loss causing depression plunged her back into the early experience of an unsafe environment. We are hopeful but not confident that a confiding relationship with a bereavement counselor or therapist will assist her recovery (in conjunction with an antidepressant if deemed necessary); but what are her risks of further relapse particularly now that her mood disorder is complicated by dementia?

Research tells us that although attachment styles tend to be robust, they do change significantly in two particular ways (Van Assche et al., 2013). Citing a number of studies, Van Assche stresses that, with advancing years, secure attachments can seem to increase, in that security can be earned or learned. It follows that anxiously attached individuals can become more secure (Barbara's husband ceased his infidelities in the latter years and as they grew closer together; Barbara never had another relapse until his death).

Anxiety and interpersonal dismissiveness

It also appears that an avoidant/dismissive attachment style also increases with age (Magai, 2008). People who have more negative interpersonal experiences may be less willing to engage in a trusting relationship. They may become more at risk because of a failure to recruit the help they need and desire.

Case illustration – Ron

Ron is physically ill from a severe chest infection and living alone. He had few relationships of any note in his life, tending to avoid closeness other than with his mentally ill and abusive late mother. As he grew up he displayed a "disorganized attachment" style, often seeking comfort from unsuitable and untrustworthy types. He was schooled in Borstels and when he left, he pursued a life of manual work and petty crime. His relationships with women were always problematic. Now that he is becoming physically and mentally frail, his awareness of the threats are acute and he reverts to old habits, displaying all the disorganized behaviours of his earlier years.

He is confused because of physical frailty and the additional burden on his brain of the infection. He is demanding of and abusive to nursing staff in the acute inpatient ward where he is being treated for his pneumonia. His breathing difficulties give rise to real anxiety and occasional panic, but he will not be reassured even when the nursing staff are attentive. He cannot recall anything that is said to him and remains panicked and distressed. He is like a man drowning in his own fear and is unable to make use of any of the metaphorical life-belts being thrown to him. It is as though he is not even aware that they exist.

Discussion

In an extension of the sea-rescue metaphor, Ron needs to be picked up and "taken in hand". It is likely that, at this point, only medication will calm him and that once he is well, he will dismiss further attempts to address his health and psychological needs. A district nurse or his own General Practitioner (GP) is most likely to be his closest attachment figure. A constant and reliable professional person to whom he can turn when in danger is what he will need in the future to try to reduce any further serious episodes; attachments are essential for improving resilience and maximizing the resistance to the vicissitudes of ageing and confusion (Cicerelli, 2010).

Attachment relationships in old age

Cicerelli (2010), investigated the changes in numbers and identities of attachment relationships in older people's support networks.

Some of his findings are to be expected; older people have relatively fewer attachment relationships due to the number of long-term friends and family dying, moving away or becoming too frail to maintain previous closeness. They make fewer new attachments, partly due to diminished opportunity, but partly due to the apparent increase in dismissive attachment styles developing in widowhood (Magai, 2008), which may in itself represent an extended period of bereavement in older widows (Sable, 1991). There is an known inverse relationship between secure childhood attachment and distress at the loss of a partner, (Parkes and Weiss, 1983; Sable 1989). Widowed men had by far the least number of attachment figures in Cicerelli's study. We are aware of the risk of suicide in older, widowed men who become depressed and physically ill. *(Our patient Ron may be a significant suicide risk if not adequately supported.)*

The increase in importance of symbolic attachment in old age

Less obviously, there appears an increase in two types of symbolic attachment, the first being a continued attachment to the deceased attachment figure (Mikulincer and Shaver, 2008). The attachment needs are met partly by a kind of self-soothing through memories and talking about the deceased object. Being able to re-create feelings of security and the ability to regulate affects from an internalized and remembered attachment figure certainly suggests the continued benefits of achieving secure attachment.

Spiritual attachment

The other symbolic attachment is to a God. Cicerelli, 2004 explores the possible reasons for this, suggesting perhaps a disengagement with the earthly world in extreme old age and looking to the next. It however may be a cohort or a population effect. Various communities within London Boroughs and parts of South-East England where I have worked, have strong attachments to their God from which they derive great comfort and resilience. Many a Mosque or Church-goer has greeted the news of their dementia diagnosis with "In sha-Allah" or "God is my fate". They are attached as much to their faith as they are to their families. The diagnosis confirms their faith and appears to strengthen the symbolic attachment. There is also the positive benefit of the *very real* religious community who behave in a quasi-familial manner and the paternal ministrations of the Pastor to whom many older ladies with dementia are determinedly and securely attached.

Attachment and adversity

The last remaining cohort of older people who have lived through one or even two World Wars, may have participated in combat or may have lost parents at critical times in their personal development. Many of my East End patients were evacuated during the Blitz although the experience they had was by no means uniform. This highlights the need to understand the patient's own perspective of an event rather than to draw conclusions based on an assumption of the effect of an early separation. Some as adults, are still traumatized by feelings of abandonment and seem never to have recovered a sense of security, while others had secure attachments at home and then developed solid, loving relationships with the host families with whom they were "billeted" and continued to visit them long after the war was over.

In a critical review paper by Van Assche and colleagues (2013), studies found that up to 42% of Holocaust child survivors showed disorganized attachment typical of childhood trauma survivors. Only the quality of post-war care arrangements predicted well-being in older age.

Attachment-focussed therapeutic interventions in late life and dementia

There is little outcome research specifically targeting this age group looking reliably at psychotherapeutic interventions. There are accounts of successful individual and group-based treatments but few, if any, that meet an RCT standard.

Attachment-based interventions, particularly for people in the early stages of dementia such as reminiscence therapy (RT) and simulated presence therapy (SPT) where a voice recording of the lost or absent attachment figure is played in order to sooth and calm distress, have been shown to be effective in their aim. Pet therapy can also be useful in some anxious individuals. It is understood that caressing an animal or receiving strokes and hugs from another (warm-blooded creature) also releases oxytocin. This may in turn add to feelings of improved well-being. These proxy attachments may be fulfilling at least in part in for the need for human (or mammalian) company. Increasing the physical contact for people with dementia in institutional or hospital care may appear a minefield of ethical and safeguarding concerns. One could of course argue that starving people of physical manifestations of affection is neglectful and so a pragmatic, problem-solving approach needs to be taken.

Lastly the peptide Oxytocin is showing some potential. Not only has it been used effectively (albeit short-acting) to improve empathic relating in patients with young-onset fronto-temporal dementia, but endogenous oxytocin levels have been noted to be positively associated with the amelioration of the experience of an adverse event in older people (Emeny et al., 2015), but only in securely attached older people. Caressing emotive slow touching has been demonstrated to raise oxytocin levels in people and will likely be the subject of further research in dementia care in future contributes to the send of body ownership, and by implication to the psychological self (Crucianelli et al., 2013; Lloyd et al., 2013).

Summary and conclusion

Bowlby's work, particularly his observation that attachment styles are robust through the life span, including old age and now to some extent in dementia (mainly Alzheimer's Disease), provides a foundation upon which further neuropsychoanalytic research into dementia is occurring. Of special note is interest in object-seeking, relationship forming and maintaining aspects of the human mind, which although driven by chemicals is experienced by the individual as love, or in the absence of love, by pain. It is noteworthy because it is rarely memory failure which causes a breakdown in care at home. It is the distressing behaviours and family carer difficulties, often due to interpersonal difficulties which precipitate the need for institutional care.

Research into understanding and into the care (Livingston et al., 2017) of existing patients with dementia now is imperative as is the improvement in skills and education of the existing care work force. Sharing the knowledge and understanding already gained needs to be done formally and informally and is best transmitted to others by demonstrating good practice, inspiring nursing and medical students to do the same.

References

Ainsworth, M.S., Blehar, M., Waters, E., and Wall, S.N. (2015). *Patterns of Attachment: A Study of the Strange Situation*. New York: Psychology Press.

Andersson, L., and Stevens, N. (1993). Associations between early experiences with parents and well-being in old age. *Journal of Gerontology*, 48(3), 109–116.

Ardern, M., Garner, J., and Porter, R. (1998). Curious bedfellows: Psychoanalytic understanding and old age Psychiatry. *Psychoanalytic Psychotherapy*, 12(1), 47–56.

Bateman, A., and Fonagy, P. (2010). Mentalization based treatment of borderline personality disorder. *World Psychiatry*, 9: 11–15.

Bowlby, J. (1969). *Attachment and Loss*, Vol. 1. London: Hogarth Press.

Brooker, D. (2007). *Person-centred Dementia Care Making Services Better*. London: Jessica Kingsley Publishers.

Brown, G.W., and Harris, T. (1978). *The Social Origins of Depression*. London: Tavistock.

Burns, A. (2017, February). *Older People Are Losing Out on Psychological Therapy*. NHS England Older Person's Tsar Blog.

Cicerelli, V.G. (2004). God as the ultimate attachment figure for older adults. *Attachment and Human Development*, 6, 371–388.

Cicerelli, V.G. (2010). Attachment relationships in old age. *Journal of Social and Personal Relationships*, 27(2). Sage.

Coan, J. (2016). Attachment and neuroscience. In J. Cassidy and P. Shaver (eds.) *Handbook of Attachment*, 3rd ed. New York: Guilford Press, 242–269.

Crucianelli, L., Metcalf, N., Fotopoulou, A., and Jenkinson, P. (2013). Bodily pleasure matters: Velocity of touch modulates body ownership during the rubber hand illusion. *Frontiers in Psychology*, 4, 703.

Emeny, R., Huber, D., Bidlingmaer, M., and Ladwig, K.-H. (2015, March). Oxytocin-induced coping with stressful life events in old age depends on attachment: Findings from the cross-sectional KORA Age study. *Psychoneuroendocrinology*, 56, 132–142.

Evans, S. and Katona, C.L.E. (1991). Treatment of Anxiety Disorders in the Elderly. In The Anxiolytic Jungle; Where Next?. Ed D. Wheatley. John Wiley. London.

Evans, S. (1998). Beyond the mirror: A group analytic exploration of late life depression. *Aging and Mental Health*, 2, 94–99.

Evans, S. (2004). Attachment in old age: Bowlby and others. In S. Evans and J. Garner (eds.) *Talking Over the Years: A Handbook of Dynamic Psychotherapy in Older Adults*. London: Routledge.

Evans, S. (2006). Where is the unconscious in dementia? In R. Doctor and R. Lucas (eds.) *The Organic and the Inner World*. London: Karnac.

Evans, S. (2008, September). 'Beyond forgetfulness': How psychoanalytic ideas can help us to understand the experience of patients with dementia. *Psychoanalytic Psychotherapy*, 22(3), 155–176.

Evans, S. (2015). What the national dementia strategy forgot. *Psychoanalytic Psychotherapy*, 28(3), 321–329.

Finger, E., MacKinley, J., Blair, M., Oliver, L., Jesso, S., Tartaglia, M., et al. (2015). Oxytocin for fronto-temporal dementia: A randomized dose-finding study of safety and tolerability. *Neurology*, 84(2), 174–181.

Francis, R. (2012). *The Mid-Staffordshire Enquiry*. DH

Freud, S. (1895). Project for a scientific psychology. In *SE 1*, 295–397.

Freud, S. (1896). Studies on hysteria. In *SE 2*.

Gabbard, G. (2000). A neurobiologically informed perspective on psychotherapy. *British Journal of Psychiatry*, 177, 117–122.

Garner, J. (2004). Dementia. In S. Evans and J. Garner (eds.) *Talking Over the Years: A Handbook of Dynamic Psychotherapy in Older Adults*. London: Routledge.

Garner, J., and Evans, S. (2000). *The Institutional Abuse of Elderly People*. CR 84, College Document, Royal College of Psychiatrists.

Health Education England. (2015). *Dementia Core Skills Education and Training Framework*. HEE

Ingebretsen, R., and Solem, P.E. (1998). Death, dying, and bereavement. In I.H. Nordhus, G.R. VandenBos, S. Berg, and P. Fromholt (eds.) *Clinical Geropsychology*. Washington, DC: American Psychological Association, 177–181.

Karantzas, G., Evans, L., and Foddy, M. (2010, September 1). The role of attachment in current and future parent caregiving. *The Journals of Gerontology: Series B*, 65B(5), 573–580.

Kitwood, T. (1997). *Dementia Reconsidered: The Person Comes First*. Maidenhead: Open University Press.

Livingston, G., et al. (2017). Dementia prevention, intervention, and care. Lancet, 390 (10113), 2673–2734. http://dx.doi.org/10.1016/S0140-6736(17)31363-6

Lloyd, D.M., Gillis, V., Lewis, E., Farrell, M.J., and Morrison, I. (2013). Pleasant touch moderates the subjective and not objective aspects of body perception. *Frontiers of Behavioural Neuroscience*, 23(7), 207.

Lowenthal, M.F. (1965). Antecedents of isolation and mental illness in old age. *Archives of General Psychiatry*, 12, 245–254.

Magai, C. (2008). Attachment in middle and later life. In J. Cassidy and P.R. Shaver (eds.) *Handbook of Attachment: Theory, Research, and Clinical Applications*, 2nd ed. New York: Guilford Press, 532–551.

Markiewicz, D., Reis, M., and Gold, D.P. (1997, September 1). An exploration of attachment styles and personality traits in caregiving for dementia patients. *The International Journal of Ageing and Human Development*. Sage, 45 (2), 111–132.

Martindale, B. (1989). Becoming dependent again: The fears of some elderly persons and their younger therapists. *Psychoanalytic Psychotherapy*, 4, 67–75.

Miesen, B. (1993). Alzheimer's disease, the phenomenon of parent fixation and Bowlby's attachment theory. *International Journal of Geriatric Psychiatry*, 8, 147–153.

Miesen, B., and Jones, G. (2006). *Care-giving in Dementia: Research and Applications*, Vol. 4. Routledge London: Taylor & Francis.

Mikulincer, M., and Shaver, R.P. (2008). An attachment perspective on bereavement. In M.S. Stroebe, R.O. Hansson, H. Schut, and W. Stroebe (eds.) *Handbook of Bereavement Research and Practice: Advances in Theory and Intervention*. Washington, DC: American Psychological Association, 87–112.

Murphy, E. (1982). The social origins of depression in old age. *British Journal of Psychiatry*, 141 (2), August 1982, pp. 135–142.

Ovid. *Elegy II-Tristia. Five Books of Mournful Elegies* (printed for Arthur Bettelworth-Red Lion on London Bridge (1713).

Parkes, C.M., and Weiss, R. (1983). *Recovery From Bereavement*. Colin Parkes & Robert Weiss. New York: Basic Books.

Perelberg, R.J. (2006). The controversial discussions and après-coup. *The International Journal of Psychoanalysis*, 87, 1199–1220.

Psychological Therapies: Annual Report on the use of IAPT services England, 2014/15 Published by Files.Digital.NHS.UK.

Robertson, J., and Robertson, J. (1967). *Young Children I Brief Separation*. Film Series. London and New York: Tavistock Institute of Human Relations.

Sable, P. (1989). Attachment anxiety and loss of a husband. *American Journal of Orthopsychiatry*, 59(4), 550–556.

Sable, P. (1991). Attachment, loss of spouse, and grief in elderly adults. *Journal of Death & Dying*, 23(2), 129–142.

Schore, A.N. (2001). The effects of a secure attachment relationship on right brain development, affect regulation, and infant mental health. *Infant Mental Health Journal*, 22, 7–66.

Shore, A.N. (2014). The right brain is dominant in psychotherapy. *Psychotherapy*, 51, 388–397.

Solms, M. (1995). Is the brain more real than the mind? *Psychoanalytic Psychotherapy*, 9, 107–120.

Strathearn, L., Fonagy, P., Amico, J., and Montague, P.R. (2009). Adult attachment predicts maternal brain and oxytocin responses to infant cues. *Neuropsychopharmacology*, 34, 2655–2666.

Van Assche, L., Luyten, P., Bruffaerts, R., Persoons, P., Van de Ven, L., and Vandebenbulke, M. (2013). Attachment in old age: Theoretical assumptions, empirical findings and implications for clinical practice. *Clinical Psychology Review*, 33, 67–81.

Vega-Roberts, Z. (1994). Till death us do part: Caring and uncaring in work with the elderly. In Anton Obholzer and Zega Roberts (eds.) *The Unconscious at Work: Individual and Organizational Stress in the Human Services*. East Sussex: Routledge.

Chapter 10

The fragile thread of connection

Living as a couple with dementia

Andrew Balfour

> *How could the complexities of being, the mechanics of our anatomy, the intel-*
> *ligence of our biology . . . the thoughts and questions and yearnings and hopes*
> *and hunger and desire and the thousand and one contradictions that inhabit*
> *us at any given moment – ever have an ending that could be marked by a date*
> *on a calendar?. . . . My father is both dead and alive. . . . He is in the past,*
> *present and future.*
>
> Hisham Matar, The Return[1]

Introduction: the ubiquity of loss

For all of us, living with dementia or not, loss is at the centre of our experience. Discovered in those everyday moments of change and transition, in the return to school or work after a holiday, in the coming to an end of an intense experience, and inescapable in the pain and long-term aftershocks of the death of someone close. It is the knowledge of our limited time, of the inevitability, one day, of the loss of those at the centre of our emotional lives which shadows everything; each separation, each change or development in our lives gains part of its shape, the outer edge of its definition, by the finitude it reveals to us. Even if we choose not to apprehend it, or can do so only partially, lest it spoil the life that is there, this is the contour of our experience. Not just the ultimate horizon-line of the end of life, but the current lived shape of experience, determined by loss and by the prospect of loss. How do we manage this? Most obviously by denial, by refusal to believe it can be true. For others maybe, but not for us, or those we love. Yet even if we try to hold onto this notion, it cannot last. Eventually, sooner or later, the limits that give life its shape confront us inescapably.

But, in a sense, loss is not 'over' – in death even, not a definitive full-stop; the presence of the person who is lost continues with you, in the interior of your living being, and in your experience of the world, as it goes on. Writers on dementia have talked about 'anticipatory grief' (Garner, 1997); perhaps an aspect of experience which this illuminates is the loss that is current alongside the presence of the person who is being lost in dementia, and the new relationship which has to be negotiated, even as the trajectory of change is towards increasing incapacity and death. Dementia brings a physical and emotional confrontation with a progressively changing person; who is the same, yet the person as they were is being diminished in their capacity and posing challenges and demands that are new and increasing as time goes on. At the same time as facing loss there is the need to adapt to these new challenges; entailing mourning as well as adjustment to the person as they are now in their changed and changing state. Despite the profound challenges of this situation, I have often been very moved in my work with couples living with dementia at witnessing the life that can be possible, adjustments, adaptations and connections between people that can be maintained and developed in new ways. Being with someone with dementia encompasses the sense of the person as they were in the past, which is part of who they continue to be; the present tense of how they are now and the shadow of the future – how they will be as the dementia progressively takes hold. These different, overlapping dimensions of time and identity are composite and are part of the emotional encounter with the family member or friend who is living with dementia.

Something like one in five people over 80 develop dementia and the way in which this is experienced will be as different in breadth and scope as the individual differences of the people inhabiting the illness. There is no 'account' of *the* experience of dementia (and of course there are a number of different types of dementia). But to respect the vastness of the range of such experience by a retreat into nomothetic data, into distanced and objective description, is to take away humanity from the account of the disease. And illness is illness – its objective fact and character render it an 'entity' with its own recognisable shape, which means that all who experience it also share something in common. As I shall discuss, personal relationships are of crucial importance in dementia and are profoundly challenged by the illness. In this chapter I shall explore the emotional challenges facing couples, drawing on research and clinical thinking to look at what may help to sustain relationships and support the resilience of people who are living together with dementia.

Attachment in old age and dementia

First, to look at some background, what does research into the psychological experience of dementia have to tell us? Perhaps the most important concept, which has gathered increasing interest in recent years, is that of 'attachment' – which is generally associated with early, not late, life. However, as adults we do not outgrow our need for security, and attachment encompasses the whole lifespan and is particularly relevant in dementia. Attachment relationships are thought to function as a protective resource in later life (Magai and Passman, 1997; Sloggett et al., 2007) and attachment theory is important in understanding the experience of people with dementia. The process of dementia can be characterised by experiences of loss and separation from attachment figures (or the fear of this) and feelings of insecurity, as an unwilling separation and disruption of attachment bonds can be a common part of the experience (Browne and Shlosberg, 2006).

Looking at the impact of dementia upon the 'attachment system' of individuals with the illness, Miesen (1992, 1993) reports a high incidence of 'attachment seeking' behaviour in people with dementia, including those in later stage dementia. Other researchers have also found that 'attachment seeking' behaviour was evident in people with dementia across the range of the illness, including those with greater cognitive impairment (Browne and Shlosberg, 2005). As Van Assche et al. (2013) point out, there is a convergence of evidence from studies in this field that insecure attachment is related to higher levels of BPSD (behavioural and psychiatric symptoms in dementia) and in caregivers it is associated with higher levels of caregiving burden, negative appraisals of the situation, and less satisfaction with perceived support, as well as higher levels of depression and anxiety. By contrast, secure attachment appears to make it easier to achieve a more accepting state of mind in relation to the losses and changes associated with dementia, and to sustain the capacity for emotional contact with the partner with dementia (Ingebretsen and Solem, 1998).

Developmental research

Given the importance of attachment in dementia, what does research have to tell us about what may help with anxieties and insecurities linked to this? Van Assche et al. (2013) point out the need to link the study of attachment in dementia with the extensive research on attachment at the other end of the lifespan and, as I shall discuss, the learning from developmental research has implications for our thinking about how to respond to the attachment needs of people with dementia. In order to explore this, we need to begin with the earliest attachment relationships we form, looking at research which helps us to understand how relationships in early life are established securely and what relevance this may have to thinking about dementia.

The fundamental message of developmental research in attachment is the importance for the infant of contact with the caregiver's mind, and of experiencing the caregiver's 'mind-mindedness', which are crucial for cognitive and emotional development and for establishing secure attachment. Ainsworth (1978) demonstrate that parental sensitivity and responsiveness to infant affect is a key determinant of secure attachment; the infant needs to encounter a mind, a mindfulness of its own internal state in its primary care givers: "it is not gratification of need that is at the heart of bonding, rather, it is the caregiver's capacity to create in her mind the infant's mental state" (Fonagy et al., 1993). This is not only at the heart of secure attachment, but also is the key to the infant's healthy emotional and cognitive development. Indeed, developmental researchers, such as Tronick (2004), have shown that when the infant's caregiver does not respond to their attempts to engage them, the coherence and complexity of their self-representation is disrupted and they move closer to states of both emotional and cognitive disorganisation, turning away and withdrawal (see also Fonagy et al., 2007; Beebe, 2015). This description of the infant's reaction to the disengagement of its object is reminiscent of observational work in dementia care settings, where the 'warehousing' of patients who, left for long periods without personal interaction, show a similar picture of disengagement and withdrawal (Davenhill et al., 2003).

Attachment needs are activated by dementia, with progressive cognitive impairment likely to cause both cognitive and emotional dis-integration in the context of the loss of opportunity for shared understanding and 'inter-subjectivity'. Partners of people with dementia often express the impact of the loss of emotional contact and reciprocal communication within the couple, and one researcher writes: "the feeling of the loss of the partner is associated with the loss of sharing or interaction with the partner". Some carers expressed this loss of communication as: "if only I knew what he/she was thinking" (Bull, 1998; see also Lewis, 1998; Murray et al., 1999). The evidence from developmental research of the importance of mutuality and 'inter-subjectivity' (Fonagy et al., 2007) for security of attachment may therefore have particular implications for people with dementia, whose attachment relationships are changing as anchorage in their familiar relational and social world is progressively under threat. Transposing this evidence from attachment research of the importance of the 'joining of minds' may have important implications for the relationship between the person with dementia and their partner, indicating how vital may be the carer partner's sensitivity or 'going on thinking' about the experience of the partner with dementia.

Linking developmental research with psychoanalytic models: 'containment'

The research finding of the importance of the caregiver's responsiveness to the infant's mental state brings us close to a core concept in psychoanalysis, that of 'containment'. Both researches in infant development as well as psychoanalytic studies show us that, in good enough circumstances, our closest relationships can be the crucible of emotional growth throughout our lives. At the different developmental stages that we traverse, what is crucial is the sense of connection that comes from emotional contact with another mind that can understand and give words to our experience, or find other articulations or connections that go beyond words. As we are growing and developing as infants, we need this connection with our mother or primary attachment figures to enable our minds to grow, and, throughout our lives, such emotional contact with others allows us to experience our thoughts and feelings in ways that enhance our sense of understanding, as of feeling understood. This is expressed in the concept of 'containment', which is a word that is often used in health and social care settings, but what does it mean in psychoanalytic terms? According to its originator, Bion (1962), if the mother is able to take in and think about her baby's distress, it can become 'detoxified' and the baby may be able to take back in its feelings in a more manageable form. As it does so, over time, the range of feelings that the infant can encompass in its own mental apparatus, expands – and the capacity of the caregiver to take in, think about, and give meaning to experience is internalised. As I shall discuss, this model of 'container-contained', with its roots in the earliest relations of infancy can be extended to other relationships throughout the lifespan. 'Containment' is closely linked to another concept, that of 'projective identification'. This is a process that is also described in terms of early development, but again, which persists through-out life, whereby feelings, particularly frightening and disturbing ones, which the infant cannot express verbally, are got rid of by projecting them out into others, who then become identified with what has been projected into them. The recipient of these projections, such as the mother, then, if she is open to them, in her 'reverie', has the chance to experience the baby's feelings, and so such 'projection' is both a communication about, as well as a defence against, feelings and experiences which are felt to be unmanageable.

From a psychoanalytic perspective, the common element in the emotional task facing family and other carers of people with dementia may be the importance of providing containment. In dementia, increasingly the carer partner becomes the witness, whose mind can register and think about what is happening to the person with dementia whose own capacities are progressively diminished.

> If the caregiver can offer a mentally receptive state of mind, conscious or unconscious, the communication can be received, modified if it is one of pain and rage, appreciated if one of love and pleasure, and recommunicated ... The caregiver's mind functions as a container for, and a sorter of, the projected emotional fragments, which, as a consequence, become the 'contained'.
>
> (Waddell, 2000)

This highlights the importance of trying to understand the communications of individuals with dementia, as often conveyed through projective processes. Win-dows of clarity, of a briefly more integrated state, may be opened for the person with dementia by trying to understand them, thereby making emotional contact and finding some way – either in words or action – of conveying that understand-ing. Waddell (2007), drawing on the disquisition on the Seven Ages of Man from *As You Like It* by Shakespeare, points out that, even in the profound losses of dementia, there might be moments of recovery, of "ripening" amidst the "rotting". To what extent, as the pressure of the illness increases and capacities are lost, more persecuted states of mind may begin to dominate is unclear – but the clini-cal case study evidence is that, to some degree at least, this depends on how much containment can be offered by the partner without dementia.

Understanding and the importance of emotional contact in dementia

The historian and philosopher Theodore Zeldin comments in his book *The Hidden Pleasures of Life*, "how well others understand you and you them, makes more difference to your life than what you own". Whilst there may be evidence of the importance of emotional contact, of the act of seeking to understand in dementia, the situation is different from that of infancy where there is development of mind and growth towards separation and greater somatic and psychic integrity. Needless to say, the situation of dementia reverses this developmental trajectory; what is ahead is increasing dependency, loss of autonomy and mental functioning and, ultimately, death. Consequently, the context for emotional contact and awareness of the mind of self and other is different; now it is loss that is at the heart of things, not developmental gains and pleasure at this, as is the prospect in infancy. Whilst recovered understanding and moments of mutuality and emotional contact may be of crucial importance in dementia, they can be difficult to achieve, facing the individual – both person with dementia and their partner – with considerable psychic challenges. Most particularly, the capacity to bear and contain feelings such as loss, anger and – for the carer partner in particular – frustration and guilt, may be necessary in order to support engagement with the emotional realities of the situation; and such feelings can themselves be brought to life and amplified by emotional contact in the relationship between the partners living with dementia. This raises the question of what supports may be needed to help the couple facing such a challenging emotional situation at this stage of life, which does not contain the hope for the future, which sustains the 'nursing couple' of mother and infant. For both partners in couples living with dementia, containment is crucial to support continued thinking and engagement with experience and to help the carer to contain the emotional needs of the person with dementia.

The challenges can be profound, both for the person with dementia and their partner, and it is understandable that carers who are themselves less contained may be less able to tolerate emotional contact with the person with dementia. In order to provide such 'containment', partners without dementia need considerable support, respite and containment themselves. It is very difficult for any of us to take in and think about the experience of someone else, if we ourselves are not feeling understood and 'taken in' emotionally. To borrow a phrase from mother-infant psychotherapy: "the mother whose cries are heard hears her infant's cries" (Fraiberg 1987). This is a crucial issue in working in this area: not simply to exhort the partner without dementia to think more closely about what is happening in their partner's mind, but to think with them about their own feelings in order that, once they themselves are feeling better understood, they may 'think their way' into their partner's shoes better and tolerate greater engagement with both their own and their partner's emotional experience.

Emotional engagement with the experience of dementia

One woman described her husband's ability to help her with disturbing and frightening states of mind and the importance of being with someone felt to have the capacity to take in her fears, and help her with her feelings:

> I was having hallucinations – my husband was able to put my mind at ease. They were awful – but he would rescue me – bring me back. . . . I could hear him coming up the stairs and I wasn't afraid because I could hear it was him. If it hadn't been for him telling me that I was seeing things I would have been

terrified – I have feelings or sensations or dreams that are genuinely frightening. On the whole he is the one person who can calm me down . . . he is the only one who wanted to understand.

Another person living with dementia conveyed how holding onto her anchorage in herself and her sense of what she could do was easily lost in the face of the difficulties that she faced as she tried to manage ordinary activities of life. It was hard for her to keep on struggling to remember, to think, to recover what she could – and she said that thinking about it could make it worse, at times. She told me she had seen some rabbits in the park and had asked herself, what do the rabbits think and feel? What capacity do they have to reflect – to feel emotions? She asked, how is her mind now and how will it be in the future? The rabbits will probably get devoured and killed off, these are cruel losses, she said, thinking of her self being devoured by the disease which was eating away her mind. She remembered a lot but saw evidence all the time of what she was not remembering, of what had got lost. It seemed that she was trying to hold onto her connection with the world, to a state of mind where she felt there were things which could still be enjoyed. However, the difficulty with engaging in thinking and staying involved exposed her more to what she could not do, confronting her with the realities of her illness. All the time, she said, she had reproachful thoughts like 'I should have known that'. This seemed to be the dilemma of her continued engagement and thinking, and trying to do things confronted her with what she could no longer manage – with the reality of new limits and loss of capacity. However, her experience of emotional contact with her partner and with the therapist in their joint discussions seemed also to lead to a shift in her state of mind. She went on to say, at other times – and she felt it could change quite quickly – she could feel more hopeful.

> "There are things I look forward to – seeing people, family – walks", and she said she had thought of taking up music again, " . . . there are things I can do to hold back the AD, not to give up", she said. "If I could find a teacher who would take someone like me, with my difficulties – what could be recovered and held on to?"

She said that she used to work with people who had been recovering from drug addiction, helping them rehabilitate – trying to bring their minds to life, and she spoke of how important this had been to her. In our work, it seemed, she felt that there was an interest in her and her feelings and perhaps the experience of this helped her to feel her mind to be alive; for a moment in time she could hold onto the music inside herself, so to speak. What felt to be of significance in the work was her experience of others seeking to understand her – and that it was the act of trying to understand, rather than of any special 'understanding', which enabled an atmosphere of emotional contact and meaning-making to emerge as part of a shared communicative endeavour. In encountering her experience at such close hand, I felt I was the recipient of hard-wrought communication of her continued struggle to stay emotionally engaged, despite the profoundly difficult feelings this confronted her with, in facing the depredations of dementia.

The couple with dementia

It has been said that the physical and psychological health of older couples is linked 'for better or for worse'. Researchers have found strong associations between depressive symptoms and 'functional limitations' (the physical inability to perform basic tasks of everyday living) between the partners in older couples: spouse's symptoms wax and wane closely with those of their partners (Hoppmann et al., 2011). Such findings show how interdependent emotionally and physically older couples are, and highlight the need for a health and social care system that does not just focus on individuals in isolation.

There is now a building evidence base indicating that the quality of the couple relationship affects carers' well-being and, in particular, the continued sense of connection between partners is linked to lower distress levels, lower burden, and higher caregiver competence (Lewis et al., 2005). Research studies converge in their findings that dementia impacts upon the couple's relationship in terms of diminished companionship, communication, reciprocity, and intimacy (Evans and Lee, 2014). However, some studies have also emphasised continuities that can be maintained within the relationship and individual differences between couples in their response to dementia. Despite the losses and changes found by many studies, the qualitative literature in particular highlights case examples where feelings of belonging, reciprocity, and continuity within close relationships in couples living with dementia were both important and sometimes possible to maintain (Hellstrom and Lund, 2007; see Wadham et al., 2016 for a review). Forsund et al. (2014) found that couples' experiences fluctuated dynamically, with recovered moments of connectedness, reciprocity, and interdependence which were reported as being invaluable for the spouses of people with dementia. These authors point out the importance of identifying, understanding and validating the shared experiences of both partners in order to support the sense of inter-connectedness in the couple relationship in dementia.

For couples, the experience of dementia occurs in the context of a relationship which pre-dates the dementia often by the best part of a lifetime, and the pre-morbid quality of the relationship affects how dementia is experienced (Ablitt 2010). Carers who report lower relationship quality prior to the onset of dementia report greater depression, distress, and emotional reactivity to the challenges of caring (Gilleard et al., 1984; Knop et al., 1998) and strain (Morris et al., 1988). However, even if things up to now have been good enough, the couple living with dementia are losing a relationship in which they have provided containment for each other. In a relatively healthy adult relationship where projections are not too fixed, partners may be able to act as containers of difficult feelings for one another in a flexible way. In a relationship where one partner has a dementia, the burden will increasingly shift to the partner without dementia to act as container for their spouse. Carer partners, particularly men, often speak of this as a 'reversal' of how things had been before. One man said:

> It used to be me who was the one who was more shut down. Now it has switched around and she is the one who is more like I used to be . . . now we are crossing over into opposite places.

For the couple with dementia we are not just talking about losing the person as they once were nor of a reversal of a projective system, but the person with dementia may start to project feelings in a way which is very persecuting, and this may become amplified as the disease progresses and projection replaces language. The carer partner may increasingly be needed to be the container in the relationship, but they are likely to be filled with feelings of loss, frustration – fears and anxieties – and so it may be very difficult for them to take in their partner's projections or state of mind. As I have said, offering containment for the partner without dementia is crucial, so that their capacity to be emotionally available is supported. The presence of a third containing figure, someone the carer partner is able to talk to about the reality of their feelings, can be very important.

In summary, the person without dementia may be struggling with their own feelings of loss, frustration and other feelings – and the stage is set for a difficult situation.

- How things were in the past is likely to colour very profoundly the experience of the intrusion of dementia into the relationship.
- We all use projective identification all of the time – and in this model, it is also the basis of empathy, and testing out your understanding of what the other person is feeling.
- In well-functioning relationships, an important factor is the flexibility in the couple's projective system, partners 'taking projections back'/reality testing their perceptions of one another.
- Under optimal conditions, in a relationship there will be a flexible interchange of projections between the partners, for example, the looking-after role in the relationship.
- The difficulty for the couple living with dementia is that where projections may once have been more fluid, this is inevitably changed by the illness.
- Encroaching dependency and loss of capacity can carry with it fears of a state of traumatic return to earlier states of dependency.
- The person with dementia loses more and more their anchorage in the world. 'I get frightened when he goes out of the room' is a comment often made, expressing the insecurity felt by many people with dementia.
- The partner without dementia can feel tremendous pressure when faced with their partner's vulnerability and need, where the memory of the reassurance that they will be back soon is lost a few minutes later.
- As language is lost so increasingly projective processes replace verbal communication.

- Now increasingly the burden shifts to the carer partner to provide a containing mind.
- This can entail a very significant emotional burden for the carer partner.
- There is a need to 'contain the container' – to help the carer partner to process their experiences, so that they are able to be emotionally available to their partner with dementia.
- Dementia can, in a sense, feel infectious – and the concept of projective identification is useful as a way of understanding this; how the dementia is also a couple experience, with unconscious as well as conscious areas of experience that are held within the couple.

Case example: working with a couple who are living with dementia

Dementia lands on the dynamics of the relationship which were there before the illness, and often its impact will be felt on familiar 'fault lines'. A dilemma which couples of all ages can struggle with is the threat of loss of individual identities in the relationship and, for this couple, this longstanding difficulty had been exacerbated by the dementia. At the start of the work, they said they felt like 'Siamese twins' – as they were 'thrown back upon themselves' by the dementia. This was a claustrophobic situation which was familiar, although the dementia had robbed them of their established defences, their previous 'escape routes' – having had separate bases, often working for long periods apart. Although these old 'solutions' were lost, the familiar dynamic was re-established in their new situation of dementia – and their lack of psychic separateness, which previously had been managed by physical distance and separation, now felt more claustrophobic than ever.

He was immersed in her world of dementia – he said that he wanted to live through it alongside her, but felt he was struggling to keep his head above water. He felt submerged at times, he said, and was strongly identified with her experience. He described how he was trying to keep his own mind alive, through reading – though he struggled to write or engage in his creative work anymore. Now he felt it was as though he didn't exist anymore. His role was gone and at times he felt that she was the one who seemed more content and to be coping better – he felt anxious, cut off from people – displaced from his old roles, from himself. It seemed that for both of them there was a feeling of being displaced. He was struggling with his identity which she was also doing. He was not working on a writing project and he had lost his anchorage in his sense of creativity and purpose. He had health problems of his own, requiring treatment and he was frightened of that, he said. The old struggle, of how to manage each of their individual needs, which were felt to threaten to negate the other's, had not gone away, appearing now in a new guise of whose health would take priority. On one occasion, they'd had a row about whose needs should prevail and he'd felt she was 'putting the knife into him'. This is perhaps an image that captures the projective identification, of how her state of mind was projected into him, and was infectious, as he put it.

Over time, in the therapeutic work, there were shifts, most notably a lessening of projective identification within the couple; as there was more containment of their feelings in the work with the therapist, he became more able to tolerate his feelings and to face the losses which confronted them. As this became more established, there was evidence of more capacity in him to recover his thinking. At one session, he commented on how, before, he had been talking of being overwhelmed and fearing that he couldn't manage things and was unable to think clearly or work in a creative way. On reflection, he said, these were feelings that one might expect her to be having, and somehow he had been having them. He thought more about this and began to recognise that whilst these feelings of losing his sense of identity, his capacity to work and his connection with the world were part of his own experience, they were also perhaps feelings which were hers as well. The intensity with which he felt them gave him an understanding of what she might be going through, he thought. As he reflected more on this, he felt he had an insight into her mind, into her experience. It seemed that he wasn't so much in that state of mind now and had recovered more his sense of himself, his own mind, and intellectual life – and he started writing again. It seemed that, as he felt he had more internal and external support and that he was more anchored in his own, separate mind, he was then more able to be alongside her and to engage with her without withdrawing so much in anger or frustration.

His identification with her had maintained the lack of psychic separateness between them and perhaps functioned to avoid the experience of loss, though it had compounded the resentment and claustrophobia of the situation. As more psychic separateness emerged, they were more in touch with the emotional pain of the losses they faced. At one session, he spoke about the loss and the changes that they had to adjust to as a couple, and added that it also made him think of the past – how there had been real costs of his decision to live away from her for all that time when they were younger. There had been impacts on her, on the family – losses, and time that they could not have back.

> I always thought that there would be more time, but some things are lost and that's it – they don't come back and you don't get a second chance.

He was faced by his guilt and by the limits of reparation that were possible at this point, now that the dementia was in process, and things could not, in reality, be 'made better' anymore. What emerged more clearly was how such guilt impoverished the emotional contact that might still be possible between them; amplifying the difficulty in facing the losses that confronted them, and fuelling his defensive retreat into anger and withdrawal from her. Anxiety about his aggression, and his frustration with her, made it harder for him to be close to her; he feared that he would be damaging towards her – and this compounded the guilt he felt. As he became more able to tolerate these feelings, and to articulate them, he spoke of his wish to make it up to her, for his unavailability before; and although the clock could not be turned back, there was the sense of reparative processes beginning to emerge, of the wish to make some repair whilst there was still time. He began to engage with her more closely when he was with her, allowing more emotional contact between them. She seemed to recognise this:

> The other night, we were going to sleep with our fingers linked together – touching our hands, and that hasn't happened for a few weeks

It seemed that when he engaged with her and did things together with her, he was more painfully in touch with the losses which faced them. He said, each time he thought of something they could still do, he asked himself, would this be the last time? Would she be able to work with him, alongside him again, in the garden next spring? At the same time, he conveyed the preciousness of the moments of 'togetherness' with her, which were still possible, even as he mourned their loss:

> We are trying to find ways to manage to hold onto things we can do, not to give up, though it is very painful. . . . What if the link that we have now gets lost? . . . I am afraid that the fragile thread of connection that we have, that we have held onto, will get lost forever.

The toleration of these losses allowed more emotional contact between them and, over time, greater capacity to bear this enhanced their intimacy and shared involvement in everyday activities with one another. Although such contact is very important, as I have tried to show, it can be very hard to sustain, raising the question of what is an optimal 'adjustment' to the illness? What should the aim of psychological intervention be? Perhaps one answer might be in helping to support the couple so that they might be helped to avoid premature foreclosure of emotional involvement and connection with one another, which research shows to be so important, even as this becomes more difficult as capacities are lost as the dementia unfolds.

Conclusion

Historically, there has been a neglect of the experience of dementia as a focus of study that could help shape our understanding of how best to help those living with the illness, and this has only begun to change in recent times. This may be a reflection, at the group or societal level, of the difficulty in allowing close emotional contact with the experience of those living with dementia that has been explored here at the level of the couple; an example of our human tendency to withdraw from things that we would rather not know about, dementia facing us, as it does, with the prospect of the loss of capacities that we think of as fundamental to who we are, to our very personhood. This neglect matters because if an understanding of the experiences of people with dementia and those living with them is not more at the heart of our approaches to dementia care, then we will fail to learn how best to support people with the emotional challenges they face. Significant change in the quality of our services will only be achieved if the experiences of people living with dementia can be brought out of obscurity into the open, or if the 'private lives' of these more intimate aspects of experience can be put at the centre of our thinking about dementia, allowing us to develop greater understanding of the emotional supports that are needed to help sustain relationships and to hold people in their familiar relational context, supporting the resilience of couples and families living with the illness.

To this end, we need to draw on what we know from research and clinical practice about the importance of emotional contact and containment in mitigating attachment insecurity and supporting the person with dementia's anchorage in the world of meaning and human relationships. From the beginning of our lives, we need to be understood, to link with others whose capacity to take us in and understand our emotional states enables us to develop emotionally, and to feel secure. Whilst this is crucial at our beginning, it continues to be true throughout our lives and becomes truer again as we move towards our end. The presence of another, understanding mind is vital as the mind is lost in dementia. In developing this idea, this chapter has discussed the evidence of attachment research across the lifespan, linking this to the psychoanalytic concept of containment in dementia care and the importance of this for supporting the emotional resources of couples and families and enabling them to live more emotionally satisfying lives together, with dementia.

Note

1 Reproduced by permission of Penguin Books Ltd.

References

Ablitt, A., Jones, G.V., and Muers, J. (2009). Living with dementia: A systematic review of the influence of relationship factors. *Aging and Mental Health*, 13(4), 497–511. http://doi.org/10.1080/13607860902774436.

Ainsworth, M. (1978). Patterns of attachment: A psychological study of the strange situation. Hillsdale, N.J.: Lawrence Erlbaum Associates.

Balfour, A., Morgan, M., and Vincent, C. (2012). *How Couple Relationships Shape Our World: Clinical Practice, Research and Policy Perspectives*. London: Karnac.

Browne, C.J. & Shlosberg, E. (2006). Attachment theory, ageing and dementia: A review of the literature. *Ageing & Mental Health*, 10 (2): 134–142.

Baradon, T., Broughton, C., Gibbs, I., James, J., Joyce, A., and Woodhead, J. (2005). *The Practice of Psychoanalytic Parent-Infant Psychotherapy: Claiming the Baby*. UK, USA and Canada: Routledge London.

Beebe, B., and Lachman, F.M. (2015). The expanding world of Edward Tronick. *Psychoanalytic Enquiry*, 35(4).

Bion, W.R. (1962). *Learning From Experience*. London: Heinemann.

Browne, C.J. & Shlosberg, E. (2005). Attachment behaviors and parent fixation in people with dementia: The role of cognitive functioning and pre-morbid attachment style. *Aging & Mental Health*, 10, 134–142.

Bull, M.A. (1998). Losses in families affected by dementia: Coping strategies and service issues. *Journal of Family studies*, 4, 187–199.

Davenhill, R. (2007). No truce with the furies: Issues of containment in the provision of care for people with dementia and those who care for them. In R. Davenhill (ed.) *Looking Into Later Life: A Psychoanalytic Approach to Depression and Dementia in Old Age*, Tavistock Clinic Series. London: Karnac.

Davenhill, R., Balfour, A., Rustin, M., Blanchard, M., and Tress, K. (2003). Looking into later-life: Psychodynamic observation and old age. *Psychoanalytic Psychotherapy*, 17(3), 254–266.

Evans, D., & Lee, E., (2014). Impact of dementia on marriage: a qualitative systematic review. *Dementia* 13, 330–349.

Evans, D., & Lee, E. (2014). Impact of dementia on marriage: A qualitative systematic review. *Dementia*, 13, 330–349.

Fonagy, P., Steel, M., Moran, G., Steele, H., Higgitt, A. (1993). Measuring the ghost in the nursery: an empirical study of the relation between parents' mental representations of childhood experiences and their infants' security of attachment. *J Am Psychoanal Assoc*.41(4): 957–89.

Fonagy, P., and Target, M. (2007). Playing with reality: 1V. A theory of external reality rooted in intersubjectivity. *The International Journal of Psychoanalysis*, 88, 917–937.

Forsund, L.H., Skovdhl, K., Kiik, R., and Ytrehus, S. (2014). The loss of a shared lifetime: A qualitative study exploring spouses' experiences of losing couplehood with their partner with dementia living in institutional care. *Journal of Clinical Nursing*, 24, 121–130.

Fraiberg, S. (1987). Ghosts in the nursery. In L. Fraiberg (ed.) *Selected Writings of Selma Fraiberg*. Columbas, OH: Ohio State University Press.

Garner, J. (1997). Dementia: An Intimate Death. *British Journal of Medical Psycology*, 70(2), 177–184. https://doi.org/10.1111/j.2044-8341.1997.tb01897.x.

Gilleard, C.J., Belford, H., Gilleard, E., Whittick, J.E., and Gledhill, K. (1984). Emotional distress amongst the supporters of the elderly mental infirm. *British Journal of Psychiatry*, 145, 172–177.

Gutstein, S. (2005, Winter). Relationship development intervention: Developing a treatment programme the address the unique social and emotional deficits of autism spectrum disorders. *Autism Spectrum Quarterly*.

Hellstrom, I., and Lund, U. (2007). Sustaining 'couplehood': Spouses' strategies for living positively with dementia. *Dementia*, 6, 383–409.

Henderson, J., and Forbat, L. (2002). Relationship-based social policy: Personal and policy constructions of 'care'. *Critical Social Policy*, 22, 669–687.

Hoppmann, C., Gerstorf, D., and Hibbert, A. (2011). Spousal associations between functional limitation and depressive symptom trajectories: Longitudinal findings from the study of Asset and Health Dynamics Among the Oldest Old (AHEAD). *Health Psychology*, 30(2), 153–162.

Ingebretsen, R., and Solem, P.E. (1998). Death, dying, and bereavement. In I.H. Nordhus, G.R. VandenBos, S. Berg, and P. Fromholt (eds.) *Clinical Geropsychology*. Washington, DC: American Psychological Association, 177–181.

Knop, D.S., Bergman-Evans, B., and McCabe, B.W. (1998). In sickness and in health: An exploration of the perceived quality of the marital relationship, coping and depression in caregivers of spouses with Alzheimer's disease. *Journal of Psychosocial Nursing*, 36, 16–21.

Lewis, R. (1998). The impact of marital relationship on the experience of caring for an elderly spouse with dementia. *Ageing and Society*, 18, 209–231.

Lewis, M. L., Hepburn, K., Narayan, S and Kirk, L. N. (2005). Relationship matters in dementia caregiving. *American Journal of Alzheimer's Disease & Other Dementias*, 20, 341–347.

Matar, H. (2017). *The Return*. London: Penguin Books Ltd.

Magai, C., & Passman, V. (1997). The interpersonal basis of emotional behaviour and emotion regulation in adulthood. In M. P. Lawton & K. W. Schaie (Eds.), *Annual Review of Gerontology and Geriatrics* Vol. 17, pp. 104–137.

Miesen, B. M. (1993). Alzheimer's disease, the phenomenon of parent fixation and bowlby's attachment theory. *Int. J. Geriat. Psychiatry*, 8: 147–153. doi:10.1002/gps.930080207 Gemma Jones and Bere M. L. Miesen (eds), Care-Giving in Dementia: Research and Applications, Routledge, London, 1992.

Morris, L.W., Morris, R.G., and Britton, P.G. (1988b). Factors affecting the emotional wellbeing of the caregivers of dementia sufferers. *British Journal of Psychiatry*, 153, 147–156.

Murray, J., Schneider, J., Banerjee, S., & Mann, A. (1999). Eurocare: A cross-national study of co-resident spouse carers for people with Alzheimer's Disease: II- A qualitative analysis of the experience of caregiving. *International Journal of Geriatric Psychiatry*, 14, 662–667.

Sloggett, A., Young, H., Grundy, E. (2007). The association of cancer survival with four socioeconomic indicators: a longitudinal study of the older population of England and Wales 1981-2000. http://www.ncbi.nlm.nih.gov/pubmed/17254357 BMC Cancer. 25; 7:20.

Van Assche, L., V., Luyten, P., Bruffaerts, R., Perssons, P., van de Ven, L., & Vandenbulcke, M., (2013). Attachment in old age: Theoretical assumptions, empirical findings and implications for clinical practice. *Clinical Psychology Review*. 33, 67–81.

Waddell, M. (2007). Only connect – The links between early and later life. In R. Davenhill (ed.) *Looking Into Later Life: A Psychoanalytic Approach to Depression and Dementia in Old Age*, Tavistock Clinic Series. London: Karnac.

Wadham, O., Simpson, J., Rust, J., and Murray, C. (2016). Couples' shared experiences of dementia: A meta-synthesis of the impact upon relationships and couplehood. *Aging & Mental Health*, 20(5), 463–473.

Chapter 11

Maintaining boundaries

Counselling in a care home

Susan Maciver, Chris McGregor and
Tom C. Russ

Last scene of all/That ends this strange eventful history.
As You Like It (2. 7.163–4)

The start

Emma, 73 years old, referred herself to our counselling service, although it
emerged that she had been encouraged to do so by psychiatric services. She made
it clear from the outset that she could pay only a minimal fee and that she would
have to be seen at the care home where she resided. Because of an interest in
working with older people it was agreed to offer her a time-limited contract at a
greatly reduced rate. The potential counsellor (C) had a professional background
as a psychiatric social worker and Mental Welfare Commissioner, and had visited
many people in their home settings including hospitals, nursing and residential
homes but had never done so as a counsellor, and so felt a little apprehensive and
wondered how she would manage in this different role.

Initial contact was made to assess the feasibility of working together. C's
telephone call was answered by an articulate and decisive person who politely
requested that they should meet. She gave clear instructions about travel and her
room location, and she emphasised that she would inform the staff that she was
expecting a visitor and that they should not be disturbed. C took from this conversation that she was not to reveal her identity and purpose and should not speak to
staff. At this stage Emma was laying down the ground rules, but C experienced
this as reassuring in that it might indicate an understanding of the counselling
process and it did indicate a person with personal authority.

The first visit in arrival terms went as she had outlined. Entrance was gained
through a security system and a visitors' book was there to be signed. C was able to
locate Emma's room without seeking staff help, finding on her open door a notice
saying "Please do not disturb," which C correctly assumed was for her arrival.
Emma was waiting, a plump, attractive woman linked to an oxygen machine
because of chronic obstructive pulmonary disease (COPD), a chronic respiratory
condition. Her room was spacious, accommodating her health treatment equipment and her personal effects – a computer, printer, phone, books, TV, and radio.
There were comfortable chairs and the room overlooked the garden.

Emma immediately impressed as intelligent, socially at ease and – despite her obvious ill health – verbally skilled. She was a graduate who had followed a successful professional career until she had become too ill to continue. After a brief introduction from C, Emma explained her wish to have counselling as a need for help with unresolved "traumas" and the daily distress of being in care. She said she was struggling with bitter disillusionment brought about by three main happenings in her life: (1) her husband had "dumped" her in the care home and seldom was in contact; (2) a few years ago she had found out that her greatly loved late father had abused both her daughter and her niece in childhood. This had come out when her niece committed suicide in adulthood; and (3) her daughter was now agoraphobic, had major emotional problems and had been rejected by her father, Emma's husband.

The day-to-day problems were about a deep anxiety that the staff could not cope with her frequent breathing emergencies and oxygen machine failures. She was also scathing about what she alleged was their lying to cover up inefficiency, their poor level of education, and management incompetence. It was clear that Emma was in continuous conflict over her dependence on the staff for keeping her alive, her mistrust of their ability and commitment to do so and her regular feelings of contempt. It was also not difficult to see that she had a strong need to be liked and valued. Her account of her plight included graphic examples of apparent failures to care and alarming incidents of when she had been left untended.

Decision time

C listened and tried to keep track of her thoughts. She liked this woman despite her autocratic tendencies and her flashes of harshness towards others. Emma seemed to have the ability to reflect and to have a measure of self-awareness. Seeing her for counselling would be interesting and challenging – but what could be achieved in time-limited therapy given the likely depth of the distress, disappointment and abandonment Emma was displaying? The losses were evident: marriage, health, career, expectation of what her daughter might achieve, the long-time integrated image of a loving father and perhaps more. C also suspected that death might be an unspoken – if not spoken – theme. Being an older person herself might present difficulties or might it be an advantage; either way the transference and counter-transference dimensions were potentially powerful.

When asked what she would like to get from counselling, Emma replied "someone who will understand." C replied by asking, "how about someone who might help you to understand?" and Emma smiled, saying "that'll do." C outlined her background and experience in brief terms and rather expected that Emma might question her credentials more and get her to justify "being educated enough." She did not, however, and conveyed her approval.

C suggested that they should work on her day-to-day difficulties while acknowledging that her past was influencing her present and C would try to be mindful of what had happened to her. Emma agreed but then revealed that her GP had referred her to psychiatric services but the waiting list to see a psychologist was likely to be six months. The psychiatrist had suggested through a community psychiatric nurse that she try counselling "meantime." Now being a stopgap had to be added to the agenda.

A contract of six sessions was agreed, preferably weekly at a fixed time lasting for an hour with no tea or social niceties – a working period. Emma had already shown that she did not want interruptions and could try to provide a safe space. A primary responsibility of a therapist is to provide and maintain a therapeutic setting. In this case, the consequences of not being able to do so would require to be monitored. C indicated that she would liaise with anyone else involved only with Emma's agreement. She decided, exceptionally, to give Emma her e-mail address as she suspected that the telephone was not always easy because of her breathing problems. She thought that normally clients coming to her space had the freedom to control their attendance, to cancel, or not turn up and she wanted Emma to have that same freedom.

Preparation

C's experience of brief psychodynamic counselling was largely with employment assistance clients of a much younger age. Her experience of working with older people was longer term and took place in consulting rooms. She was currently involved in the field of dementia but in governance rather than therapy although she had regular interaction with people with dementia and their carers. Unlike many of the other residents, Emma did not herself have dementia. However, C's experience of dementia was relevant in recognising the difference between Emma and her co-residents and the impact of the environment. What can be stirred up in people who do not have dementia through living alongside people who do is worthy of noting. There are likely to be reactions such as fearfulness ("I may become like that"), superiority ("they are all stupid"), empathy ("poor souls"), being incorporated into the residual memory set of co-residents ("she thinks I'm her mother") and there has to be understanding of how individual responses may be affecting the behaviour of the non-impaired person.

Brief psychodynamic counselling has considerable coverage in the literature (e.g., Searle et al., 2011). However, working short term with older people specifically remains less well covered, but what there is however suggests that it is possible to have a measure of success (e.g., Evans and Garner, 2004). The supervisor of this work gave enthusiastic ongoing support and there were opportunities to discuss the issues with colleagues in the Human Development Scotland (HDS; formerly the Scottish Institute of Human Relations) Working with Older People Group.

The sessions

The second session gave a powerful experience of what Emma disliked about residential living. Some 20 minutes into the work, the door opened and a cheery worker said "Want a cup of tea?" despite notice on the door. Emma exploded and in an imperious tone shouted "Can you not read?" but quickly followed with "Please, I have a visitor – no tea." The worker backed out and C knew she had witnessed a regular dynamic – exasperation followed by regret that she had reacted so strongly. Doubting if the staff member had heard the softer tone, C acknowledged the incident "I think we are both a bit shaken by that interruption." Emma, looking sad, replied "they drive me mad – they are so stupid." "You look sad despite your angry words." "I get fed up being cross with them.'" At this stage it seemed enough to recognise that they had shared in their own ways what had happened.

The themes of this session were further examples of being let down by the staff, the support she received from her sister who visited regularly, her pride in her grandchildren, and her sorrow at her husband's apparent indifference to her ("I have not seen him for 40 weeks.") She revealed that she was angry with her GP and a social worker who had been allocated to her; they were described as being "in cahoots with the staff." There was a move to transfer Emma to nursing home care and she was resistant. Despite her criticisms of the place, she wanted to stay. She articulated the positives in terms of her being able to manage all her own personal care apart from oxygen emergencies, liking the accommodation, and, surprisingly, having a role. She had been asked to produce and edit a home magazine, to organise some activities and to write letters on behalf of the residents. She introduced an acerbic note by adding "They are happy to use me when it suits them." C countered by making the point that it was probably recognised that she had skills and that she could do things that other residents no longer could. In offering this, C was aware of a need to make things better and to enable Emma to have an alternative and more positive way of interpreting the actions of others; she was experiencing being put in the role of a "good parent."

In the weeks that followed, they met another four times. Emma did not avoid the fact that the work was time-limited and was keen to see C's input as a way forward. Emma requested early on that C write to the psychiatrist confirming that she had been in counselling and was worthy of further help. They wrote the letter together. She did not abuse the fact that she had C's e-mail address. Throughout their contact she was engaged, thoughtful and, although sad and angry from time to time, she did not show any level of psychiatric disturbance.

The work on Emma's relationships with the staff was foremost but felt constrained by C not being able to speak to them. In other professional capacities she would have been able to attempt some bridging work. However, Emma's ability to trust that others would be loyal was fragile – she even had a moment of mistrust about her beloved sister who was "buttered up" by the social worker and was perceived to have formed a short-term alliance with her.

Emma had worked with young people with learning difficulties and spoke of them respectfully. C noted privately that then Emma had had the control and others were dependent on her. Nevertheless, Emma was able to act on a comment that the skills she had learned in that work were still available to her – patience, recognition of the struggles people had with language and understanding, fears of apparently complex matters such as medical needs and lack of educational opportunities. She did amend her scornful reactions to the staff to some extent and got involved in staff training sessions on the intricacies of her breathing equipment. However, these gains could be easily obliterated by any behaviour experienced as crass or unfair. The spectre of her rejecting husband was ever present and unbearable at times, bringing the powerful urge to externalise her bad objects.

A major setback was a case conference when she experienced the GP, social worker and staff as attacking her unjustly. She was told "The staff are all scared of you and don't want to work with you." Although very hurt, she was prepared to reflect on this and accepted that it could be frightening for some staff to try to help when she was having a breathing crisis. They also knew she could be articulate about any failure on their part. She had the capacity to make them feel bad about themselves and therefore they hated her at times. However, it seemed that no one in the setting worked with this dimension and without direct contact with the staff and management, C was unable to establish facts about the operational system, staff support and the general ethos of the care home.

This situation had echoes of Menzies Lyth's work published in 1959 where she highlighted the defences nurses (in this context, careworkers) developed in the face of working with patients they found demanding (Menzies, 1959). A recent edited volume revisits Menzies Lyth's paradigm "of a psychoanalytically informed approach to the practical understanding of institutions" (Armstrong and Rustin, 2014). In a series of scholarly and well-researched papers, her "original insights" are shown to stand the passage of time and massive changes in institutional structures. Unconscious mental activity still fosters defences against anxiety and has an impact on behaviour in work situations as in wider life.

The case conference recommendation was to expedite the move to a nursing home. C was surprised that Emma did not welcome the idea of trained nursing care being on hand to meet her medical needs but could see how much it mattered to have her existing abilities respected and her independence valued.

A continuing puzzle was that apparently her husband, who seemed to be in an affluent position, was not making any financial contribution to her care and the only places being considered for her were NHS hospital facilities. This aspect made no sense to C yet she had to work with what Emma was reporting to be the situation. Inconsistencies had to be borne but evaluated for what they could tell, despite the social worker in her being frustrated.

In their time of working together, there were some positives. Emma converted her hurt and anger about the case conference into a measured request to be assessed by a geriatrician who eventually confirmed she did not need nursing home care and that her needs could be met by the staff in her current home. She continued to respond to requests to organise some activities and events in the home and to help some senior staff in unfamiliar situations, for example preparations for a special church service. She also successfully applied to her high school charitable fund for a grant to pay for a holiday for herself, a friend and a carer. A grandchild left University in the midst of a teenage crisis. Emma appeared to be the only one in the family who kept in contact and this proved to be a vital link. She was unfailingly polite and warm towards C although they had some frank and potentially wounding conversations.

The issues

The limit of six sessions was difficult and C felt Emma needed sustained support to consolidate her gains. The psychiatrist confirmed she was on the psychology service waiting list. With her agreement, C put her in touch with a mental health charity who had a pilot programme of CBT for older people. They agreed that C would return to see her "socially" in few months time, though C knew this was largely the dimension of her countertransference which shared Emma's anxiety about what the future might hold.

Emma's story included a mother who was vain, distant and almost rejecting of her two little daughters. She described her father as their loving protector and carer so that the revelation of his later life came as a huge shock and raised unbearable questions of whether she had to rewrite her childhood. In the time they had, Emma looked at being able to continue to value the experience of a loving father despite subsequent events and speculated about the dynamics of the parental marriage and change emerging.

The hurts she had had to bear were considered; some had come with ruthless suddenness and she recognised that she fiercely defended herself from any more coming out of the blue – better to attack, even though she might pay the price of not being loved. She could see that her defences embraced projection and that the staff were the recipients of her own negativities. This was, however, an academic recognition and her powerful feelings won through in the reality of daily interplay.

There was also a suggestion that Emma was suffering from depression. She had been treated for puerperal depression after the births of her two children and there was a hint of her feeling that she had failed as a mother. She felt that these illnesses were the start of her husband withdrawing – his mother cared for the babies until Emma was well. She did not herself think that she was now depressed, although this has been suggested by nursing and medical staff though without any specific treatment being recommended. C wondered if this was a convenient label for an old person whose complex inner world was unexplored.

Emma was well aware of the precariousness of her life. She spoke of her fears of not being helped in time to save her in emergencies. Some nights she would sit in her armchair rather than risk being in bed where she was less able to help herself.

Her husband figured greatly in her conversation. She had ambivalent and conflicting feelings, angry and critical of his apparently full life yet still harbouring hope that he would support her and visit. She desperately wanted to believe that he still cared.

For C, a sadness of this case was that it was not possible to do continuous work of any depth with this woman to help her integrate her life experiences in a way that gave her a chance of accepting her losses and achievements with coherence and meaning. In therapeutic work with older people, it has to be accepted that time factors will have an impact and the limits on what can be achieved will be real and sometimes painful. However, Quinodoz (2009) states

> Our awareness as psychotherapists of our helplessness when it comes to the brevity of a treatment that we should like to have continued without any limit being imposed on it from outside is, perhaps, a way of letting our patients feel less alone when faced with the brevity of a life that they would have liked to see go on without any limit being imposed on it. If as therapists we can take that helplessness fully on board instead of looking on it as a handicap, it becomes a way of silently accompanying the patient. The patient will sense this, too.

Ending

The mood of the final session was rather flat and Emma seemed distant. She spoke of her sadness that her husband had not attended a recent relatives' meeting in the home in spite of her encouraging him to do so by email. There had been a bout of norovirus in the home and although Emma had not been directly affected, there had been repercussions in the form of curtailed visits and reduced contact with the outside world. They reviewed the work they had done which Emma acknowledged in positive terms. She was clear about the programme they had arranged together but there was no avoiding the difficulty of the ending and the symbolism of C leaving her unloved in a "sick place."

Emma emailed a report of the CBT pilot programme breaking down due to a combination of her having an emergency hospital admission and the sickness of the CBT therapist. C visited her once more, as promised, and found her still struggling with care and attention issues but strong and positive on some fronts. Her holiday had been a happy experience, she now had a great granddaughter and the young father was taking an interest in his child, her sister continued to be attentive, and her daughter was visiting from time to time despite being largely reclusive. She had an appointment to see a clinical psychologist the following month. Some weeks later, she phoned C twice from hospital where she was being treated in failing health. She seemed calm and was appreciative of the care she was receiving for what seemed to be an unpleasant but not life-threatening condition.

C was still considering the appropriateness of visiting her in hospital, when Emma's sister, Julia sent an email saying that she had died and had wanted C to know the arrangements for her funeral. Julia expressed her deep admiration for Emma's forbearance in the face of pain and discomfort, hiding her distress from her visitors.

Concluding thoughts

C attended the funeral service which she found an uncomfortable experience. Emma had written her own eulogy which was read out by her sister. She had chosen to convey thanks for a happy and fulfilled life without any rancour. This idealised state was in contrast with the real woman C had encountered but she accepted that, in death, Emma wanted to be remembered positively and chose to emphasise what she wanted to be her story.

There were a number of recognisable careworkers present, but it was hard to know if this denoted a regard for Emma or if attendance at residents' funerals was standard practice. The row of identifiable family members in the front pew stirred strong feelings which C acknowledged were her reactions to what Emma had brought to therapy. There had however been little time to use the feelings in direct work with Emma. Supervision was essential in the processing of these unresolved conflicts and discussion with the HDS Working with Older People Group allowed C to round off the experience with learning and acceptance of what had been achieved.

Commentary – psychiatric

The setting of this chapter is very familiar from clinical practice and the simple offer of a cup of tea is often the sign of a care home which is looking after its residents well. However, given the specific reason that C and Emma had for meeting, the simple – and probably well-intentioned – solicitousness of the staff proved a substantial hurdle to the work being done. My reaction to this episode wavered between exasperation – that a simple message could not be read and followed – and amusement at the alien intruder into the first meeting between Emma and C. However, directly experiencing it, as either counsellor or client, must have been extremely surprising, almost bizarre, and have taken some time to recover from and to return to the work at hand. The safe space which is aimed at may not have felt particularly safe for Emma or C.

This was one of many ways in which these counselling sessions were atypical. However, C's flexibility in seeing Emma in her care home allowed her to have six hours to think together with C about her current situation and link this to her earlier experience. A rigid requirement that she attend an outpatient clinic or consulting room would have denied her this.

Another unusual feature about the counselling – even in the context of older adults in general – was Emma's severe COPD requiring supplementary oxygen through a mask in her own home. The impression conveyed is of a fragile situation with the daily possibility of emergencies, rescues from which depended on the care home staff – who were thought of as anything but dependable. This daily awareness of every breath must have had a profound psychological effect on Emma and her sense of mortality must have been very real. This perhaps makes her tendency to paranoid thinking more understandable. Her chronic health complaints coupled with the stresses of living somewhere she felt was far from ideal may have made the projection of some less acceptable parts of herself a ready solution to make her situation a little more bearable. The staff seem to have identified with this role and, in turn, singled her out as being particularly difficult. It is extremely sad when someone's paranoid thinking develops a parallel basis in reality through the actions of staff who lack the emotional support to reflect on their own reactions.

While Emma did not have dementia, we have noted that the fact that many of the other residents in the care home will have would have affected her in a variety of ways. Thinking more generally, though, there are many parallels which could be drawn with counselling or therapy with a person with some element of cognitive impairment or dementia. Flexibility as to the setting – as here – may be necessary. Indeed, the format of sessions may need to be altered to make allowances for an individual's cognitive state. For example, a therapeutic "conversation group," which used to take place on an old age psychiatry ward, mixed in terms of the sex of the patients and their illnesses, including people with dementia and functional mental illness, was flexible in a number of ways to take into account the particular needs of the participants. Participation was optional, but patients were encouraged and helped to the room more than would normally be the case. There was a break halfway through the meeting when the ward domestic brought tea and coffee in for the patients. These relatively minor alterations allowed patients to participate in wholly unexpected ways, including one patient with dementia to describe her experiences memorably like an archipelago in which the islands (of memory) seemed to be drifting further apart.

Emma also imposed slightly unusual boundaries on the work. C was not permitted to make contact with the psychiatric team also involved in her care (and presumably her GP). In addition, C was not allowed to speak to the care home staff and had to enter and leave incognito. This must have altered the dynamic of their relationship but was probably important to Emma being one of the few things she was able to have some control over.

However, my main impression from the preceding case description is how important, insightful and of continuing relevance is the work of Isabel Menzies (1959). Virtually no front-line staff of any seniority – with the exception of psychiatrists who may have the opportunity to attend a Balint group – receive adequate support to process and cope with the difficult and unsettling emotions stirred up by working with suffering, sick and dying people. We discussed the relevance of Menzies (1959) to working with older adults in detail in a previous chapter (Maciver and Russ, 2014), but suffice to say that there is substantial danger in not providing emotional support for care staff – particularly those who work intensively and intimately with people as in a care home. Individuals who cannot process the negative emotions stirred up through this caring relationship may instead act them out and one can speculate whether this may partly be responsible for such extreme failures of care as were seen in Mid Staffordshire NHS Foundation Trust (Francis, 2013). Even in a time of funding shortages throughout the public and charity sectors this must be seen as a priority.

Commentary – psychodynamic

> *Love fled*
> *And paced upon the mountains overhead*
> *And hid his face amid a crowd of stars.*
>
> *Yeats*

On reading this moving case study, my first response was of how potentially over-whelming this was for the counsellor. As C says, she had six sessions to work with a client who used fairly rigid defences to hold herself together in the face of overwhelming losses and considerable fear for her own survival. With a longer therapy one would expect that as the defences softened in response to the containment provided by the counsellor there would be a time of immense sadness as well as the anger that was more obvious. So what could C responsibly do in the time she and the client had together? I think that undertaking this work called for a great deal of courage as well as compassion from C.

She made full use of her capacities to listen and to bear witness and this was what her client longed for – to be taken seriously, to be met with kindness by an intelligent, curious and understanding mind, to be seen as the person behind the oxygen "mask." The narratives we weave for ourselves at different times of our lives are of great interest to psychodynamic practitioners; indeed, we accept truth as a subjective and emotional truth as distinct from a preoccupation with what actually happened. Emma was able to tell C of her great hurts and disappointments, her anguish and her regrets. By way of contrast, in the funeral eulogy that she wrote for herself, we see the ego ideal at work, describing the life she would have liked to live, the person she wished she had been. The fact that she wrote it herself reveals a desperate anxiety and lack of trust in how others saw her – of course this was very painful for C. Interestingly, although knowing that C knew the more honest version, Emma wanted her to be informed of her death and no doubt to be at her funeral, trusting C to respect and keep faith with what she had shared with her.

C mentions her potential disquiet at what Emma might make of her, a woman older than Emma but fit and well and engaged in productive work with others. Emma's sister, of course, was also healthy enough to live independently, to come and go as she pleased. Any envious feelings towards C seem to have been repressed; I am assuming that they were there as I do not understand how they could not be. She seems in the transference to have turned C into a wise older sister or colleague who could be trusted in an unsafe world. There is an element of "we two against the world (world of the home)" and a strong invitation to C to collude with this. C had to tread a careful path in not taking up this invitation but also not conveying disapproval for the rather high-handed way Emma behaved towards the staff. One can hypothesise that Emma, because she was so frightened of her oxygen failing, of not being helped when desperately in need, became frightening. She was unconsciously giving the staff the experience of being her via projective processes. Of course, staff were not emotionally equipped to understand this and so reacted in a retaliatory fashion which added to the gulf between them and her and added to her enormous anxiety.

C succeeded in helping Emma think about this, especially after the wounding case conference at which Emma was left in no doubt as to what the carers felt about her. C knew that a deal of splitting was going on with the hatred Emma felt towards her neglectful husband compounding her hurt at the actual carelessness of some of the staff. Because of the short contact, C handled this with an appropriately light touch.

One can speculate that in a longer piece of work a different more parental transference may have come into play. Holidays may have felt like an abandonment and Emma may well have seen C as the rejecting object or the unreliable one, like her father, who was not what he seemed. Where a longer therapy may have provided an opportunity for this to be worked through, it would also have run the risk of giving more pain to a woman whose life was full of it. Perhaps the brevity of the work suited Emma's needs?

This story has a sad but not tragic ending: Emma died before her planned therapy started and after her happy holiday. But she did not die in bitterness and that is a moving testimony to the work C and she did together.

References

Armstrong, D., and Rustin, M. (eds.). (2014). *Social Defences Against Anxiety: Explorations in a Paradigm*. London: Karnac.

Evans, S., and Garner, J. (2004). *Talking Over the Years: A Handbook of Dynamic Psychotherapy With Older Adults*. London: Routledge.

Francis, R. (2013). *Report of the Mid Staffordshire NHS Foundation Trust Public Inquiry*, 3 Vol. London: The Stationery Office.

Maciver, S., and Russ, T.C. (2014). A plea to 'see into the life of things': Thinking psychoanalytically about later life. In K. Cullen, L. Bondi, J. Fewell, E. Francis, and M. Ludlam (eds.) *Making Spaces: Putting Psychoanalytic Thinking to Work*. London: Karnac.

Menzies, I.E.P. (1959). The functioning of social systems as a defence against anxiety: A report on a study of the nursing service of a general hospital. *Human Relations*, 13, 95–121. (Reprinted in Menzies Lyth IEP (1988) *Containing Anxieties in Institutions. Selected Essays*, Volume 1. London: Free Association Books, pp. 43–99).

Quinodoz, D. (2009). *Growing Old: A Journey of Self-Discovery*. London: Routledge.

Searle, L., Lyon, L., Young, L., Wiseman, M., and Foster-Davis, B. (2011). The young people's consultation service: An evaluation of a consultation model of very brief psychotherapy. *British Journal of Psychotherapy*, 27, 56–78.

Shakespeare, W. (2004). *As You Like It*, edited by Cynthia Marshall. Cambridge: Cambridge University Press. ProQuest Ebook Central.

Chapter 12

Music as mirror in the care of elderly people with dementia

Rachel Darnley-Smith

> *No noise nor silence, but one equal music.*
> *John Donne, from 'At our last awakening', 1628.*

Introduction: music and music therapy

Lullabies, the music of infancy, are not simply sung to soothe the child; as Donald Winnicott observed they also serve an emotional function for the Mother who sings (1949, p. 74). When considering the meaning of music throughout life, it would seem to be of significance that our earliest communication is based upon sounds and song occurring in relationship with others. The capacity for such engagement between newborn infants and their carers has in recent years been given new understanding, encapsulated in terms of an innate capacity for 'communicative musicality' (Trevarthen and Malloch, 2000; Malloch and Trevarthen, 2009). On this account, music, emotion, meaning and our relationships with others are axiomatic, most probably laying the foundations for a lifelong relationship with the art of sound. Our relationship to music can be seen as paradoxical: whilst individual and personal, it is also 'culturally dependent' in a totally boundary-less way upon our experiences in the wider communities into which we were born, live or visit, including the ubiquitous access now provided by the internet.[1] In all, music is not a passive art form: music is always music in action, it is not an isolated entity without people: a perspective encapsulated in Christopher Small's notion of 'music*king*' (Small, 1998, italics added). We express ourselves through music, and also encounter the expressions or musicking of others: through listening, improvising, composing or playing, not forgetting of course moving and dancing. Generalising from a Western and European perspective, these opening assertions about music could be said to underpin the various approaches to music making that have developed specifically as a form of help, companionship or enlivenment. Music therapy is one such form and in common with what can be considered in the UK as related practices of community music and arts for health, there is a growing tradition of people in later life taking part in music making, including those with a diagnosis of dementia (Spiro, 2010; Bowell and Bamford, 2018).

Music and dementia

It is well known that in the late stages of dementia illnesses, many people still respond to music. Music appears to retain meaning and pleasure whilst cognitive faculties such as facial recognition declines. Within the music therapy literature and elsewhere there is a wealth of clinical case study material which presents the impact of music as a medium which can still be recognised and enjoyed by elderly people with moderate-severe dementia (see Aldridge, 2000; Darnley-Smith, 2002; Odell-Miller, 2002; Ronse and Maes, 2014; Pavlicevic et al., 2015; Freeman, 2017). Whilst there are specific challenges to cognitive research in dementia, some researchers have hypothesized that certain abilities such as musical memory, which enables the type of responsiveness to known tunes, may be 'spared in dementia' (Cuddy and Duffin, 2005, p. 230, Simmons Stern et al., 2010, p. 3164). The determinants of this phenomena are complex to establish, however, with the recent advent of neuroimaging technology, music neuroscience now has the practical tools 'to examine brain structures and processes that allow us to experience it' (Clark and Warren, 2015, p. 2122, see also Fächner, 2016; O'Kelly et al., 2016). One recent study found there to be an 'overlap of musical memory regions [of the brain] with areas that are relatively spared in Alzheimer's disease' thus explaining 'the surprising preservation of musical memory in this neurodegenerative disease'. This, the authors conclude, 'may well underlie the observed preservation of musical memory in Alzheimer's disease although this evidence is so far indirect' (Jacobsen et al., 2015, p. 2448).

Music therapy practice

In the UK, through the recent work of the UK Commission on Music and Dementia, there is now collected together a wealth of research and anecdotal evidence for the benefits of live and recorded music. (Bowell and Bamford, 2018). Musical practices accounted for in this report include performance, listening and song writing. Music therapy emerged from out of a wide range of similar practices in the post war years of the late 1940s–50s in tandem with developments in special education and the founding of organisations such as the 'Council for Music in Hospitals' the work of which still continues today as Music in Hospital Care, see https://mihc.org.uk/ (Darnley-Smith, 2013). The new practice that defined itself as distinct from conventional performance or educational work gradually shifted in emphasis from playing or performing music *to people* towards playing and especially improvising music *with* people The music therapy practice that began to develop in the 1970s and 80s was loosely based upon a notion of musical improvisation as expressive of feeling and intention.

As noted, during the past two decades music therapy practice has been supported by new observational research into the non-verbal communication which occurs between parent and infant in the first months of life. Trevarthen and Malloch have observed how parents and infants make use of the musical elements of pulse, pitch and timbre, 'to form vocal narratives of shared emotion and experience'(2000, p. 6). Two conclusions from this area of research are significant for music therapy practice. First, a parallel is suggested between the capacity for meaningful communication involving sound prior to language and the expressive/communicative possibilities in music making that music therapists intuitively draw upon in their work with people of all ages (Trevarthen and Malloch, 2000; McDermott et al., 2013). Second, it can be considered that making music of any kind, with another, can be experienced as form of inter-subjectivity engendered at any stage of life. On these terms a rationale for music therapy as integral to the care of people with dementia is not difficult to establish. We know from experience and through emerging research studies that music making is meaningful between people and has impact in relation to people with dementia (Hsu et al., 2015; Ridder, 2016). How though might it take place? In this next section I describe clinical casework. The focus here is not just upon the content of the music making, but also upon my perspective of the experience of being with each client: in each instance, through the musical and (where possible) spoken medium, some insight into the emotional world of the client is described. Whilst such an approach that relies upon the subjectivity of the therapist is always speculative, the understanding from psychoanalysis and elsewhere is that it is possible to have a conscious and unconscious experience of another person and to derive meaning from this, whether or not there is a possibility of spoken language. In the work that I will now describe, I have found Winnicott's theory of mirror to be particularly relevant as a way of reflecting upon the varied experiences of making music with older people with dementia and the way in which the therapist is involved and part of the meaning making process. I will provide some discussion of this later in the chapter.

Two case studies

Case study 1

This first case study is described in the form of a diary over the period of a calendar year: this is in order to convey a sense of the period of time, rather than specific events or goals met. I worked with Mrs G. in an inner city social services day centre for elderly people with dementia. The day centre was based on the ground floor of a large care home. The full-time staff, many with a background in nursing or social work, were always busy and often fraught as they were constantly faced with the challenge of meeting the needs of different people at once. In turn the elderly people who attended the day centre were frequently confused and not always happy to be in the company of strangers, or people who appeared to them to be strangers. However my colleagues here were extremely experienced in meeting such needs and providing a reassuring presence, and they were friendly and helpful towards me. This was supportive and enabled me to provide the open-ended and concentrated work with Mrs G. She was a white British woman in her late 80s with symptoms of moderate to severe dementia. I knew little about her life except that it had been mostly lived in the locality in which we were based. She lived at home with her husband, although it was her son who was actively in contact with the centre. She could walk slowly with help, she had virtually no spoken language. Her demeanor was one of genuine *bonhomie*, she seemed and felt to me to be content but possibly lonely and without enough social contact. I was asked to work with her because she evidently enjoyed the music from the radio that formed part of the day in the mornings and at lunchtime. My own aim in working with her became finding a way on a weekly basis simply to respond to her expressive smiles, the nods of her head and touch of her hand.

January

In the first session I saw Mrs G. for about 40 minutes: I was struck by her level of concentration and how time seemed to go very quickly. As a way to find out about her, I either played tunes on the piano or sang British and American songs that judging by her age I thought she might know: the *Skye Boat Song, My Old Man, Blueberry Hill, Amazing Grace*. I gently encouraged her to make sounds herself using her hands and fingers on the cymbal, djembe drum and other small hand-held percussion. Where she vocalised or spoke I responded in sound also. I felt that even though she hardly said anything, her attention was much sustained during the time I spent with her and she seemed to be enjoying the music. She indicated this through her eye contact and change in body posture where the music became more expressive or more relaxed. In all she seemed quite at ease with me.

March

Two months after I began to work with her, I wrote:

> [Mrs G] stayed for about 30 minutes: she joined in with singing, making tiny sounds, but didn't seem to recognise the songs I sang. So I improvised songs around her vocalisations incorporating the musical pitches she sang and occasional words and we moved our arms in time to the music: she seemed very responsive to this, and together with the eye contact she made and the timing of her responses I felt there was a meaningful connection through musical sounds.

May

Very alert this morning, she said one or two words. She seemed to like exploring the cymbal with her fingers and joining me in the songs I sang with a note as she breathed in and out. I improvised at what I felt to be her pace, as simply suggested by her presence – which was often slower than I expected but there was something very clear in her communication of this – I also sang around her note and this seemed to enhance the sense of interaction.

She said 'nice' and I think pointed at my bag but I thought she was pointing at the cymbal at first so I brought this over to her as it was on the other side of the room. I improvised a wordless song in a modal key which seemed to fit. She took my hand, not for the first time, moving it in time to the music [maybe] its reassuring, I asked myself.

September

Mrs G seemed at ease with my singing and spent much of the session speaking, apparently in response although mostly I did not understand what she was saying to me. She didn't hold my hand or touch the instruments as previously but at the end she said quite clearly 'that was very good'. This was the first time we had met for a month, and it seemed to me possible that something about the sessions was still sustained for her in her memory.

October

Mrs G seemed very lively today, even after a gap of three weeks. She communicated with me closely in different ways throughout the session, she seemed to enjoy herself, playing with the cymbal, smiling to the songs and talking. We sustained this activity for about 40 minutes, which seems like a considerable length of time.

November

Mrs G was very responsive as usual. I missed last week as I was on leave, my experience of her was different and she seemed a little different to me. For the first 20 minutes of the session she held my hand very tightly almost to the point of pinching it, I found myself asking out loud, was she thinking about her family? She held my hand and swung it in such a way that rhythmically it felt natural to sing to her the *Skye Boat Song*. The question is how much can my experience of Mrs G inform my knowledge of her, or assessment of how we are engaging with each other? She says words and sometimes these seem to fit. When I sang or played the piano she seemed to recognise the music, or at least that it was music, and to indicate that she wanted to play. I wrote

> there is an intensity to this work: the interaction feels authentic, I feel half the time like I am interrupting her as she speaks, so I sing around what she is saying leaving gaps but incorporating her words at the same time. We sang: '*I could have danced all night*', and '*Only You*'. I wonder how frustrated and sad she feels and whether she is thinking about people, her memories, and the daily concerns of life? In all I am wondering, in the parlance of everyday life, just what is going on for her?

December

Mrs G seemed bright in mood today and was very alert and responsive: I considered that since I started working with her last January she still seems just as eager to come to sessions and her ability to interact with me has not diminished, even though this is of course limited; it is not possible for me to comprehend most of her spoken words, but she still speaks. She takes part in the music making through speaking, making sounds, smiling and making eye contact with me as I in return speak and sing. She appears to enjoy both the music and the time spent in company. I gain a sense of this through her facial expression, the way in which she holds my hands and sways, and the way in which she speaks, which feels like authentic communication even though her words do not always make sense. I continued working with Mrs G for a further six months until I left the day centre: her son started to bring in CDs so that I could learn a wider repertoire of songs that she knew.

Discussion

There are some defining features of working with Mrs G that I shall briefly mention here. First, over the course of a year, there was little change in either form or content of sessions other than the specifics I have just noted: there is very little narrative here or markers that might indicate 'progress'. Mrs G seemed to enjoy the sessions, and furthermore seemed pleased to see me each week, possibly even there being some recognition from her that she had met me before. Whilst I was usually exhausted at the end of sessions, as mentioned earlier, time always passed quickly. Part of the communication was via touch: Mrs G would take my hand and direct us both in a kind of dance using our arms. I usually sang in these moments and deliberately but quite spontaneously sang at the tempo at which my hand was being moved by her. Most of the time she held my eye closely, often smiling and nodding. Sometimes sighing. The firm grip of her hand and the physical control in these moments that she exerted over me may have expressed something of her need for closeness and acknowledgement. What I understood as my countertransference experience were feelings of warmth and success and the impression that I was able to offer her something that she wanted.

In all this, work was focussed in a series of near weekly 'musical encounters' and demonstrates the strength of working with people in the later stages of dementia in artistic media where words are not required. As might be supposed the strength lay not only the music making itself, but in the intensity of the music making as a shared experience. Shared musical experiences though are more complex than this and, in this instance, it felt as though something of the quality of that experience manifested in the consistency with which Mrs G would look and smile at me as I sang, or the way in which she held my hand and we danced. Indeed this aspect of her presence is what remains in my memory of working with her beyond the written notes. For Winnicott the role of looking is key to the way in which the infant develops a sense of self through another also indicating a parallel of this process in the adult patient in analysis. I now want to extend this notion to suggest how a similar process might also take place in shared musical experience occurring between people at any stage of life, including where one has dementia.

Mirror and meaning

Winnicott's mirror is an account of the role of the Mother's looking, and what the infant looks at, sees and absorbs in/from Mother's face, together with the meaning of seeing or not seeing themselves 'reflected'. The underlying idea is that through our relationships with others we gain a sense of ourselves, in other words, the self is inherently dependent on the relation to other selves, and in our earliest months this has special meaning.

The baby's act of looking around and seeing, for Winnicott, is fundamental to this first relationship. It is of course not a literal mirror that replicates the face of the infant that Winnicott has in mind. Rather, as he states he is using the term figuratively, as a metaphor. This is so that, to paraphrase Roger Scruton, 'we respond to it in a different way' (1999, pp. 84–85). Winnicott's notion of mirror is explicitly that of a dynamic mirror*ing* between mother and infant. He writes,

> What does the baby see when he or she looks at the mother's face? I am suggesting that, ordinarily, what the baby sees is himself or herself. In other words the mother is looking at the baby and *what she looks like is related to what she sees there.*
>
> (Winnicott, 1986, p. 131. Italics in original)

Taking the case study just outlined, I want to suggest that my intuitive response as therapist to Mrs G, not only entailed my listening and hearing, but also my looking and seeing. I felt that her often powerful engagement of me in this process was reciprocal, this was an experience that we were actively sharing and taking part in. On the one hand, my attention to Mrs G. was almost total: she compelled me to listen to her, even if she wasn't speaking or making sounds, even if she was silent, she was looking at me, frequently nodding and smiling. Simply put, there was too much 'going on' for my mind to wander, her presence felt total. On the other hand, such was the strength of her presence and facial expression, I had a sense of pace and of tempo: frequently I found myself needing to slow down, to sing or to play slower than was necessarily comfortable. Through such an encounter, I was able to draw upon the music making, including Mrs G's listening, to both structure and lend communicative meaning to the time went spent together. As therapist I was able to outwardly make sense of Mrs G's evident wish to be present in company through my musical response, a mixture of improvisation and the improvisation of known songs, her gestures and sounds, that in my role as therapist I felt was drawn from me.

Case study 2

This second case study describes another sustained piece of work over a period of about 15 months which took place in the same day care setting. I want to provide some contrast to the previous example, demonstrating how in music, and words, the process of listening, looking and seeing could be profoundly difficult and uncomfortable.

> Mr P had grown up in a Caribbean country but had lived most of his adult life in the UK. He had been the youngest child of a large family and during his school years had often found himself at home alone in the company of his Mother, whilst he saw little of his Father who became a pilot in the RAF and was away on active military service in Europe during the war years 1939–45. His Mother was deeply religious, and he spoke frequently of how she would only allow Pentecostal hymns to be sung in the house. But he readily spoke about his love of singing and how he sang in a choir as a boy, and later in a band as a tenor, then bass. He seemed a little anxious about and by his voice, he would frequently say that he didn't sing much now and that his voice wasn't as good as it had been once. He sang with me though if I started the music; he would also play a drum from the selection of drums available, again if I began. He always warmed to music that had a religious tone, particularly Christian hymns such as the contemplative, *'Grace tis a Charming Sound'*, or the more lively *'Go Tell it on the Mountain'* or *'Michael Rowed the Boat Ashore'*. Sometimes during sessions other group members would not be present, usually due to their health. Mr P would talk repeatedly about his early life during these sessions. His life was most interesting but at the same time difficult to hear about. This was not only because I heard the same stories told many times over the 12 or so months that I worked with him, but also because of the content, and the grief and anger he conveyed in talking about his childhood in another country. In particular he would speak of the life decisions he had made as a young man, firstly to stay with his Mother to care for her whilst she was sick rather than to marry, and subsequently his decision to leave his country with two friends for England. He expressed much guilt at having left his Mother whom he never saw again. His guilt it seemed was not only unresolved, it was certainly unresolvable.
>
> When there were other group members present, who also had dementia and significant memory problems, he would often lead the music making, especially the singing, as though we were at school or in a religious service. Whilst there was a feeling that we were under his control as he sang, there was also a warmth and generosity in his leadership. At other times he became agitated and impatient and would angrily criticise other members of the group, as a teacher might, especially those whom he felt should be 'trying harder'. This included a woman who frequently complained about the day centre during sessions and another who would fall asleep. Mr P would become angry

with me too when my attention was directed towards other group members with whom he seemed to feel little in common with, and who he felt didn't take the session seriously enough. Over time, particularly as Mr P and some of the other members of the group markedly began to deteriorate cognitively, the sessions became harder and the music making less flowing. I began to feel increasingly uncomfortable and disconnected during the music making. There was a sense that with Mr P's deteriorating memory, his ability to make use of the sessions as a place to reminisce through music, and through conversation to reflect upon his life, also deteriorated. The music no longer felt like an expressive fluid exchange. This latter period coincided with members of Mr P's family taking him away on an extended holiday and whilst we were able to say goodbye before he left, when he returned, I was in the process of leaving the day centre and our work together came to an end.

On reflection, whilst the deterioration in Mr P's use of sessions could be described and explained in terms of what was happening to him organically, I also felt that the very fact of his deterioration activated something very painful to do with not his feeling psychically *held*, reflected also in his increasing need to control both myself and other group members in terms of what we sang or played and how we might go about this. Winnicott writes how

many babies . . . do have to have a long experience of not getting back what they are giving. They look and they do not see themselves. There are consequences. First, their own creative capacity begins to atrophy, and in some way or other they look round for other ways of getting something of themselves back from the environment . . . second, the baby gets settled into the idea that when he or she looks, what is seen is the mother's face. The Mother's face is not then a mirror. So perception takes the place of apperception, perception takes the place of that which might have been the beginning of a significant exchange with the world, a two-way process in which self-enrichment alternates with the discovery of meaning in the world of seen things.

(1986, p. 132)[2]

My experience of Mr P. in the later sessions was one of rigidity, of feeling controlled and unable to play; I mean play in both senses of the word. I felt increasingly disconnected when playing music: a kind of musical countertransference, an experience that was useful to me in the sense that I could gain some experience of his inner world. Through my musical experience of 'looking' I felt that what I 'saw' was someone who needed me to direct and control me. Incorporating into Winnicott's mirror, the notion of hearing, my experience of the musical and verbal dialogue provided me with a direct way of 'knowing him' as lonely and isolated but also with the need to shut me and the other group members down, and to keep me at a distance. As Mr P. declined, it seemed harder for him to feel held and seen, it was as though a negative transference towards myself became more real for him and took over our exchanges, although there were also still moments of humour and mutual appreciation.

Conclusion

In this chapter I have considered a music as a form of meaningful shared encounter with older people who have dementia. As one approach to forming an understanding of some of the particular encounters I experienced as a music therapist, I have considered aspects of Winnicott's theory of the role of the mirror function is the development of the self. I have suggested that it is this mirror function that may be explicitly evoked through the moment by moment experience of free music making, whether this music is freely improvised or entails unplanned song.

Ultimately, for Winnicott the task we have throughout life is 'the striving towards being seen, which is at the basis of creative looking' (1986, p.134). He makes this comment in relation to the painter Francis Bacon, whom he describes as 'the exasperating and skillful and challenging artist of our time who goes on and on painting the human face distorted significantly. . .[Bacon is] seeing himself in his mother's face, but with some twist in him or her that maddens both him and us' (1986, p.134). As Winnicott quotes the art historian, John Rothenstein, 'to look at a painting by Bacon is to look into a mirror, and to see there our own affliction, our fear of solitude, failure, humiliation, old age, death, and of nameless threatened catastrophe' (Rothenstein, J., 1964, in Winnicott, 1986, n. 137).

This raises the question of the role of art in processes of healing that there may be some cathartic experience of self, mirrored in the artwork itself, even if where like in the case of music there is a less explicit narrative evoked than in the example from Bacon. However in the music making described previously, I have illustrated how it may be possible for patient and therapist to experience each other in an immediate way, that allows for the possibility of an inter-subjective looking, seeing and hearing. It maybe through shared music making that elderly people with a degenerative syndrome such as dementia can gain access to an experience of themselves via another and, most importantly, the experience of being seen and heard.

Notes

1 Rachel Beckles Willson (2009) in her discussion of the notion of universality of music as central to the conception of the West-Eastern Divan Orchestra cites from an interview with the Arab Israeli musician Khaled Jubran, 'Some say music is an international language. It isn't. It is the most culturally dependent thing I know'. Beckles Willson (2009), p. 320. For further discussion, well beyond the scope of this chapter, see also P. V. Bohlman (1999).

2 Abram elucidates this particular meaning of 'apperception' as 'the term Winnicott gave to the infant's subjective experience of merger with mother [and it] thus involves relating to subjective objects. Consequently apperception means seeing oneself through being seen by mother'. See Abram, Jan (2007), p. 240.

References

Abram, Jan (2007). *The language of Winnicott: A dictionary of Winnicott's use of words*. London: Karnac Books.

Aldridge, D. (2000). *Music Therapy in Dementia Care*. London: Jessica Kingsley Publishers.

Beckles Willson (2009). The Parallax Worlds of the West – Eastern Divan Orchestra, *Journal of the Royal Musical Association*, 134 (2), pp. 319–347, DOI:10.1080/0269040090031009109.

Bohlman, P. V. (1999). 'Ontologies of music', in N. Cook and M. Everist (eds.), *Rethinking music* (New York: Oxford University Press, 1999), pp. 17–34.

Bowell, S., and Bamford, S.M. (2018). *What Would Life Be, Without a Song or Dance, What Are We: A Report from the Commission on Dementia and Music*. London: International Longevity Centre, UK. Available at www.ilcuk.org.uk/index.php/publications/publication_details/what_would_life_be_without_a_song_or_dance_what_are_we [accessed 12 April 2018].

Clark, C.N., and Warren, J.D. (2015). Music, memory and mechanisms in Alzheimer's disease. *Brain*, 138(8), 2122–2125. https://doi.org/10.1093/brain/awv148 [accessed 12 April 2018].

Cuddy, L.L. and Duffin, J., (2005) Music, memory, and Alzheimer's disease: is music recognition spared in dementia, and how can it be assessed?. Medical hypotheses, 64(2), pp.229-235. https://doi.org/10.1016/j.mehy.2004.09.005

Darnley-Smith, R.M.R. (2002). Group music therapy with elderly adults. In A. Davies and E. Richards (eds.) *Group Work in Music Therapy*. London: Jessica Kingsley Publishers.

Darnley-Smith, R.M.R. (2013). *What Is the Music of Music Therapy? An Enquiry into the Aesthetics of Clinical Improvisation*. Available at http://etheses.dur.ac.uk/6975/

Fächner, J.C. (2016). The future of research in music therapy and neuroscience. In C. Dileo (ed.) *Envisioning the Future of Music Therapy*, 139–147. Available at www.temple.edu/boyer/documents/ENVISIONING_THE_FUTURE.pdf [accessed 20 April 2018].

Freeman, A. (2017). Fathoming the constellations: Ways of working with families in music therapy for people with advanced dementia. *British Journal of Music Therapy*, 31(1), 43–49. https://doi.org/10.1177/1359457517691052 [accessed 20 April 2018].

Hsu, M.H., Flowerdew, R., Parker, M., Fachner, J., and Odell-Miller, H. (2015). Individual music therapy for managing neuropsychiatric symptoms for people with dementia and their carers: A cluster randomised controlled feasibility study. *BMC Geriatrics*, 15(1), 84.

Jacobsen, J.H., Stelzer, J., Fritz, T.H., Chételat, G., La Joie, R., and Turner, R. (2015). Why musical memory can be preserved in advanced Alzheimer's disease. *Brain*, 138(8), 2438–2450. https://doi.org/10.1093/brain/awv135.

McDermott, O., Crellin, N., Ridder, H.M. and Orrell, M., (2013). Music therapy in dementia: a narrative synthesis systematic review. International journal of geriatric psychiatry, 28(8), pp. 781–794. doi: 10.1002/gps.3895

Malloch, S., and Trevarthen, C. (2009). Musicality: Communicating the vitality and interests of life. In S. Malloch and C. Trevarthen (eds.) *Communicative Musicality: Exploring the Basis of Human Companionship*. Oxford: Oxford University Press.

Odell-Miller, H. (2002). Musical narratives in music therapy treatment for dementia. In L. Bunt and S. Hoskyns (eds.) *The Handbook of Music Therapy*. Hove: Bruner Routledge, 149–155.

O'Kelly, J., Fachner, J.C., and Tervaniemi, M. (2016). Dialogues in music therapy and music neuroscience: Collaborative understanding driving clinical advances. *Frontiers in human neuroscience*, *10*, 585.

Pavlicevic, M., Tsiris, G., Wood, S., Powell, H., Graham, J., Sanderson, R., Millman, R., and Gibson, J. (2015). The 'ripple effect': Towards researching improvisational music therapy in dementia care homes. *Dementia*, 14(5), 659–679.

Ridder, H.M. (2016). The future of music therapy for persons with dementia Hanne Mette Ridder. In C. Dileo (ed.) *Envisioning the Future of Music Therapy*, 88–95. Available at www.temple.edu/boyer/documents/ENVISIONING_THE_FUTURE.pdf [accessed 20 April 2018].

Ronse, L., and Maes, R. (2014). The walking bass. In J. Sutton and J. De Backer (eds.) *The Music in Music Therapy: Psychodynamic Music Therapy in Europe: Clinical, Theoretical and Research Approaches*. London: Jessica Kingsley Publishers, 200.

Scruton, R. (1999). *The Aesthetics of Music*. Oxford: Oxford University Press.

Simmons-Stern, N.R., Budson, A.E., and Ally, B.A. (2010). Music as a memory enhancer in patients with alzheimer's disease. *Neuropsychologia*, 48(10), 3164–3167.

Small, C. (1998). *Musicking: The Meanings of Performing and Listening*. Middletown, CT: Wesleyan University Press.

Spiro Neta (2010). 'Music and dementia: Observing effects and searching for underlying theories', Aging & Mental Health. 14 (8) pp. 891–899, "https://doi.org/10.1080/136078 63.2010.519328"10.1080/13607863.2010.519328

Trevarthen, C., and Malloch, S. (2000). The dance of wellbeing: Defining the therapeutic effect. *Nordic Journal of Music Therapy*, 9(2), 3–17.

Winnicott, D.W. (1949). Hate in the counter-transference. *International Journal Psycho-Analysis*, 30, 69–74.

Winnicott, D.W. (1971/1986). The mirror role of mother and family in child development. In *Playing and Reality*. Harmondsworth: Pelican Books, 130–138.

Chapter 13

Groups for people with cognitive impairment and with dementia

What should we be doing?

Sandra Evans

> *What, then, is a 'group'? How does it acquire the capacity for exercising such a decisive influence over the mental life of the individual? And what is the nature of the mental change which it forces upon the individual?*
>
> Freud, S. (1921) Group Psychology and the analysis
> of the ego. SE, Vol.XVIII, p. 71

Introduction: why groups?

Dementia awareness is growing and, as a result, its stigmatising potential may be losing its grip. There is strength in numbers; people find it easier to fight back and rehearse new arguments together. Thanks to the National Dementia Strategy UK 2009, growing numbers of people have a dementia diagnosis following a professional assessment, including medical investigations which unfortunately often end with only a prescription for an anti-dementia drug. Commonly, this is followed by nothing at all in terms of ongoing support – although that too is changing. In a connected world, information is available which can be empowering for people. Persons with dementia and their families mostly desire such information; even with a condition that currently has no cure. Few people eschew any kind of help, although some will need time to come to terms with the dementia before they accept what is offered.

More of those who have this horrible illness are actively asking for support to take some control and make their own decisions about how services are organised and delivered (Cantley et al., 2005).

Services for people with a new diagnosis of dementia need to change with the times (Clare, 2003). There is much more expectation of a good experience of the communication of the diagnosis and for information subsequently (Dooley et al., 2015). The numbers of patients in the early stages of dementia who are in a position to benefit from support services included in after care are in the hundred thousands (Mental Health Foundation, 2007). Strategies involving the use of groups to involve, educate and support people make economic sense (Knapp et al., 2006) but also satisfies the need to manage peoples' reasonable expectations.

Group interventions from the psychological perspective

The group is key. In Freud's later works, he moved away from the solitary ego-based psychology and started to think more about man (and woman) in relation to social groups and social functions including the role of religions (Freud, 1922). He also looked at intergenerational issues and examined some of the aggressive behaviours towards the parental object in terms of an aspect of the social. He was followed in his theoretical deliberations by the object relations theorists who explored human psychology mainly in the dyadic relationship with mother, but who also invoked the role of the third, usually father, who supported the dyad but also frustrated it by opening it up and creating a space for social interaction. The first social interaction is within the family. Family therapy regards problems in persons as having been initiated or potentiated within a system: forces as much against change for the better are present in systems which have reached a dynamic equilibrium, such as situations of chronic illness such as dementia. Family therapy is well developed in old age psychiatry settings and in dementia care (Benbow et al., 1993). The original group analysts such as Foulkes (1964) and Bion (1961), along with the other Northfield psychiatrists, performed pioneering work on combat-fatigued men during the Second World War. Change, recovery and support can all be made possible or accelerated in group settings.

The premise upon which all these theoretical standpoints and modalities are based, it is reiterated here, is that distress or psychopathology which occurs in families and small groups can and should be revisited and ameliorated in a small group therapy setting (Pines, 1984). Moreover, for people with dementia, whose very identity and sense of self is under attack, groups can help reconstruct something of the person's identity (Boyd, 1991). It is in the groups we belong to that identities are continually constructed and reconstructed (Hutchinson, 2017). As Erikson (1968) himself put it so eloquently "the whole interplay between the psychological and the social, the developmental and the historical, for which identity formation is of prototypical significance, could be conceptualised only as a kind of psychosocial relativity".

Clinical illustration

In a cognitive stimulation therapy group for patients with a new diagnosis of dementia, some had their first experience of a group therapeutic space, shared with others with the same diagnosis. The clinician who had made their original dementia diagnosis found the experience of being more present in the group setting as herself was particularly interesting and humbling. For her, there was a changing experience in identity from professional to social to which the group members also responded. They demonstrated a shift in behaviour and affect. The members seemed to appreciate being seen as people in a more three-dimensional and less patient-like manner. Instead, they responded to the group facilitators with great warmth and affection. They easily shared reminiscences. Most of them seemed able to experience themselves in the group space as people with a competent past by re-inhabiting that self and having it witnessed and reflected rather than being cast in the role of sick people, severely disabled by dementia.

Positive aspects of the small group

Yalom (1985) was among the first to describe the group-based positive effects of a small group that meets regularly and retains a core membership. It is now accepted that groups which are well run (Evans, 2001) can provide emotional support and security for its members, sufficient for them to explore deeper feelings within themselves and also between them and other members. Even relationships with people outside the group can, through interactions within the group, be analysed appropriately; this is achieved through careful listening and interpretation of group transferences by the group conductor (Foulkes, 1964).

Groups strengthen ego and sense of self (Brown, 1994). The ego is particularly at risk in dementia (groups challenge super-ego forces, freeing people to face and accept changes). A harsh super-ego or unrealistic ego-ideal may encourage feelings of anxiety and shame in a person with the early signs and symptoms of dementia. This is exemplified by the self-berating behaviour which often occurs in people who can no longer meet the high standards they used to achieve but still demand of themselves. They are also likely to insist that no one else should have to meet similar standards. This holding of two standards, one for the self and a kinder one towards others, can within a kindly but challenging group lead to a softening of attitude. The group in this scenario would be acting as representative of another part of the patient's self. Unchallenged, these feelings of shame and self-doubt are likely to be followed by social withdrawal or reduced activity. Peers in a group can be mobilised to counteract these negative feelings and encourage people with dementia to brave that party, or the swimming baths (lane swimming can be a particularly harsh environment for someone with dementia and spatial disorientation) or whatever is their personal challenge.

Groups reduce emotional isolation. A 'slow-open' group (one where the memberships changes slowly over a long period of time, mirroring changes in the natural world), which promotes trust between people by maintaining a constant membership, encourages disclosure and grows intimacy; a benefit which many people with dementia ordinarily lose due to common social embarrassment.

Groups model and reinforce adaptive behavior. Social forces encourage change (Festinger, 1955) and while people inter-react in a group setting they learn about themselves in relation to others, particularly as they experience how others respond to them. This powerful learning experience (Bandura, 1977) shapes people's behavior and can build on itself as the new influences alter existing perceptions, making fears less potent and reduce projections. This is also where people with dementia can learn from others how to manage their condition for a little longer and, to some extent, this also explains the cognitive benefits of cognitive stimulation therapy (Spectre et al., 2003). Group therapy can reduce maladaptive behaviours such as denial of dementia (Clare, 2002); group interventions tend to be more powerful that a single voice. Groups are democratic. Other persons with dementia in a therapeutic group may have more impact than the therapist or group facilitator. The locus of control can move from the therapists to the group as a whole and on occasions to the members themselves. People can leave a group feeling empowered and energised.

Negative aspects of groups

What also needs to be considered is the group's potential for harm. Groups amplify feelings and if there is too much negativity or hopelessness in a group, people may be affected adversely. Fear of attending small groups or clubs for older people may be born from an implicit knowledge or fear of this phenomenon. The author is aware that malignant mirroring (Zinkin, 1983) can put people off attending in the first place: being mistrustful of anywhere that is 'full of old people' – i.e. 'just like us' – with all the negative projections and grotesque stereotypes imaginable (Evans, 1998).

With respect to the amplification of feeling, we are aware of what occurs in a large crowd, when capacity for logical thought and individual responsibility becomes much more difficult and emotions can take over. This has been demonstrated repeatedly as a catalyst for people to do things they would not ordinarily countenance, let alone act out. People who have a looser grip on reality by dint of their brain disorder may be more vulnerable to this kind of group-think. They may also be more vulnerable to an unsupervised therapist who may lose sight of the dynamic in the group. For example situations such as encouragement by other group members, which may reinforced by the therapist, may risk becoming too enthusiastic, particularly should the subject of the encouragement feel bullied or harassed.

Dynamic administration (thinking and anticipating the logistics of group times, meeting spaces and absences) needs to be tightly managed in a setting where group members may lose their skills at a faster rate than others and be unable to keep up. The danger is that the feelings of being left behind and of social isolation would be re-created or exacerbated in the group setting and become worse than anti-therapeutic; it would have the capacity to harm. Cognitive stimulation therapy group conductors equally have to monitor patients' abilities closely or ensure that there are additional staff available to give one or two patients close attention for the duration of the group in order to keep them engaged and part of the activity.

Therapists could easily exercise undue influence and must therefore be properly regulated and supervised. For this reason alone, it should never be assumed that untrained and unsupervised staff could run a therapy group. People, however, should be encouraged to convene social groups and activities for those who are not vulnerable, who retain capacity for their own decisions and who can voice objections as required (Mental Health Foundation, 2007).

Benefits of groups for people with dementia

A review of published work largely demonstrates that groups for older people with deteriorating conditions are potential spaces for mutual support, self-awareness and personal growth. Notwithstanding the important caveat that researchers and group enthusiasts are less likely to publish work that achieved negative outcomes, it appears that bringing people together is a worthwhile venture.

Joan Hunter (Hunter, 1989) included people with cognitive problems in a therapy group with older adults. She identified that her patients did not waste time worrying about the usual neurotic concerns but got on with the business of therapy due to their awareness of the need to make use of the limited time they had. This was echoed in the experience of Canete, Stormont and Esquerro where their patients seemed to abandon the usual rivalries and defensiveness seen at the start of groups for younger patients (Canete et al., 2000). The positive aspects of finding acceptance among fellow sufferers of long-term conditions and the instillation of hope (Jones et al., 2002) in the group were also iterated as beneficial factors in groups where death and dying became a primary preoccupation. Groups can be safe spaces in which to provide psychosocial support and will include themes commonly expressed among friends. For example, people may talk about loneliness, sex or the lack of it and fears of dependency. Other themes which may emerge are the dementia diagnosis itself, acceptance of it and the attitudes of others including stigma and lack of respect shown to the sufferer (Hawkins and Eagger, 1999; Clare, 2002).

Cognitive stimulation therapy

CST groups developed from a concerted effort to find the best and most effective mixture of activities for people with a new diagnosis of dementia. Reality orientation therapy and reminiscence-based work became popular in the late 1990s and were thought to be useful. These techniques were combined and assiduously researched; they were found to be at least as effective as the anti-dementia drugs in reducing the rate of decline of cognitive function (Spector et al., 2003). The mark of a good memory service (MSNAP) currently includes one which provides post diagnostic support and education. Cognitive stimulation therapy is one such method with a significant evidence base. It is relatively simple to organise in a clinic where there is a steady stream of people with a new diagnosis needing support, provided there are sufficient qualified staff and the infrastructure in place to make it happen.

What is clear from turning theory into practice is that the group dynamics and the dynamic administration of the conductors remain critical therapeutic and cohesive factors in the success of the enterprise. The conductors must be ever-vigilant to the needs of the group and responsive to the shifts in moods and content.

Clinical illustration

A CST group was organised in a memory clinic setting. The group was co-run by two people, a man and a woman. The group members had all been through the clinical assessment and had been recently given a new diagnosis of dementia. Some had been first assessed at home and most of them had been seen by one of the clinical staff prior to the group. The group was run for seven consecutive weeks and material was prepared prior to each group by Anton, an occupational therapist who took responsibility for the dynamic administration – letters to patients and carers, refreshments, room bookings and timing.

There were six patients in the group. As each person arrived in the third group of the series, they greeted each other, removed their coats (poignantly to the tune of Bob Marley's "Get up, stand up (stand up for your rights)" and waited expectantly. They seemed to assume they would be well looked-after as most recalled enjoying the previous week. After teas and chocolate biscuits, they were shown a smart screen and asked questions about the day's weather. Since this was easy for most, it had the advantage of making people feel relaxed and removed potential for threat and the unknown.

(Of course, for those who might function at a higher level, the potential risk of them feeling demeaned is very real, however, moving things on quickly can maintain interest and engagement.)

The next exercise was for each to write down details of their own birth-place, siblings and something they remembered about their childhood. Each person was asked to read out their answers, including both the facilitators. This democratic way of running the group bonded people together so that group cohesion seemed to form quickly: 'staff' and 'patient' categories were soon broken down and there emerged a curious feeling of exhilaration in everyone being on first-name terms, and talking easily about the past and the present. The air of pleasant expectation persisted.

The next game was to use various items to create new things. Playdoh, beads, puzzles and jigsaws were attempted. Two women made things together and chatted about childhood friends, scholarly triumphs and early years in foster care. The vicissitudes of the years were recounted without rancor or self-consciousness. One person needed help as their spatial awareness was particularly affected by dementia – a sharp reminder to all of the reality of the vicious effects of the disease – so one of the facilitators moved to lend individual interaction. It was very delicate, the line between encouraging independence and abandoning that person to their muddle.

Groups for MCI

There is no question of a need for support and psycho-educational groups for people with a label of MCI (mild cognitive impairment), or a diagnosis of 'minimal cognitive impairment' (ICD-10). People with a condition of memory loss with this label often need guidance and reassurance – although reassurance is not always appropriate and should be honest, as some people do progress to develop dementia. MCI is a description of a state which could be both a snapshot of functioning along the road to increasing impairment, i.e. dementia, or it could be a static state that does not progress further (Burns and Zaudig, 2002). It is possible that this mild memory problem can improve due to changes in physical health or improvement of social interaction; for some, MCI is reversible. CST groups are likely to be of benefit to people in each of these three categories for reasons given earlier.

Memory services providing groups for MCI are less common than those for established dementia. Some would argue that this should be the domain of primary care (general practice), given that it is a kind of primary prevention strategy. Irrespective of any agreement about who should take responsibility for this kind of work, while we wait for decisions to be made about evidence-base and commissioning intentions, there are people in need of information and guidance who are not getting it as standard.

This is an area of health-related work which needs considerable creativity and which is often supported initially by charitable organisations which are aware of the need and may have the flexibility to pump prime an innovation for a year or two (Alzheimer's Research UK, 2018). Once such a service is established, sustainability is key. Services that have proved themselves useful to a population will need then to be adopted by statutory commissioning. Such interventions are more likely to be taken up and to succeed if they are embedded in existing services and compliment them. They will of course need to comply with regulatory standards that are both necessary and which risk the stifling of innovation.

It seems worthwhile at this juncture to think of the national and organisational approach to service provision for older patients generally and for people with dementia more particularly. In a country like the UK with a National Health Service which serves the demands of multiple needs, there will always be a ranking according to perceptions of necessity and deservedness. That public servants are vulnerable to the 'colossal forces' of our society, both conscious and unconscious (Foulkes, 1964) is undeniable, and whereas NICE is in place to consider funding for evidence-based treatments and economic viability; politicians and to a lesser extent charities respond also to the 'will of the people'; or perhaps the press. Suffering infants in this kind of contest will always rank ahead of the very old. MCI may not meet the criteria for national funds but could be an important stage in researching the development of dementia. It is therefore also a potential moment to implement public health awareness. Considering a group-based strategy need not be costly.

Activity groups

Charities such as Alzheimer's Society and Age Concern host and support group-based social activities which are never badged as 'therapy' and which can therefore maintain the innovative quality and support diverse groups. Groups such as the LGBT community who might otherwise struggle to feel comfortable in the usual settings can meet together to discuss their worries (e.g. Opening Doors London). Jewish Care and specific ethnic groups can offer similar social activities with a shared culture and an embedded, group adhesiveness.

Carers support groups

There are probably more than 800,000 people living with dementia in the UK. Most of these live at home and are cared for by friends or family members as unpaid care-givers, of whom there are an estimated 670,000 (Carers Trust, 2014). It has been estimated that unpaid care-givers contribute 11.6 billion pounds of work (Alzheimer's Society, 2014) to support the economy. The care-givers of people with dementia are often elderly themselves and are at greater risk of health problems as a result of their caring responsibilities (Zarit et al., 1986; O'Hanlon et al., 2004).

Education alone of informal care-givers has not produced the positive effect hoped for; in some cases they had a negative effect (Selwood et al., 2007). Respite also does not always hold the desired effect of improving the well-being of carers. A review of trials undertaken demonstrated a poor evidence base and the positive and negative effects of respite care remain unclear (Maayan et al., 2014). It is conceivable that many factors confound any benefit from a short period of respite including the distress caused for both parties by separation, guilt and increased confusion. Carer burden and distress is recognised to be greater in young onset dementia when the problems may be more challenging due to the unexpectedly youthful appearance of the sufferer, their physical robustness and an increase in psychiatric morbidity (Freyne et al., 1999)

Supportive interventions of a more informal type for carers reduce the rate of nursing home placement (Mittelman et al., 2006). Improved support may hold benefits not just for the carers, but the people with dementia.

It is important to note that carer stress has been shown to be reduced significantly upon the person's admission to a care home. (Gage et al., 2015). Support and information about when other care services could be sought is important in the well-being of carers. (Pinquart and Sorensen, 2003). This is particularly worrying as there is an increase in risk of abuse of people with dementia by their carers if their carers are anxious or depressed (Cooper et al., 2010).

There is considerable evidence of the benefits of support groups for the carers and spouses of people with dementia (Steuer and Clarke, 1982), including a controlled trial (Kahan et al., 1985). The effects of caring for people with dementia living at home was well documented in the last century (Gilhooly, 1984; Gilleard et al., 1984) when the care landscape was very different from the present day and was being provided well before there was any significant treatment for dementia. The anti-dementia drugs have changed dementia from being a 'social problem' (i.e. one which demanded social care), for which there was little medical intervention possible, to becoming very medicalised. Assessments usually involve brain imaging, sometimes spinal fluid assays and, more rarely, genetic counseling. Treatment involves medication and evidence-based interventions such as cognitive stimulation therapy – mainly in groups. Including the partners in interventions is still relatively rare, despite the knowledge that they too are suffering and that sustaining them in caring for people at home, particularly when the carers are also old and frail; supports the well-being of both parties.

Currently it is the third sector which provides the bulk of carers' groups through charitable funding. Sustainability of this important work is an ongoing concern to clinical services unable to fund similar groups through clinical commissioning. Proportionally fewer people go into care home settings than previously and, when they do so, it is later in the illness. For those who do go into institutional care, relatives and partners may suffer significant feelings of guilt, separation and with the added stress of visiting and all that entails. Ironically, institutional care settings can also offer opportunities for people to come together as patient groups, carers' group and a mixture of both. The demise of the institutions can remove some of these opportunities for meeting and challenge us to find new and creative ways for people to meet for their mutual benefit (Evans, 2015).

Evans, Ong and Glover worked on a group for the spouses of people in long-term care at a time when the National Health Service provided hundreds of local hospital beds for people with dementia. Their support group was seriously under-powered to demonstrate any evidence of benefit and was unpublished. They were however able to describe themes developing in the group over time. These are outlined in the following clinical example.

Clinical example

In a group designed to support the spouses of people with dementia, the co-therapists were a junior doctor and a senior nurse who both worked on the dementia ward where the other spouse resided.

The group was held at the hospital and was offered only to those spouses who made regular visits, thus demonstrating their ongoing commitment to their partnership. A number of identifiable themes emerged.

The first was the spouses admitting that there was a problem. This was more than relentless hospital visiting. The healthy partners were there for a relatively long-term commitment of regular visits, which were tiring and not always rewarding. In a group they found a voice to express grief and anger for their loss.

As the group began to feel a safer and more supportive space, guilt was expressed at having put their spouse in institutional care. They often berated themselves, describing feeling helpless and worthless. They also berated the group for being helpless and useless and indeed the co-facilitators often felt useless, occasionally feeling tempted to abandon the group altogether. They may have picked up in their counter-transference the unconscious wish to flee the negative emotions and abandon the dependent spouse. Both spouse care-givers and co-facilitators continued meeting nonetheless.

Eventually some of the members accepted help for themselves although others did not find they were able to achieve acceptance.

The group became angry with the ward staff for not being caring enough and for not doing things as well as they would have done for their partners. This clearly developed with the theme of guilt but also with anger with the patients themselves for the way they had become. This might have been the hardest to express and it needed the critical mass of others to say, but also the understanding of the group to air such unacceptable feelings. It suggested the group were forgiving themselves and each other for their use of institutional care.

The theme of the spouses' own physical frailty emerged from the anger. Their own health and well-being was being put at risk by taxing visits to partners who may be enviably physically robust but may struggle to remember them or make sense of the visit. The group members started to look at death as a blessing and as an acceptable exit for their spouses and for them. When one member was widowed during the course of the group, there was much talk of death but then also the possibility of new beginnings. There might even be a new life for themselves after their own spouse died.

Once able to face the death of their partners, the group members echoed the sense of the value of the group by consolidating the value of their visits. There would come an end at some point, but, in the meantime, they would be the holders of the meaning of their relationships and the custodians of the memories of their spouses. The group ended on a lighter note; perhaps the death of the group mirroring the end of suffering for the spouses and the relief that they could stop the painful introspection, even though it had been of value.

Conclusion

Once medical interventions per se come to an end, attending to the emotional and social needs is an important factor in sustaining patients and carers alike. Clinicians too struggle with having to let go of patients whom they know have grown attached through the process of diagnosis and sharing information. We doctors, nurses, occupational therapists and social workers are well aware that people with dementia need a link to the possibility of further treatment and support after diagnosis. That it is potentially very expensive should not deter us from trying to find ways of maintaining healthy, helpful links in a cost effective way. Groups go a long way to deliver such a model of care. Long term ill-health, declining abilities and being left feeling helpless can be ameliorated through the universality of humanity that is expressed and experienced through meeting in small groups. Groups are more than the sum of their parts and are powerful tools in themselves as therapeutic interventions and as ways of delivering information, skill-sharing and making the unconscious, conscious. Additionally, they are also good spaces for self-reflection and airing feelings initially feared to be unacceptable.

Groups are also places to re-identify with identity and reconnect with lost aspects of the self. The author argues that groups are therefore also positive places for people with early dementia when identity and sense of personal integrity is under threat.

References

Alzheimer's Research UK. (2018). *Thinking Differently: Preparing Today to Implement Future Dementia Treatments*. London: AS Publications.

Alzheimer's Society. (2014). *Dementia Update 2014*. Available at www.alzheimers.org.uk/site/scripts/download_info.php?downloadID=1491.

Bandura, A. (1977). *Social Learning Theory*. New York: General Learning Press.

Benbow, S., Marriott, A., Morley, M., and Welsh, S. (1993). Family therapy and dementia: Review and clinical experience. *International Journal of Geriatric Psychiatry*, 8(9), 717–725.

Bion, W. (1961). *Experiences in Groups and other papers*. London: Tavistock.

Boyd, J. (1991). The matrix model. In R. Boyd (ed.) *Personal Transformations in Groups: A Jungian Perspective*. London and New York: Routledge Group Therapy.

Brown, D. (1994). 'Ego training in action'. Self-development through social interaction. In Denis Brown and Louis Zinkin (eds.) *The Psyche and the Social World*. London: Jessica Kingsley Publishers, 107–123.

Burns, A., and Zaudig, M. (2002). Mild cognitive impairment in older people. *The Lancet*, 360(9349), 1963–1966.

Canete, M., Stormont, F., and Ezquerro, A. (2000). Group analytic psychotherapy with the elderly. *British Journal of Psychotherapy*, 17(1).

Cantley, C., Woodhouse, J., and Smith, M. (2005). *Listen to Us: Involving People With Dementia in Planning and Developing Services*. Newcastle upon Tyne: Dementia North, Northumbria University.

Carers Trust. (2014). *A Road Less Rocky – Supporting Carers of People with Dementia*. Available at www.carers.org/sites/default/files/dementia_report_road_less_rocky_final_low.pdf.

Clare, L. (2002). Developing awareness about awareness in early-stage dementia: The role of psychosocial factors. *Dementia*, 1(3), 295–312.

Clare, L. (2003). 'I'm still me': Living with the onset of dementia. *Journal of Dementia Care*, 11(2), 32–35.

Cooper, C., Selwood, A., Blanchard, M., Walker, Z., Blizard, R., and Livingston, G. (2010). The determinants of family carers' abusive behaviour to people with dementia: Results of the CARD study. *Journal of Affective Disorders*, 121, 136–142. Netherlands, 2009, Elsevier B.V.

Dooley, J., Bailey, C., and McCabe, R. (2015). Communication in healthcare interactions in dementia: A systematic review of observational studies. *International Psychogeriatrics*, 27(8), 1277–1300.

Erikson, E.H. (1968). *Identity: Youth and Crisis*. New York: Norton & Company.

Evans, S. (1998). Beyond the mirror: A group analytic exploration of late life and depression. *Ageing and Mental Health*, 2(2), 94–99.

Evans, S. (2001). Group analytic psychotherapy: A realistic treatment for older adults? *CPD Bulletin Old Age Psychiatry*, 3(1), 9–12.

Evans, S. (2015). What the national dementia strategy forgot: Providing dementia care from a psychodynamic perspective. *Psychoanalytic Psychotherapy*, 28(3), 321–329.

Festinger, L. (1955). Social psychology and group processes. *Annual Review of Psychology*, 6, 187–216.

Foulkes, S.H. (1964). *Therapeutic Group Analysis*. London: Allen & Unwin.

Freud, S. (1921). Group psychology and the analysis of the ego. In *The Standard Edition of the Complete Psychological Works of Sigmund Freud, Volume XVIII (1920–1922):*
Freud S. (1922). Group Psychology and the analysis of the ego. Standard Edition 18 65–143. London & Vienna. International Psychoanalytical Press.

Freyne, A., Kidd, N., Coen, R., and Lawlor, B.A. (1999). Burden of care in carers of dementia patients: Higher levels in carers of younger sufferers. *International Journal of Geriatric Psychiatry*, 14(9), 784–788.

Gage, H., Cheynel, J., Williams, P., Mitchell, K., Stinton, C., Katz, J., Holland, C., and Sheehan, B. (2015). Service utilisation and family support of people with dementia: A cohort study in England: *International Journal of Geriatric Psychiatry*, 30, 166–177.

Gilhooly, M. (1984). The impact of care-giving on care-givers: Factors associated with the psychological well-being of people supporting a dementing relative in the community. *British Journal of Medical Psychology*, 57, 35–44.

Gilleard, C., Bedford, H., Gilleard, H., Whittick, J., and Gledhill, K. (1984). Emotional distress among the supporters of the elderly mentally infirm. *British Journal of Psychiatry*, 145, 172–177.

Hawkins, D., and Eagger, S. (1999). Group therapy: Sharing the pain of diagnosis. *Journal of Dementia Care*, 7(5), 12–14.

Hunter, J. (1989). Reflections on psychotherapy with ageing people, individually and in groups. *British Journal of Psychiatry*, 154, 250–252.

Hutchinson, S. (2017). *The Times They Are a Changing*. Foulkes Lecture.

Jones, K., Cheston, R., and Gilliard, J. (2002). *Group Psychotherapy for People with Dementia: Development, Facilitation and Evaluation of Psychotherapeutic Support Groups*. Bristol: Dementia Voice.

Kahan, J., Kemp, B., Staples, F., and Brummel-Smith, K. (1985). Decreasing the burden in families caring for a relative with a dementing illness: A controlled study. *Journal of the American Geriatric Association*, 33, 664–670.

Knapp, M., Thorgrimsen, L., Patel, A., Spector, A., Hallam, A., Woods, B., and Orrell, M. (2006). Cognitive stimulation therapy for people with dementia: Cost effectiveness analysis. *British Journal of Psychiatry*, 188, 574–580.

Maayan, N., Soares-Weiser, K., and Lee, H. (2014). Respite care for people with dementia and their carers. *Cochrane Database Systematic Reviews*, 1, CD004396.

Mental Health Foundation. (2007). *Getting on with Living: A Guide to Developing Services for People with Early Dementia*. London: Mental Health Foundation. ISBN 978-1-903645-96-

Mittelman, M.S., Haley, W.E., Clay, O.J., and Roth, D.L. (2006). Improving caregiver well-being delays nursing home placement of patients with Alzheimer disease. *Neurology*, 67, 1592–1599. United States.

O'Hanlon, A., McGee, H., Barker, M., Garavan, R., Hickey, A., Conroy, R. et al. (2004). *Health and Social Services for Older People II (HeSSOP II) Changing Profiles from 2000–2004*. Dublin Council on Aging and Older People.

Pines, M. (1984). Mirroring in group analysis as developmental and therapeutic process. In T.E. Lear (ed.) *Spheres of Group Analysis*. London: Group Analytic Society, 118–136.

Pinquart, M., and Sorensen, S. (2003). Differences between caregivers and noncaregivers in psychological health and physical health: A meta-analysis. *Psychology and Aging*, 18, 250–267.

Selwood, A., Johnston, K., Katona, C., Lyketsos, C., and Livingston, G. (2007). Systematic review of the effect of psychological interventions on family caregivers of people with dementia. *Journal of Affective Disorders*, 101, 75–89.

Spector, A., Thorgrimsen, L., Woods, B., Royan, L., Davies, S., Butterworth, M., and Orrell, M. (2003). Efficacy of an evidence-based Cognitive stimulation therapy programme for people with dementia: Randomised controlled trial. *British Journal of Psychiatry*, 183, 248–254.

Steuer, J., and Clarke, E. (1982). Family support groups within a research project on dementia. *Clinical Gerontologist*, 1, 87–95.

Yalom, I.D. (1985). *The Theory and Practice of Group Psychotherapy*. Chapter 1, New York: Therapeutic Factors in Groups.

Zarit, S., Todd, P., and Zarit, J. (1986). Subjective burden of husbands and wives as caregivers: A longitudinal study. *Gerontologist*, 26, 260–266.

Zinkin, L. (1983). The malignant mirror. *Group Analysis*, 16(2), 113–126.

Chapter 14

Disintegration and integration in dementia care

Mentalization as a means to keep whole

Stephanie Petty, Michelle Potts and Daniel Anderson

> *Are not the sane and the insane equal at night as the sane lie adreaming?*
>
> *Are not all of us outside this hospital, who dream, more or less in the condition of those inside it, every night of our lives?*
>
> *Charles Dickens (1860)*

Introduction

If you allow yourself to notice, it is apparent that emotions are commonplace in dementia care. We can understand that emotions become stronger and more prevalent when the experience of dementia is of fragmentation: that is, losing a sense of yourself and losing familiar relationships that help you to find congruence. Yet this is not the predominant discourse. In this chapter we offer an exploration of emotion in dementia care, employing the method of psychodynamic observation.

There is repeated exclamation that the model of care for individuals with dementia is failing and unsatisfactory (Obholzer and Roberts, 1994; Department of Health, 2012; Francis, 2013). An individual's most human, intimate needs become dismissed and are unable to be prioritised. It is curious that the care offered to infants or loved ones in times of need does not seem to extend to individuals later in life who become dependent on others for physical and emotional safety. What is so intolerable about dementia?

To explore this, we set the research question of 'where is the emotion in dementia care?' We made no directional hypotheses, instead beginning with the aims of neutrality and curiosity. The method of psychodynamic observation offers a more intimate and relational viewpoint of an environment. An observer is orientated towards their emotional experience in connection with the environment. In this way, we share a curiosity about more than what is visible. This is in contrast to more distancing methods that place the observer as disconnected from their environment, counting or categorising behaviour. Thirty hours of reflective observations were carried out by one staff member over a four-week period. Immediately following each observation period, the observer made written entries into a reflective diary, which formed a qualitative data set. The setting was two inpatient units for people predominantly with dementia diagnoses and a level of complexity requiring hospital care, typically described as 'challenging' to services.

Here we provide an overview of this observation, offering quotes from the diary as brief illustrations of the observer's experience, with discussion throughout. Themes of integration, disintegration and seeking integration became apparent, which are explored to offer an attempt at understanding 'where emotion is'. Finally, we present some ideas about an approach towards dementia care that utilises the concept of mentalization as a means to equip the carer with psychological tools to enable safe and meaningful interactions.

Towards a different approach to care in dementia

You could be forgiven for misunderstanding the author of the reflective diary; the misunderstanding would be to suspect that the diary is written by a person with dementia. This offers a striking viewpoint; there is a lack of clear differentiation between the professional and the patient.

In attempt to organise something that felt disorganised, we present three broad 'themes': towards disintegration, seeking integration and integration. 'Disintegration' represented avoidance and extreme fragmented emotions without a dialogue that was considered necessary. In 'seeking an integrated self' in this context, use of metaphor, grounding and seeking attunement with others were predominant themes. 'Integration' became the sense of a whole self that is ambivalent and thinking.

This is not meant to suggest a linear model, or discrete experiences, but is organised as such in attempt to communicate the felt experience of the observer in a manageable way. The three themes were experienced repeatedly, and fluidly, throughout the observation. This intuitively communicates an often intangible experience of dementia.

Towards disintegration

"The TV was the only sound I could hear as the rest of the unit it was quiet. I didn't feel quiet."

"I felt sadness, or maybe not sadness but a sense that something wasn't quite right?"

"Nothing here feels constant except maybe the constant fluctuations."

"My words can't be heard or understood so I tried to be understood through my face or my body language."

"It isn't always easy to second guess what others are thinking or I don't find it easy and I must get it wrong all the time."

"Conversations are sort of always laced with confusion."

"– very strange, completely incongruent. I found it hard to concentrate on our conversation, what was around us just didn't make sense."

"True understanding doesn't exist anymore, not only for the client but for me too and it doesn't matter. . . . I had a conversation that had really no start, middle or end and it was still a conversation and we both seemed content to have it."

The author is a staff member: a young, well, un-dementing person, employed to care for others. Yet the experiences of feeling 'disintegrated' were vivid and shared.

"There is real sadness when I think about it because things that have been stolen or that have disappeared won't ever come back."

"– but in that moment at the window, with the clock reminding me of how slow time can be I felt sadness, or maybe not sadness but a sense that something wasn't quite right?"

'Disintegration' captures a crumbling away of the self. Largely there was a distance between emotional experiences and the necessary dialogue to make sense of them. It describes the experience of extreme fragmented emotions and the temptation to avoid feeling the fragmentation. Dementia is an integrated state becoming disintegrated.

In later life, there is a mixture of myth and truth about emotions becoming less salient and therefore less deserving of attention. There is a robust evidence base of cognitive theory and neuroscience showing that older adults experience less negative emotions as emotions become more regulated with aging (Mather et al., 2004; Reed and Carstensen, 2012; Mather, 2012), notably anger (Kunzmann et al., 2014). The idea being that, as we get older, we become more skilled at regulating our emotions and therefore may appear to express less intense emotions. Yet according to theories of emotional aging, emotional regulation requires cognitive resources for self-reflection and life-reflection, to prioritise and engage with certain relationships and find meaning (Carstensen, 2006). This is desirable; it may help to ease the anxiety of ageing and provide some reassurance when caring for an older person. As desirable or convenient as it may be, it is not the complete picture.

Miesen (2004) describes the likely experience of dementia as

it is as if they are landed in a 'strange situation' in which they experience feeling unsafe for long periods of time, powerlessness and having no structures to hold on to. They are constantly wrestling with feelings that they do not belong, that they do not feel at home and that there is a barrier between them and their nearest and dearest.

(pp. 184)

De Masi (2004) describes the idea of 'nothingness' being unimaginable to humans. A person living with dementia will experience a gradual annihilation of the self as they begin to forget their loved ones and themselves; this becomes the 'nothingness' that is traumatic.

In this observation, the 'strange situation' was felt by the author, but it was only felt when the author was mindfully observing. It was easy to forget the 'strange' reality of the workplace. There was temptation to avoid the difficulty of the work, though temptation implies choice. The author experienced a lack of thinking and lack of choice.

> "their despair is so loud, I get this lump in my throat – the thing that's like a silent cry."

> "Things can instantly feel anxious in the office, anticipating something bad is going to happen, when there isn't really anything to warrant such anxiety, or there wasn't this morning."

> ". . . and then looking at this lady sat beside me in despair – very strange, completely incongruent. I found it hard to concentrate on our conversation, what was around us just didn't make sense."

Task orientation and working with older adults is common place; in Obholzer and Roberts' (1994) writing in *The Unconscious at Work* they describe the tendency of staff teams to focus time and energy on physical health, on tasks with a clear beginning and end, to the extent that quality of life is second place or even forgotten. Anxiety and fear can be stirred up, fears about our own fate as we become older and perhaps it evokes memories of our relationships with older people in our lives (Obholzer and Roberts, 1994). Perhaps the fear and anxiety feel more extreme when dementia is also a factor? Staff need to find ways to cope with the emotional pull and challenging feelings that are prevalent in the work. A metaphor of a mask is used by Sheard (2010), where he describes the real task as to be able to remove the mask that places barriers between staff and patients, the mask providing some kind of emotional distance and therefore making it difficult for staff to just 'be'.

> "Physical stuff is around a lot, or it kind of always is but at the moment it feels more apparent and more of a worry for the team, me included. There is quite a lot of stuff to remember, who has what done and how often they need it doing and most importantly where you write down to say you've done it . . . The folder with all the sheets in that we have to fill in (food, fluid, engagement obs, turning, physical obs and I probably missed some) is packed!"

> "Occasionally when I'm assisting someone with their meal I think about what I would do if they started to choke, it fills me with panic."

> "It's odd really, once someone's dead – they literary disappear, I know that actually they do disappear, well their body does but also them, no one talks about them much, unless they're referring to their bedroom."

> "Someone died recently and I was surprised how much sadness I felt about him passing away and how much he was on my mind. So when I heard this other guy had been sent to hospital I quite quickly and quite irrationally thought he

was going to die. When the phone rang this morning my first thought was – it's the hospital ringing to say he has passed away in the night. . . . Death is obviously completely out of anyone's control but I think because we have so much control of our guys and ladies it's hard not to find the inevitability of people dying difficult to comprehend. . . . Another client had to go to the hospital this morning – another! I decided to officially declare in my mind that no-one is allowed to die until next year, I'm doubtful that saying this to myself will make any real difference but that's what kept running through my head this morning – no death allowed here!"

Coping strategies such as task orientation and humour serve a purpose, and to an extent help to maintain staff wellbeing (Blagg and Petty, 2014). The trick appears to be recognising the moments when such strategies are needed and useful, whilst also being fluid, moving positions depending on what feels the most helpful in the moment.

"I was glad to be leaving though, the noise was still there and this might make me the bad person but I was so grateful that I got to leave and didn't have to try and fall asleep listening to the noise."

"I was kind of trying to avoid being around people for too long."

"If I'm only around for an hour or two and it gets me a bit het up – maybe I'd be even worse if I was on all day – the pressure."

"I was uncomfortable again really wished I had something to do . . . I think really I was thinking if I want time to speed up so I can go back to doing what I know . . . outcomes, sessions all that, and leaving to go home"

"honesty compels me to acknowledge that I have three databases, ordered and colour co-ordinated"

"The rush of the day . . . at half 7. Staffing was a bit short and there ensued the panic, there was lots of talk about how we were going to get people up if there are only 5 people on! Luckily and quite predictably no one was awake and raring to get up at 7.30 in the morning . . . panic over."

"There's a hierarchy of jobs at lunch time, at the top is 'the server' – the person who is in control of the trolley and dishes up, 'the runner' – the person who doles out the dishes, 'the assisters' – the people who help feed people who struggle to feed themselves."

The disintegration of experience, of emotion existing on islands for the individual with dementia and those connected to them, means an 'us and them' culture continues to exist in dementia care because the 'source' of difficult emotion needs to be managed. Sheard (2009) describes how this is to the detriment of patients as they are not receiving a true reflection of person-centred care but instead a surface level version. This culture can lead to the dehumanising of people and is part of the wider of picture of what happens when care goes wrong, and instead becomes abuse. There are recent examples of care going wrong: Winterbourne View Hospital (Department of Health, 2012) and the failings of Mid Staffordshire NHS Trust (Francis, 2013) were heavily reported by the media. Abuse in care can happen when the people being cared for are not seen as human beings, when a culture of emotional detachment exists; the results of such cultures are at best hollow care and at worst criminal.

Seeking integration

> "I want to my feet firmly on the ground on one side of the fence."

From the experience of disintegration, the observer sought to feel differently. This included seeking another person to feel connected to, the use of metaphor and literature to find temporary meaning, and grounding within the present moment.

When feeling estranged and alienated, as when experiencing dementia, the human response is to seek safety through people that provide comfort (Bowlby, 1979; Adshead, 1998; Jones, 2004) and by taking action to establish some meaning and control over the situation. As the observer, as a member of staff, we can appreciate the demand placed on another to bear with the person. "Because the parent is offering an integrated-enough experience then the infant also internalises this – is able to offer themselves a good-enough integrating voice" (Leiman and Sutton, 2004, p.30). Yet here there is difference from an infant learning an integrating voice from a parent. We expect individuals in later life to remember this human connection. In contrast, dementia becomes isolating; individuals become denied the presence of others due to the struggle of communicating. There is a culture of ignoring the person (Kitwood, 1997). We are missing the moments of shared meaning, space, play.

> "I noticed myself wanting to talk or be talked to"

> "I wonder if others feel like that"

> "– but I wanted others to be sad with me, sharing in it all. It's seems harder to say what I'm actually thinking or feeling when it appears to be different to the general consensus or atmosphere . . . I was filled with a sense of disappointment"

> "I know I feel at my most useful and content when I'm with someone and I can tell they feel content and safe with me."

> "Like I really wanted others to see just how happy I was or just how much their sadness affected me."

> "We, me and the client were doing it together, almost making up some kind of fiction together"

"I honestly started to feel a little resentful and maybe disappointed that the atmosphere wasn't what I expected; I kind of wanted the place to reflect how I felt . . . a bit sad and mopey."

"A more helpful way to describe my relaxed feeling would be to use the word content, I and I think those around me appeared content in what they were doing or not doing."

When the primary system of sharing meaning, through verbal language, is degrading. Vygotsky differentiated making 'meaning' and making 'sense' through language (Vygotsky, 1986): where 'meaning' becomes stable over time with repetition and is shared culturally, 'sense' is idiosyncratic and changeable. Over time, the shared understanding communicates more complex thoughts and emotions. The sense making in dementia is of more intense and changeable emotions being shared between people, with less reliance on verbal words. In what Evans calls 'extreme dependency' (Evans, 2008), emotions are communicated through projective identification.

"To be someone's safety is a huge responsibility, not just their physical safety but their emotional safety – like a rag doll, being hugged and loved one minute and then tossed aside or nipped and punched the next . . ."

"Tears started to come to my eyes too and we just looked at one another for what felt like ages – in reality it probably wasn't that long – I felt like we were completely connected, only for a few moments."

Dialogue, the act of saying aloud or to yourself your true thoughts and feelings, helps. Winnicott (1949) highlighted the necessity to express these difficult emotions, for the good of the self and for vulnerable patients you are caring for; voicing your negative feelings prevents them from being acted out. This highlights the need for a clearly defined and boundaried space where emotional expression is encouraged and developed. It is established that although the 'thinking areas' of the brain are eroding, the 'feeling parts' remain intact (Evans, 2008), therefore things such as play, music, scent can be helpful when working in dementia care. Helpful to the client, to elicit memory (Evans, 2008) but also helpful to the staff member, enabling or giving them permission to be in the moment with someone, sharing an experience, where each person plays a crucial and mutual part.

"Wherever you were on the unit this afternoon you could hear music and smell paint, I found this soothing and kind of grounding in a way, I hope that was felt by others too."

"Surely we can do both, 'do and feel' or 'do then feel' or vice versa."

"being able to notice the moments when you can let yourself fall apart and accept that."

"Thinking about death, people disappearing, losing people – where I am now, I want to feel it – the loss and sadness, I'd be more worried if I didn't or couldn't."

Integration

Integration is the more emotionally straining and cognitively demanding position. This does not mean to imply an end-goal to be desired, but something to be aware of and move in and out of. Of course the narrator shows a consistent level of integration throughout the writing of the diary. The process of actively pausing to use pen and paper to capture an experience, eloquently and verbally is a demonstration of integration.

> "it felt long enough. . . . I felt sort of stressed really trying too hard to think and feel . . . I feel rushed and sick of noticing"

> "now I have the time and space to think and feel and I'm at a loss"

> "I've noticed that over the last few weeks whilst doing my observations, I've been kind of polarising in my thoughts and feelings, finding it hard at times to sit in the middle ground, I kind of thought the opposite would happen."

The author experienced the exhaustion of struggling to remain whole. It was exhausting to continue to feel and process the emotions that arose. The idea of not feeling, or striving to reach certainty, became desirable.

We agreed that the work is allowing yourself to notice your internal experience and bear this. For the most part there is a need to accept the ambiguity and incongruence of what is around you and be able to get lost in this. It is intriguing that this is a shared labour for staff and patients.

> "I think the things that I don't say, that I keep to myself, find a way of surfacing, whether that's through being passive aggressive or purposefully questioning."

> "not knowing where to put myself, wanting to be helpful but not quite knowing how to be unless instructed. . . . In these moments I felt stressed, probably the combination of feeling a bit on the outside and worrying I wouldn't be liked . . . or be disliked more."

> "Perhaps I was worried about being blamed or looking as if I didn't know what I was doing – which most likely some of the time I don't."

We define integration as having a sense of yourself that is whole, having the ability to feel ambivalent, to not know but to hold thoughts and feelings together. It usually carried tension.

> "It's odd because unless I'm really paying attention I forget there is confusion most of the time, it doesn't feel important that conversations or interactions are not based on what makes sense and instead rely on an appreciation of just being."

"I was looking around at ALL the tinsel and then looking at this lady sat beside me in despair – very strange, completely incongruent. I found it hard to concentrate on our conversation, what was around us just didn't make sense."

"Today was a mixed day really, I felt like things were in extremes, or my response to things were in extremes. Only in this type of work can you go from throat lump/almost crying to wandering around contently, smiling about the decor."

Miesen (2004) describes how caregivers can be a symbolic presence to someone with dementia, perhaps highlighting the importance of being a whole symbolic presence. You are mentalizing when you are attending both implicitly and explicitly to the mental processes and subjective states of yourself and of others (Bateman and Fonagy, 2010). This relates to Winnicott's (1956) idea of being 'held' or 'tuned in' to another impacting your sense of well-being.

"The whole environment felt exaggerated at times, people reactions and emotion felt amplified to me, I think I mirrored that; my words can't be heard or understood so I tried to be understood through my face or my body language. I found this a little tiring, always wondering can they tell I'm happy or do they know I'm relaxed."

Mentalization in dementia (the MinD approach)

We would like to introduce the mentalization in dementia (MinD) approach to care as a way to bring together these observations and our understanding of them. The model describes what might be termed implicit approaches to care, where there is not an obvious therapeutic intervention occurring or structural programme being followed. Rather, this description attempts to describe a cultural ethos of how behaviours and feelings are made meaningful within the care environment generally and in specific interactions. The MinD model provides the framework and the tools to work therapeutically moment by moment and is in contrast to other prevalent models of dementia care that distance the person with dementia and their experience.

mentalization is the capacity to mentalize; that is, it is the ability to focus upon the mental state of both ourselves and those of others in order to understand behaviour (Bateman and Fonagy, 2004; Fonagy and Adshead, 2012). It is an imaginative mental activity that largely happens outside of an individual's awareness unless they actively adopt a stance of curiosity. In terms of dementia care, it is seen as a core skill needed to understand your own emotions, thoughts and behaviours as a carer as well as consider, be curious about and hold in mind such states in the patient. It is a reflective capacity to hold both minds at once (Main, 1991).

This is a basic assumption of dementia care: the patient always has a mind that is present, no matter how advanced the dementia may be, and that the person's mind is trying to communicate against all odds. The essential skill of a care team working therapeutically is the orientation towards this communication and a willingness to share each moment in a genuine interaction. This is a culture of curiosity; the staff team must be curious about what a patient may be communicating in their own language or why they have presented in a particular way as a result of what they may be thinking or feeling. This applies at all times, underpinning every moment, be that during administration of covert medication, facilitation of personal cares or singing and dancing.

In dementia, we anticipate that the ability, or willingness, to trust others to expertly 'receive' your attempts at communication can be disrupted beyond any other time of life. Holding in mind the relationship history of a person with dementia, both in the here and now and from their earliest time as a child, is essential. Individuals reaching hospital care likely have experiences of neglect or hostility from a caregiver, repeated through ongoing problems in adult relationships, and exacerbated by the experience of dementia, irrespective of the severity of dementia. mentalizing requires a careful understanding of the circumstances of actions, of prior 'patterns of behaviour' and experiences that an individual has been exposed to (Ryle and Kerr, 2002; Bateman and Fonagy, 2004). mentalization theory, dementia and the realities of clinical working meet together in this model.

The experience of having dementia, and being alongside dementia, can be akin to moving from a state of feeling integrated to feeling disintegrated in both the person with dementia and their carer. This is not to suggest a predictable and linear journey. Instead, the experience of dementia can seem intangible, changeable. Emotions can come and go and are felt with intensity, but don't always seem connected to thoughts, to each other or to the surroundings. Language to communicate and join up the emotions can be absent. The person can struggle to keep hold of a whole identity whilst navigating their moment by moment experiences. There is ever more an attempt to find a different experience; to seek meaning, to establish control over the moment, to find comfort or familiarity (Miesen, 2004; Evans, 2008). This means communicating the current experience with others, having them understood and responded to by an other. The challenges of residing in a dementia unit mean there can be an absence of familiar people and familiar environment and so a searching/seeking is apparent. Just as there is a basic assumption of dementia care that the patient always has a mind that is present that is trying to communicate against all odds, there is an allied assumption that, within a therapeutic environment, there is a fundamental relational connection between people, to find shared meaning and alleviate distress.

Aims of the MinD model

To make clear an expectation of emotional openness from staff working with individuals with dementia.

To train staff working in dementia care in the necessary therapeutic skills to achieve moment-by-moment competency.

To offer a framework to understand the impact of working with fragmented states of mind and to understand the importance of care for staff.
The model supports staff to manage the emotional demands of the work in
a sustainable way.

To influence the underpinning goals of admission and expected outcomes
for individuals with dementia in inpatient care settings.

Key concepts in the MinD model

All dementia patients have their own mind. The main issue in care is how
to communicate that mind to an other, such as a carer.

There is no patient with dementia in isolation. There is always a carer and
patient interaction, a patient and family interaction, a carer and multidisciplinary team interaction and a multidisciplinary team and hospital/wider
NHS interaction. The carer needs to be mindful of these levels of systems
in their care planning.

The therapeutic stance of the carer

Humility from a sense of not knowing is important. It is not always possible to know
exactly what meaning to make of a communication, either through language or
through behaviour. Sometimes all we can do is try to validate the patient's feelings
by bearing with or suggesting a feeling state. The attempt at sense-making, though
this might not be spoken, can hold the moment together at times of fragmentation.

Patients with dementia are never to blame for their behaviours. The carer must
be able to recognise when the carer is being pulled into a disintegrated non-thinking
space and use such awareness and team support to bring themselves back into an
integrated state. Disintegrated states in a care are seen as dangerous in that there
is a real risk of the carer turning their own feelings into an unhelpful or even risky
behaviour such as neglect or aggression.

The carer must constantly be asking themselves questions in the care moment:

How do I feel right now?
Why do I feel like this?
How do I understand this for the patient with dementia?
What might it feel like for them?
Am I blind to something here such as my anger?

Theoretical underpinning of the MinD model

Care in dementia depends on universal psychological needs as well as physical
and social needs. The attachment approach is based upon attachment theory as
developed by the psychoanalyst John Bowlby in the 1950s. Originally used to
describe the patterns of attachment of infants to their parents, especially mothers,

it is useful for thinking about dementia care, particularly the move from an integrated state to a disintegrated one. Elements of feeling fragmented and dependent on others may be likened to that of a child or infant. This is not akin to treating the person with dementia like a child. It addresses how human beings respond within relationships when hurt, separated from loved ones or when perceiving a threat. Essentially, attachment depends on the person's ability to develop basic trust in their caregivers and self. In infants, attachment as a motivational and behavioural system directs the child to seek proximity with a familiar caregiver when they are alarmed, with the expectation that they will receive protection and emotional support. The most important tenet of attachment theory is that in the presence of a sensitive and responsive caregiver, the infant will use the caregiver as a 'safe base' from which to explore.

The key ideas include

1   There is a fundamental human need for relational attachment to a significant carer, at least one significant other person, which is stable and becomes more meaningful over time despite an apparent lack of conscious memory for that person. We assume that emotional memory remains and can grow for individuals with dementia of any type and of any severity.

2   Containment of distress is provided; emotions are taken by the staff member and processed (mentalized), rather than being bounced back. Such emotions are instead taken to appropriate staff supervision later on, which requires an ability on the part of the carer to be able to bear such emotions.

3   A secure base as in a carer from which the patient can move away from and return safely. We use individual and environmental nursing observations to achieve this. We also emphasise the patients' bedrooms as being private spaces that feel secure.

4   An honest and open reflection of the self in terms of emotions that may arise when giving care. This may include personal experiences both professionally and personally. These emotions may be difficult to talk about but can include shame, disgust, anger, guilt, love, erotic feelings and anxiety, and may relate to issues around death.

5   The creation of communication, to have our attempts to communicate recognised and attended to by somebody who is motivated to understand the meaning behind them. It is this quality that is captured in the term 'mentalization'. Finding the same kind of vocabulary or using non-verbal techniques such as touch or play. This may be about validating an emotional state or providing information such as an answer to 'where am I?' in an honest manner.

6   The creation of meaning and hope, and the maintenance of the patient as a human-being through valuing all aspects of these interactions no matter how apparently meaningless they may at first appear to be.

7   To belong to a family or other care-giving social group and to have a recognised and respected identity within that group.

The tools of the MinD model

Cognitive analytic therapy (CAT) advances on attachment theory whilst incorporating the principles. Whereby attachment theory is primarily concerned with describing how things are, the emotional ties between individuals and their caregivers, CAT offers the tools to the carer for dealing with emotional experiences at the point of care.

The theory recognises that individuals can behave in anticipation of responses from others, forming an internal model of relating both to themselves and others. It is derived from the psychoanalytic tradition and object relations theories, concerned with how early relationships form an individual's self, hence what an individual then seeks and expects from their relationships with others in each interaction. It incorporates understanding from infant observation. It is able to offer an explanation of distress and, importantly, suggest therapeutic change. CAT allows for change to occur through therapeutic interactions. A mentalizing stance is essential in the carer if each interaction has the potential for being therapeutic.

The 4Ps is a tool that asks the staff team to work through a reflective cycle of mentalizing; it considers the mind of the other, their own mind and how these come together in a reciprocal interaction (Figure 14.1): that is, in each moment, what is being communicated between two people. The 4Ps model was developed as a tool for reflection, drawing on the CAT concept of reciprocal roles in relationships. The 4Ps tool for reflection has been taken from an existing training package adapted specifically to focus upon clinical issues relevant for those with dementia (Petty et al., 2014). It provides a framework for individual staff members and the staff team as a whole to understand how a continuous therapeutic relationship is achieved with individuals with dementia and anticipate the emotional demands of the work.

The experience of dementia is changeable, with somebody's experience of themselves and their environment seeming fragmented. Emotions can be extreme, without the person being able to keep a continuous thread of what they are feeling and why, without being able to influence the cause of the emotions, and without being able to share their experiences through words. This changeability is true for all those in this context, for individuals with dementia and those around them. Individuals seek to feel differently, often seeking another person to feel connected to and find meaning with. Effective care in this context is better evaluated moment by moment: moment by moment competency.

Therapy on the units is comprised of moments of therapeutic engagement, whereby the individual's internal world is understood, or attempted to be understood, and responded to in a way that is respectful and compassionate, and not collusive with harmful, feared responses. In this way, there is an understanding that underlies every therapeutic intervention based on psychodynamic theory: the seen behaviour and apparent anxiety alert us to hidden and unresolved emotions, and the communication of these emotions with us in the moment replicates well-worn relationship patterns.

The skill in connecting meaningfully with another, in each moment, is labour-intensive and exhausting. This therapeutic model is in contrast to other prevalent models of dementia care that distance the person with dementia and their experience.

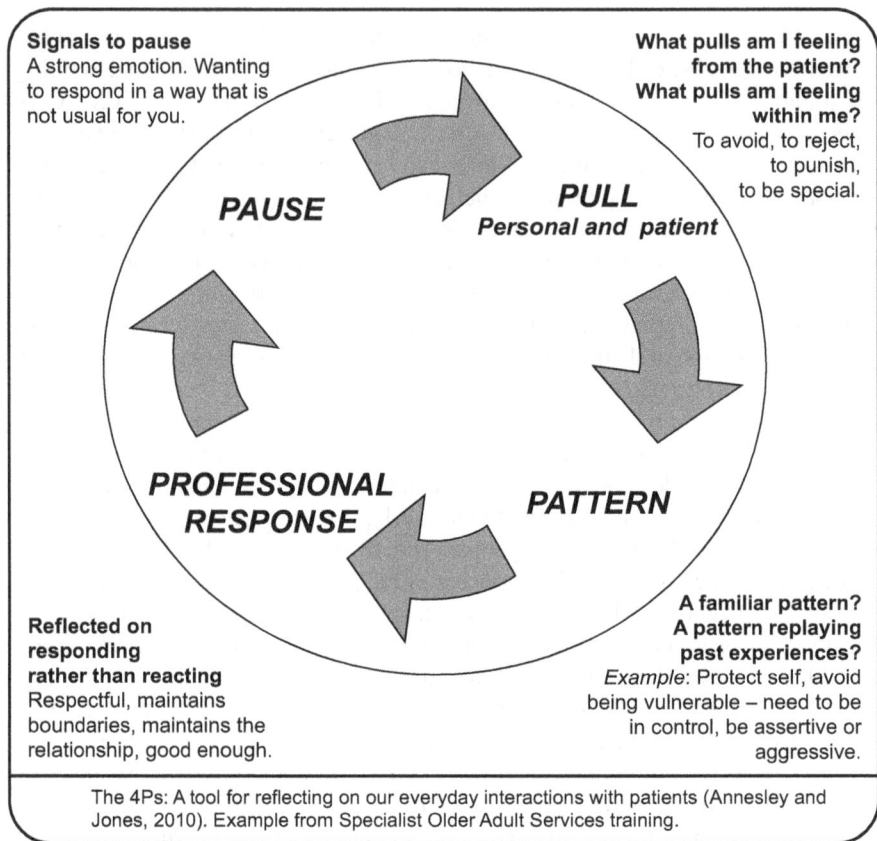

The 4Ps: A tool for reflecting on our everyday interactions with patients (Annesley and Jones, 2010). Example from Specialist Older Adult Services training.

Figure 14.1 The 4Ps

Emotional demand

As human beings, the staff team members need their own emotional support. Being with someone with dementia can be extremely emotionally demanding. The experience is one of various urges and responses, ranging from dreadful sadness through to anger. The multidisciplinary team need to be treated with the same degree of compassion as the person with dementia. This acknowledges that care is not limited to something that you do to somebody else, it is a shared, two-way experience.

For a staff team to manage this demand, there needs to be a significant investment in staff supervision. This must be taken seriously and done both at an individual level involving an understanding of the person with dementia in terms of psychological formulation and crucially at a whole team level. That bridges both worlds, both sides of the care dynamic. The staff can then understand and have a framework for understanding the person being helped, but can also understand what the experience is doing to them with their peers.

Team supervision needs to be treated with the same respect and privilege as any other psychotherapeutic intervention. It is confidential and staff are encouraged to speak openly about their experiences with the people they are caring for and with each other. This is not an indulgence but a serious attempt to engage with the whole experience of being with someone with dementia, both the caring and uncaring parts of that experience. It is acknowledged that, however difficult such feelings may be, they are a normal and an expected part of being with and being able to help the patient.

Summary

The overriding quality markers of the model can be summarised as follows:

- The main aim of a therapeutic placement for an individual with dementia is an increased understanding of emotions, thoughts and behaviours: the individual with dementia reaching a more validated and whole sense of themselves, resulting in better communicating with those around them; and carers (the professional staff team, family, the systemic care team beyond the hospital) reaching a better understanding of the emotion, thoughts and behaviours of the individual with dementia.

- Humility from a position of not knowing is important. It is not always possible to know exactly what meaning to make of a communication, either through language or through behaviour. A willingness to share each moment and commit to better understanding is required; to remain curious about the patient's internal world that may have prompted a particular presentation or communication. The creation of communication is to have our attempts to communicate recognised and attended to by somebody who is motivated to understand the meaning behind them. There is always some available 'vocabulary' or non-verbal technique such as touch or play.

- There is an expectation of emotional openness and curiosity from all involved.

- Containment of distress is provided; emotions are taken by the staff member and mentalized, rather than being bounced back. Such emotions are instead taken to appropriate staff supervision later on, which requires an ability on the part of the carer to be able to bear such emotions.

- Moment by moment competency: therapy is comprised of moments of therapeutic engagement, whereby the individual's internal world is understood and responded to appropriately. The skill in connecting meaningfully with an other, in each moment, is labour-intensive and exhausting. Care is not limited to something that you do to somebody else, it is a shared, two-way process. There is a focus on being consciously aware of the changing emotional experiences for yourself, in connection with others, and how this provides rich and valuable information about helpful ways to respond.

- Non-mentalizing: the labour-intensive nature of holding a curious and mentalizing stance is acknowledged. Times of losing hold of the curiosity (non-mentalizing) must and will exist. Supervision functions to openly discuss what makes mentalizing challenging and find ways to get back on track as soon as possible.

We would like to thank all clients and staff of Katherine Allen and George Jepson units at The Retreat.

References

Adshead, G. (1998). Psychiatric Staff as Attachment Figures. Understanding Management Problems in Psychiatric Services in the Light of Attachment Theory. *The British Journal of Psychiatry*, 172, 64–69.

Annesley, P., and Jones, L. (2010). *Developing Relational Skills in Working with People with Complex Presentations: An Evaluation of a One Day Workshop for Multidisciplinary Staff*. Poster presentation.

Bateman, A.W., and Fonagy, P. (2004). *Psychotherapy of Borderline Personality Disorder: mentalization Based Treatment*. Oxford: Oxford University Press.

Bateman, A.W., and Fonagy, P. (2010). Mentalization based treatment for borderline personality disorder. *World Psychiatry*, 9(1), 11–15.

Blagg, R. and Petty, S. (2014). Sustainable Staff Well-being within older Adult Mental Health Services, 20(2), pp. 92–104.

Bowlby, J. (1979). The Making and Breaking of Affectional Bonds. London: Tavistock Publication.

Carstensen, L.L. (2006). The influence of a sense of time on human development, Science, 312, 1913–1915.

Department of Health. (2012). *Transforming Care: A National Response to Winterbourne View Hospital*. Department of Health Review: Final Report.

De Masi, F. (2004). Making Death Thinkable: A Psychoanalytic Contribution to the Problem of the Transience of Life. University of Michigan, Free Association.

Dickens, C. (2007). Night walks. In *The Uncommercial Traveller*. Gloucester: Dodo Press, 91.

Evans, S. (2008). 'Beyond forgetfulness': How psychoanalytic ideas can help us to understand the experience of patients with dementia. *Psychoanalytic Psychotherapy*, 22(3), 155–176.

Fonagy, P., and Adshead, G. (2012). How mentalization changes the mind. *Advances in Psychiatric Treatment*, 18, 353–362.

Francis, R. (2013). *Report of the Mid Staffordshire NHS Foundation Trust Public Inquiry*. London: The Stationery Office.

Jones, G.M., and Miesen, B.M. (eds.). (2004). Towards a psychology of dementia care: Awareness and intangible loss. In B.M. Miesen (ed.) *Care-giving in Dementia: Research and Applications*, Vol. 3. Hove: Brunner-Routledge Psychology Press, 184.

Kitwood, T.M. (1997). Dementia reconsidered: the person comes first reference. Buckingham: Open University Press.

Kunzman, U., Barlow, M., Wrosch, C. & Gouin, J. P. (2014). 'Is Anger, but not Sadness, associated with chronic inflammation in older adulthood?', Psychology and Aging, 34(3), pp. 330–340.

Leiman, M. and Sutton, L. (2004). The development of the dialogic self in CAT: A fresh perspective on ageing. In:J. Hepple and L. Sutton (eds.) *Cognitive Analytic Therapy in Later Life: a new perspective on old age*. Hove: Brunner-Routledge, 6–44.

Main, M. (1991). Metacognitive knowledge, metacognitive monitoring, and singular (coherent) vs. multiple (incoherent) models of attachment: Findings and directions for future research. In P. Harris, J. Stevenson-Hinde, and C. Parkes (eds.) *Attachment Across the Lifecycle*. New York: Routledge-Kegan Paul, 127–159.

Mather, M., Canli, T., English, T., Whitfield, S., Wais, P., Ochsner, K., Gabrieli, J. D. E., & Carstensen, L. L. (2004). Amygdala responses to emotionally valenced stimuli in older and younger adults. *Psychological Science*, 15, 259–263.

Mather, M. (2012). The Emotional Paradox in the Aging Brain. Annals of the New York Academy of Sciences, 1251(1), pp. 33–49.

Miesen, B.M. (2004). Towards a psychology of dementia care: Awareness and intangible loss. In G.M. Jones and B.M. Miesen (eds.) *Care-giving in Dementia: Research and Applications*, Vol. 3. Hove: Brunner-Routledge Psychology Press, 184.

Obholzer, A., and Roberts, V.Z. (1994). Till death us do part: Caring and uncaring in work with the elderly. In *The Unconscious at Work: Individual and Organizational Stress in the Human Services*. London: Routledge.

Petty, S., Jones, L., and Annesley, P. (2014). *Communication Where All Else Fails: CAT Enables Relationship-centred Care*. Institute of Mental Health Annual Research Day. Poster Presentation.

Reed, A. E., & Carstensen, L. L. (2012). The Theory behind the Age-Related Positivity Effect. *Frontiers in Psychology*, 3, 339.

Ryle, A., and Kerr, I.B. (2002). *Introducing Cognitive Analytic Therapy: Principles and Practice*. Chichester: John Wiley & Sons.

Sheard, D. (2008). Less doing – More being person-centred. *Journal of Dementia Care*.

Sheard, D. (2009). *Nurturing: Emotions at Work in Staff*. London: Alzheimer's Society.

Sheard, D. (2010). The task is the mask: solving the riddle of being person-centred. *Dementiacarematters*, [online] 15(1), pp. 3–6. Available at: http://www.dementiacarematters.com/pdf/signpost.june2010.pdf [Accessed 8 Aug. 2017].

Vygotsky, L. S. (1986). Thought and language. Cambridge, MA: MIT Press.

Winnicott, D.W. (1949). Hate in the counter-transference. *The International Journal of Psychoanalysis*, 30, 69–74.

Winnicott, D.W. (1956 [1975]). Primary material pre-occupation. In *Through Paediatrics to Psychoanalysis*. New York: Basic Books, 300–305.

Chapter 15

A psychoanalytic and philosophical exploration of boredom and disengagement in dementia

Sandra Evans

> Nothing happens. Nobody comes, nobody goes. It's awful.
>
> (Becket, 1949)

Introduction

The experience of boredom is universal and yet hard to define. It means different things to different people but may also denote different kinds of experiences to individuals. The author's interest here is in the realm of the dementias, not simply because it is commonly complained about by carers: from the apathetic and listless boredom to the restless, agitated states when nothing is desired (perhaps the sufferer desires nothingness). By exploring what is written about it in philosophy and in literature, including the psychoanalytic, it may be possible to understand a little more about boredom. It is hard even to be confident in the assertions about boredom in healthy adults who can tell us about their experience. It is so much harder for those with dementia to explain what they are feeling; yet their experience often impacts negatively on those trying to care for them. Listlessness and apathetic boredom is perhaps easier to tolerate than restlessness and relentless importuning. Carer distress is more commonly provoked by the latter behaviour.

Restlessness and agitation therefore that is difficult to contain – and to bear – is an important factor in the decisions made to use institutional care settings (Brodaty et al., 1993). Since carers have become some of the most important, if invisible, workforce in the UK, we should consider measures to alleviate their distress. Importantly also for dementia sufferers an attempt to elucidate boredom in dementia may help them too.

Since the National Dementia Strategy UK (2009) there has been considerable success in achieving one of the desired targets: to increase the number of people with dementia who receive a diagnosis. Less well-publicised issues are about resources (Evans, 2015). Diagnostic memory clinics in the UK are currently funded by Clinical Commissioning Groups (CCGs), which also fund psychological and non-pharmacological interventions for people with early dementia. Additional services for people with BPSD, the behavioural and psychological symptoms associated with dementia are funded from extra mental health money or resourced from within existing services. There is little NHS funding for services for the majority of people with dementia who are becoming increasingly cognitively impaired, but whose illness is relatively "uncomplicated". Listlessness and quiet boredom are likely to be classified as uncomplicated. The more quiet and undemanding a person is, the easier it is to manage their daily needs – from a care-delivery perspective. Currently supports for this group come from the Social Care budget. Charities such as the Alzheimer's Society do provide such support and there are some Clinical Commissioning Groups which pay directly for similar input; however care tends to be limited and postcode driven.

Importuning and demanding restlessness, particularly that which escalates risk taking or demands on the carer, tends to be classified as BPSD – the behavioural and psychiatric symptoms of dementia. Essentially, task-based care provided by social services rarely includes time for social interaction (Age Concern, 2007). We know that social interaction (Foulkes, 1964) is an essential part of human existence and that continued social engagement reduces the malignant effects of dementia (Livingston et al., 2017). In the absence of a cure for dementia, the least we can do is to attempt amelioration of the condition, and yet it is this kind of fundamental social support which is often lacking or forgotten altogether (Evans, 2015).

The fact that it is still a problem and a growing one suggests we might examine social interaction and "being with" people with dementia at a closer level. I am not talking about ageing generally but more specifically about serious illness and frailty in later life and extreme frailty when true independence is no longer possible.

Social interactions in very late life and extreme frailty

The demise of the day hospital, day centres for the elderly, and even public libraries make it harder for older people to meet each other. Old people who are frail, even without dementia, often complain of loneliness and isolation. Once our basic needs are met; when we are fed, clothed and not in pain, we seek affection, play and sex (Panksepp, 2010). When people with dementia complain of boredom, is it the loneliness and isolation to which they are referring or something else less tangible? It is plausible that in dementia there is a return to a previously experienced existential state, which shares features with the early use of an object (Winnicott, 1969).

In his paper, "The Use of An Object and Relating Through Identifications", Winnicott writes about:

> the move away from self-containment and relating to subjective objects into the realm of object-usage.
>
> (Winnicott, 1969, p. 88)

This time, the use of an object in the context of a dementia is not for psychic growth but for psychic equilibrium.

Motivated and healthy older adults usually find their own activities and peer group. Bored and lonely adults may join meet up groups, clubs and dating websites (Wada et al., 2017). By contrast, those who are physically dependent or lacking the drive to engage due to dementia can be enormously frustrated and may escalate demands on carers by unconventional means. The so-call behavioural and psychiatric symptoms of dementia (BPSD) can include non-verbal communications and projective identifications, which have a powerful effect on carers. These can add to stress if not understood and supported adequately (Evans, 2009; Waddell, 2009, Balfour, see chapter 10).

One of the main concerns of carers is boredom. People with dementia often express ennui which can be hard to manage. Their carers also may be reluctant to admit that they too are bored by endless caring. Further examination of the concept of boredom may help us think more clearly about this phenomenon. It is likely that it is fundamentally linked to the experience of time and problems of meaning (Goldstein, 2005), both of which become distorted in dementia.

How to understand boredom in dementia

Life itself, in a debilitated state or the devastating effect of the dementia may be boring. Johnson famously suggested that to tire of London was to "tire of life"; as though if one felt insufficient interest in the UK capital city, then nothing could sustain it. Boredom in dementia isn't merely this insufficient interest in life; although it might fit well with existential philosophy and the notion of fatigue (Levinas, 1947). Levinas wrote of fatigue as "the pain of effort (that) is wholly made of this being condemned to the present". Psychoanalytic psychotherapists Lynne Ellis and O'Connor (2010) link this concept to the "restlessness of the present" when people are trapped by a mood disorder such as depression, or possibly by dementia. As clinicians we see many people suffering existential crises as a result of unceasing losses but not complaining of boredom; however boredom might be a contributing factor to an existential crisis.

If previously enjoyed talents and pleasures can no longer be appreciated and there are no substitutes, life might indeed seem dull. Feeling that there is nothing new and everything is the same is boring. Being in a sterile environment which holds no beauty or visual aesthetic (Angel Byers, 2011) is boring and dulling. For this reason, filling a home or a new room in a care home with objects of interest and meaning to the person with dementia is important (Evans, 2004a), but this many not be sufficient explanation.

Boredom through restrictions
of remaining talent

In an early dementia, a person with a poor short-term memory may face potential risks to health and safety while retaining other skills. For example, no longer being able competently to take a bus to meet friends in a music group, while still being able to play one's music beautifully. This mismatch of what a person can still do and what they can no longer manage may lead to considerable frustration; particularly if they cannot see the risk of doing the former, for example taking the bus to the music group and getting hopelessly lost in the process.

A person with dementia may be bored by these constraints and feel underutilised, particularly if there is no-one to accompany them safely to their activity, or no money for taxis. Douglas Adam's (1979) creation of "Marvin the Paranoid Android" whose planet-sized brain could never be fully appreciated gives us a humorous appreciation of this phenomenon of people with dementia frustrated by not being allowed to fulfil their remaining potential.

Boredom as a function of nothing to do

The Alzheimer's Society reminds us that:

> A person with dementia may get bored if they are no longer able to do the things that used to interest them (AS, 2010). However, there will still be lots that the person can enjoy doing that will keep them occupied and stimulated.

Of course this is essential. Much prosaic activity such as setting tables or drying dishes can maintain a routine and a sense of self and most importantly add meaning to life by continued contribution to others. The philosophy of re-ablement-in-care may seem a bit overly optimistic when referring to people with advanced dementia, but it is apposite when it comes to maintaining independence on discharging people from acute hospitals after an inpatient stay. For example, when a person is no longer able to cook for themselves either safely or competently without supervision, bringing in "meals on wheels" or equivalent should still only be a last resort. More resource intensive and therefore potentially expensive strategies, like having a companion with whom to shop, cook AND eat is likely to be superior for the person who can make use of the social interaction. "Meals on Wheels" is an answer to the basic need of supplying food (although there is no guarantee that the person will actually eat). Engaging a person with a task is nurturing, containing and supplies an auxiliary ego to the disintegrating one (containing in the Bionic sense that it is responding to a need to participate; Bion, 1962).

There should not be any illusion that this is an easy task. Being the containing container for an adult with dementia involves the full engagement of the mind and attention of the carer. Co-creating a meal with a frail person with dementia may not be very stimulating for the "carer", and it is they who may find themselves bored and disconnected. We are asking carers to be a "transformational Object" (Bollas, 1987), one that provides an experience which changes/balances the person and who may be changed in turn. Paid carers for local authorities and private services are being asked to do similar important work which requires considerable amounts of mature self-regulation for less than the minimum wage (Mary Beard, 2014). It is tragic that such important work is valued so little by our society.

Perhaps there is something dark in the "Collective Unconscious" which allows this contradiction to continue whilst expressing dismay at every care home scandal that appears in the media.

Boredom as disengagement

There are many other ways to maintain emotional contact with those suffering from dementia through touch (hand massages), shared listening to music and looking through photographs to share memories. There are also occasions when these are not enough. They may seem even to frustrate, overwhelm or upset the person with dementia. Mental states are also observed which suggest a degree of "tuning out" despite attempts to keep the person involved. Irritability may emerge, eschewing all attempts to distract or pacify. Restlessness, agitation and lassitude also might convey a sense of discomfort in the person with dementia. It is distressing to witness and we need to understand it in order be of assistance. We also need to understand it for our own sakes.

Boredom as a metaphysical state

Heidegger, controversial because of his sympathy with the Nazis, offered different ways of interpreting the term "boredom". He described fundamental "profound boredom" as the ultimate precondition for the experience of time stretching as a long shadow, "*Lange-weile*" (Heidegger, 1929). It is from this state that we can be "awakened". The author understands this as a way of experiencing time, which in *Lange-weile* stretches out inexorably as a feeling of extents, as opposed to the intensity of engaged living.

Heidegger theorised that boredom creates a specific readiness for certain experiences, and a kind of attentiveness or wakefulness in experience. This approach is based in part on the observation that although we are always in some existential orientation or other, we are for the most part not attentively in it.

Dasein – is being-there: existing in any of a variety of non-attentive, absent-minded, unfocussed modes of being. This is the background of consciousness, the default position of being present but unconsciously so, unaware without any poignant self-consciousness. Punctuated every so often by spells of lucid attentiveness, of wake- and mindfulness, which then truly deserve to be called "Being there".

Heidegger suggests this is the reason we do not have a clear idea of what boredom and other existential orientations really are. Despite these states structuring experience in pervasive ways, in order to gain an understanding of boredom, we need to wake up to it, attend to it and live it in some lucid sort of way. The author imagines this to be similar to Samuel Beckett's tragi-comedy drama – *Waiting for Godot*. The eponymous Godot does not arrive but without him nothing can be started. Godot is the object which needs to be used (Winnicott) in order to find a desire or motivation.

There is an active tendency to turn away from the experience of boredom. In boredom, just as in anxiety, the default tendency is not to be inattentively bored but actively to seek distractions in order not to be bored. For this reason, a person on the verge of becoming bored constantly engages in activities that serve the sole purpose of "passing time". Most of the time, it seems to most people that they are in fact not bored. Instead, in order to appreciate real boredom one has to inhibit the activities and distractions that routinely fill most of one's regular life. Once these are removed, boredom is revealed to be there already, lurking beneath the surface of distracting activities. This is harder than it might seem (and may be quite unpleasant – particularly if boredom holds another anxiety such as fear of abandonment or fear of death).

> Only then, in the resulting state of withholding all distractions and lofty engagements, we have a chance of getting hold of our boredom, probably in a state of ever-increasing unrest, in a conspicuous and oppressive felt emptiness that threatens to drive us insane.
>
> (Heidegger, 1927) (from Slaby, 2010)

This appears to be a good description of the observed states of unrest in a person with dementia. The author conjectures that dementia returns the sufferer to an earlier existential state due to the absence of the "shallow distractions" that would normally keep it at bay. Many of us are aware of feeling that we have "no time to be bored". We have much to do and many ideas –however – there are moments when we may perceive a lurching unrest: a disquiet that suggests a lack or emptiness. It puts me in mind of the childhood ennui on a rainy afternoon when only the engagement of an adult in play mode would do. We might ask ourselves what it is that this adult provides? Is it containment of and from an existential anxiety or is it perhaps desire itself as Adam Phillips suggests (Phillips, 1993)?

Boredom as absence of desire

Adam Phillips, a child psychotherapist has written on the phenomenon of boredom. In it he describes the ennui of childhood summed up in the existential question "what shall we do now?" This is the mood of diffuse restlessness which contains the wish for a desire. He suggests that in the boredom is an unconscious waiting for an experience of anticipation. There is a free-floating attention, an unawareness of the waiting. This resonates with Heidegger's Dasein, the half-experienced boredom of readiness for an experience. Grosz (2014) describes a clinical case of a boy whose every waking moment is filled with purposeful self-improvement activity. Needless to say, he is miserable and unable to make friends. He has "conversation", but no real connection with others and what he says is profoundly boring.

Phillips suggests that in the emotional development of a child there is a need for the adult to "hold" the experience of being bored, not to sabotage it by distraction.

In the facilitation of the child being able to experience their own boredom comes the capacity to be alone in mother's presence (Winnicott, 1958). The acquisition of the ability to regulate emotional states is a fundamental task of early life. As Winnicott explained, it is best developed within a secure attachment to an attuned caregiver in an enriching environment. Development may be frustrated in its progress to an appropriate modulatory level by many interpersonal or environmental factors. The regulatory capacity may also be challenged in later life by personal disaster or other overwhelming experience such as the catastrophic changes that occur in dementia (Raju et al., 2012)

Evans (2004b, 2008) describes a loss of the capacity to be alone, even in cases where previously it existed. It is argued that it is the process of some dementias, more likely those of a vascular nature which may destroy critical parts of the pre-frontal cortex: those associated usually with mirror neurones and the ability to internalise/introject the parental imago. This means that the individual can no longer hold on in memory, unconsciously, the image of parent/other being there providing an ongoing sense of security (Schore, 2001; Winnicott, 1958). It is this which may also contribute to the general feeling of anxiety which often predates the more obvious confusion associated with the multiple-infarct dementias (Evans, 2009).

Boredom as projective identification

Harwood (personal communication 2003; Evans, 2008), while spending time in a nursing home as part of an observation (Mackenzie-Smith, 2009 of people with advanced dementia, noted a feeling of lassitude and boredom which came over him during a time sitting among the patients in the lounge after lunch. Since he was observing, he was not interacting and was picking up an atmosphere in the room. Being self-reflective, he argued that he was not physically well at the time, but, leaving that aside, he may also have been acting as a conductor in a small group: picking up, identifying and articulating a sense of what was already there (Foulkes and Anthony). Foulkes described the role of a group analyst in a small group situation. His description of reverie is suggestive of a free-floating attention that allows the perception and appreciation of the mood state of a group. This reverie is appreciated by those who engage in participant observation. Harwood caught and conveyed that sense of listless ennui that anyone who has ever entered a residential care home will recognise. This intense form of projective identification perceived by a receptive person is a communication of a mental state probably impossible to articulate. For those residents, few had any words left to describe how they were feeling, but they were still able to communicate an affect in a powerful and visceral manner.

In healthy people also, not suffering from dementia, projective identification communicates unconscious mental states; they may say one thing and communicate quite another non-verbally. Unconscious mental states are unconscious because they have been actively repressed in the service of protecting the ego.

These residents by contrast struggle with egos that are fragmented and reduced. Much communication in residential and nursing home is unconscious and is delivered in what can be projected into a receptive audience. Harwood also noticed people "waking up" almost literally as a member of staff came into the room. The staff member was identified as a person bringing something pleasurable – which could have been interaction: a container for fragmented egos, an end to the waiting . . . a spark of anticipation that something might occur (interestingly the residents are rarely interested in each other). We see this in a video available on YouTube with a music therapist entering the room occupied by people with dementia, how they all "wake up". Their heads and shoulders raised up and they look eager and full of anticipation.

When a nurse enters the room, some people lift their heads in expectation of something. A treat perhaps, such as tea and cake? Desire? Perhaps it is a whole, functioning ego that can integrate theirs and give them the life-blood of psychic energy to feel whole again, however transiently? This is, I think, the transformational Object of which Bollas (1987) writes: one that changes or adds to us.

Foulke's idea of a gestalt is interesting here. A group is more than a sum of its parts. Small groups of people with dementia have more potential for bringing together a sense of one whole-functioning ego, particularly with a therapist present. This is demonstrated exquisitely by Marion Violets (2004), where she described her dance/movement working with whole groups of people with severe dementia. Here in Violet's group, people who rarely interacted with each other came together in a different way. They began to identify themselves again as people with a past and a present. They related to other patients and argued and even flirted. With the assistance of an auxiliary mind as in Marion's mind during the group, they were able to hold on to parts of their selves-in-relation-to-others; something that seems harder to manage when left to their own devices.

Being the receptacle of these projective identifications can be uncomfortable, particularly so for a partner or family carer of a person with dementia who is restless and dysphoric. In nursing homes in previous years these might have been the patients for whom staff asked the doctors to prescribe medication: to provide a relief for the observers as much as for the patients themselves. The carer may be followed constantly or feel put upon. It feels hard to leave dependent people alone – and maybe we shouldn't.

Boredom as denial of death

The late Danielle Quinodoz (2010) examined the phenomenon of boredom in old age in which she commented on old people who complain that life has become boring with the same old routine. She suggested that they have locked themselves into this monotonous repetition as a defence against the anxiety of the "long shadow" of death. If they see time yawning endlessly before them in the tedium of repeated dull activities, they can deny the existence of an end. The alternative is to see their lives as a completed whole viewing it, as she suggests, as if from a hilltop. As the end comes into view, new moments are greeted with interest and savoured, because they are transient. People with Alzheimer's Disease get locked into repetitive behaviour too, often caused by bilateral damage to a small area of the brain called the hippocampus. Their repetition-compulsion may be triggered less by denial than by brain damage, but the repeated questions and preoccupations with time and its passing may reveal an awareness of time running out, or even, ironically, an unending tedium of reliving day after day in similar fashion. This "ground hog day" routine may well be appreciated by the sufferer; compelled to repeat it but bored by it nonetheless.

Denial of death manifest as boredom can also be a disguised form of depression. Quinodoz asserts that some boredom may also be a manifestation of unacknowledged depression. Boredom becomes an expression of mood. In Woodward's (1991) reading of Freud, she indulges her interest in the man himself when he wrote to his friend Andreas-Salome of his aging self (Freud, 1925). Freud described feeling less sensitive to the world around him. His ennui was a detachment that Freud himself attributed to old age and a natural process that he called returning to the inorganic, the dead matter. Freud understood this is terms of a brilliant paper he had published just a few years earlier which contained an idea of a death instinct: a natural tendency of the organism to resist and protect itself from stimuli and to return to an inorganic state. In "Beyond the Pleasure Principle" (Freud, 1920) here is a balance, he stated, between Eros – love and the cathexis to others – and Thanatos – death, the detachment proper to old age which occurs when life loses its gloss. He felt that his own interest was the same, but clearly it was not. Freud may have been depressed. He describes withdrawal from others and a sense of narcissism in the ascendency. Woodward (1991) thought he was depressed as do I (Evans, 1998), but he was also ill with a very painful and invasive cancer. Illness too also demands that people withdraw – conserving their energies.

Is social disengagement and boredom inevitable in dementia?

Dementia, as people are increasingly aware, is an illness which, through attacks on the brain, the seat of our intelligent being, robs people of their ability to manage simple daily tasks of personal care. It steals whole chunks of memories even of a life well-lived, and can turn loved ones into strangers and one's home into a prison. It appears that as the external world becomes increasingly alien to the sufferer, then a retreat to an internal world may be preferable or more accessible. As Bere Miessen (1993) divined from his attachment theory–based work, people with more advanced dementia may begin to hallucinate their objects, taking refuge in a long-dead mother. They may interact less with the real people in their lives as a consequence. This may feel hurtful to families, and be experienced as a disengagement from life itself.

Social disengagement theory, (Cumming and Henry, 1961) is a now discredited idea that suggested that normal ageing resulted in a gradual withdrawal from life, activities and relationships. This disengagement was thought to begin as a kind of natural process in anticipation of death. It has a certain resonance with Freud's hesitant forays into the "death instinct". Indeed there is a certain economy in this theory in which the living organism will move towards a quieter, more low energy state. Elsewhere I have linked this disengagement with depression, which is commonly seen in older persons but may be misinterpreted as a sign of dementia (Evans, 1998).

Social disengagement theory clearly holds little validity generally and the wisdom of geriatric medicine helps us to appreciate that reducing sensory impairments, relieving pain, improving physical fitness and wellbeing can prevent older people from being excluded from a full and active participation in their community if wanted.

Disengagement from the community may however be a sign of illness

Knight (1986) cites a clinical study in which "Susan is worried that her mother is depressed because she has stopped going to bridge which she used to enjoy". On closer inspection, it seems that her mother is aware of memory problems that cause her to become confused while playing. She is aware that she finds it difficult and that her bridge partners have found it frustrating and so she stops attending. She seems less bothered by this fact than her daughter is and certainly is not depressed. She still enjoys being at home watching her TV. She is suffering from dementia and cannot manage the demands of bridge. The people most upset by this loss are the people who perceive the risk that she will become bored by this lack of activity; it is also true that this indicates a new reality for Susan. Her mother is no longer pursuing an active outgoing life and may make new demands on her daughter. The nature of their relationship may be altered forever and Susan has to adjust to a new reality. Time spent with her mother may be less stimulating and may be "boring" but may also be painful. Psychic mechanisms come into play at these difficult times, including denial.

Is there a link between detachment in dementia and boredom?

When Winnicott (1958) suggested that we learn as children to be alone in the presence of mother, he described the introjection of the object, there for use as required. I have often wondered, and at times written in previously published work, about this capacity appearing to be lost in some people with dementia (Evans, 2009) due literally to the loss of connections which somehow "hold the introjected object". Could the restless, distressing form of boredom that is so affecting to others be related to that need to use an object that is no longer reachable in the usual ways because of disrupted connections of the damaged brain.

Is the lassitude seen in the nursing home, the expectant waiting room drama, the default position of human existence? Could the residents be waiting to be woken by a spark of desire but not intrinsically distressed? Can we think about these two manifestations of a mood or metaphysical state in dementia to think about how we organise care and allocate resources in a more humane and creative way?

What I am suggesting is that "care" must be more than maintaining bodily functions. In order to survive, people need attachments, connections and meaning. Food and hygiene are important but carers should provide interactions as well. We know that time for the "human touch" is not always factored into task-based care.

Summary and concluding questions

Boredom can be related to the under-utilisation of ability, most commonly perhaps in early dementia. It could be related to a denial of aging and death leading to an inability to live comfortably in the moment and a fear of looking too far ahead because of fear of what the future might bring and therefore being stuck in a place where nothing happens.

Boredom could be seen as the default position of human existence: a Beckettian waiting room feeling, mixed with fear, expectation and boredom. One cannot get on with anything "meaningful" while "attending" to this other expedience, whether it be the effects of illness for the sufferer or for the carer who devotes their attention and energies (libidinal investments) in the support of the other. "Nothing to be done".

I do however think that boredom is most difficult to bear if it denotes the withdrawal from active life and engagement with the world. As dementia progresses, distress often seems to diminish with weakening of the ego (Evans, 2008) leading to a decathexis from mindfulness. Is this death instinct territory as in Freud's (1920) forays into existentialism (an armour of insensitivity is growing around me), detachment proper to old age and Andre Green (1997), the work of the negative, in that withdrawal leads to an absence of cathexis? As in Harwood's observation of feeling bored in a nursing home, the people in the sitting room of the residential nursing home are slumped in a state of torpor, and his counter-transference sense is one of boredom and lassitude. Harwood was picking up sensitively on a projective identification. It seems that the residents were communicating strongly to him a stupefying mental state, broken only when a designated carer arrived.

Finally, if boredom is secondary to an absence of stimulation – a state of loss of desire in which there is a disinvestment in the future – is that a problem for the person with dementia or only for those of us observing it?

References

Adams, D. (1979). *The Hitch-Hiker's Guide to the Galaxy*. Pellican.

Age Concern England (2007). Ahe of Equality?- outlawing age discrimination beyond the workplace, London: Age Concern England.

Alzheimer's Society. (2010). *Factsheet 505*. Alzheimers.org.uk

Banerjee, S. (2009). *National Dementia Strategy UK*. DH, England.

Beard, M. (2014). *The Paradox of Growing Old: A Point of View*. BBC Radio 4 Podcast.

Beckett, S. (1953). Waiting for Godot: A Tragicomedy in Two Acts. London: Faber & Faber.

Bion, W.R. (1962). *Learning from Experience*. London: Heinemann.

Bollas, C. (1987). The transformational object. In *The Shadow of the Object: Psychoanalysis of the Unthought Known*. Free Association Books.

Brodaty, H., McGilchrist, C., Harris, L., and Peters, K.E. (1993). Time until institutionalization and death in patients with dementia: Role of care- giver training and risk factors. *Archives of Neurology*, 50, 643–650.

Byers, A. (2011). Visual aesthetics in dementia. *International Journal of Art Therapy*, 16(2).

Cumming, E., and Henry, W. (1961). *Social Disengagement Theory: In Growing Old*. New York: Basic Books.

Evans, S. (1998). Beyond the mirror: A group analytic exploration of late life depression. *Aging and Mental Health*, 2, 94–99.

Evans, S. (2004a). The old self: Kohut, Winnicott and others. In S. Evans and J. Garner (eds.) *Talking Over the Years: A Handbook of Dynamic Psychotherapy in Older Adults*. London: Routledge.

Evans, S. (2004b). Attachment in old age: Bowlby and others. In S. Evans and J. Garner (eds.) *Talking Over the Years: A Handbook of Dynamic Psychotherapy in Older Adults*. London: Routledge.

Evans, S. (2008). Beyond forgetfulness' how psychoanalytic ideas can help us to understand the experience of patients with dementia. *Psychoanalytic Psychotherapy*, 22(3), 155–176.

Evans, S. (2009). Where is the unconscious in dementia? In R. Doctor and R. Lucas (eds.) *The Organic and the Inner World*. London: Karnac.

Evans, S. (2015). What the national dementia strategy forgot: Providing dementia care from a psychodynamic perspective. *Psychoanalytic Psychotherapy*, 28(3), 321–329.

Foulkes, SH. (1964). *Therapeutic Group Analysis*. London, Allen & Unwin.

Foulkes & Anthony (1965). *Group Psychotherapy: A Psychoanalytic Approach*. London: Karnac.

Freud, S. (1920). Beyond the pleasure principle. In *SE, 18*, 7–64.

Freud, S. (1925). Letter to Andreas-Salome. In *Letters of Sigmund Freud 1873–1939*, 360–361.

Goldstein, E.S. (2005). *Experience Without Qualities: Boredom and Modernity*. Stanford: Stanford University Press.

Green, A. (1997). The intuition of the negative in 'Playing and reality'. *International Journal of Psychoanalysis*, 78, 1071–1084.

Grosz, S. (2014). *The Examined Life: How We Lose and Find Ourselves*. London: Random House.

Harwood, I. (2003). Personal communication in an unpublished work while on observation in a continuing care ward as a medical student.

Heidegger, M. (1927). *Being and Time and Daesin*.

Heidegger, M. (1929). *Grundbegriffe der Metaphysik. Welt – Endlichkeit – Einsamkeit*. Frankfurt: Klostermann, 2004 [1929/30]; translated by William McNeil and Nicholas

Walker: Basic Concepts of Metaphysics. World – Finitude – Solitude, Bloomington, IN: Indiana University Press, 1995.

Knight, B. (1986). *Assessment of Psychological Disorders: Psychotherapy With Older Adults*. New York: Sage Publications, 73–93.

Levinas, E. (1947 [1986]). *De l'existence à l'existant*, 2nd ed. Paris, France: Librairie Philosophique J. Vrin.

Livingston, G., et al. (2017). Dementia prevention, intervention, and care. *Lancet*, 390 (10113), 2673–2734. http://dx.doi.org/10.1016/S0140-6736(17)31363-6

Lynne Ellis, M., and O'Connor, M. (2010). *Questioning Identity: Philosophy in Psychoanalytic Practice*. London: Karnac Books.

Mackenzie-Smith, S. (2005). Observational study of the elderly: An applied study utilizing Esther Bick's infant observation technique. *International Journal of Infant Observation and Its Applications*, 12(2009), 107–115.

Meissen, B. (1993). Alzheimer's disease, the phenomenon of parent fixation and Bowlby's attachment theory. *International Journal of Geriatric Psychiatry*, 8, 147–153.

Panksepp, J. (2010). Affective neuroscience of the emotional mind-brain: Evolutionary perspectives and implications for understanding depression. *Dialogues in Clinical Neuroscience*, 12(4), 533–545.

Phillips, A. (1993). On being bored. In *On Kissing, Tickling and Being Bored*. London: Faber & Faber.

Quinodoz, D. (2010). *Growing Old: A Journey of Self-discovery*. Hove, Sussex: Routledge.

Raju, R., Corrigan, F.M., Davidson, A.J.W., and Johnson, D. (2012). Assessing and managing mild to moderate emotion dysregulation. *Advances in Psychiatric Treatment*, 18, 82–93.

Schore, A.N. (2001). The effects of a secure attachment relationships on right brain development, affect regulation and infant mental health. *Infant Mental Health Journal*, 22, 7–66.

Slaby, J. (2010). The other side of existence: Heidegger on boredom. In Sabine Flach, Daniel Margulies, and Jan Söffner (eds.) *Habitus in Habitat II – Other Sides of Cognition*. Berlin: Freie Universität.

Violets-Gibson, M. (2004). Dance and movement therapy for people with severe dementia. In Sandra Evans and Jane Garner (eds.) *Talking Over the Years: A Handbook of Dynamic Psychotherapy With Older Adults*. Hove: Brunner-Routledge.

Wada, M., Mortenson, W.B., and Clarke, L.H. (2017, December). 'I am busy independent woman who has sense of humor, caring about others': Older adults' self-representations in online dating profiles. *Ageing and Society*. doi:10.1017/S0144686X17001325.

Waddell, M. (2009). Discussion of Sandra Evans's chapter; Where is the unconscious in dementia? In Ronald Doctor and Richard Lucas (eds.) *The Organic and the Inner World*. London: Karnac.

Winnicott, D.W. (1958). *The Capacity to Be Alone*. London: Tavistock.

Winnicott, D.W. (1969). The use of an object. *The International Journal of Psychoanalysis*, 50, 711–716.

Woodward, K. (1991). *Aging and its discontents: Freud and other fictions*. Indiana University Press.

Chapter 16

Continuing care review

A report on a thoughtful project and its untimely demise

Jane Garner

> *The true virtue of human beings is fitness to live together as equals.*
> *John Stuart Mill 1869*

This chapter reports a piece of work undertaken by an NHS multidisciplinary group also involving relatives of patients and two representatives from the local branch of the Alzheimer's Society. A review was made of life on continuing care wards in the hospital (it was an NHS project but all the discussions and conclusions are equally applicable whoever the provider). It was one of three interlinked projects, the others being 'The psychological mindedness working group' which aimed to increase psychological thinking in all interactions within the Old Age Psychiatry services (Garner, 2008) and 'Understanding institutional abuse of older patients' (Garner, 2005), what are the derivatives how may we recognise and prevent it? This was not a safeguarding agenda of protocols, registers and discipling but about thinking.

The remit of the Continuing Care Review was threefold:

- To improve the lives of patients in a continuing care setting many of whom will be there until the end of their life.
- To improve the working lives of staff on the ward, recognising they have a difficult job which is frequently undervalued.
- To improve the experience of relatives and friends of patients who may have problems coming to terms with the apparent differences over time in the person with dementia.

The emphasis throughout was on 'the individual', not just 'an old man with dementia', not only 'a care assistant low down in the hierarchy'. There was an attempt to identify a common humanity, balancing professional/patient identity with other aspects of the self; an attempt to get away from 'us and them' while recognising that we are positioned differently within the system. It felt like a journey into the sometimes forgotten corners of human commonality. We did not discuss the egregious politics of who is eligible, which form to complete, who should pay. Continuing care is far along the continuum of a condition for which there is no cure. We were looking at how to consider and improve the lives of patients in their final months, moving towards death.

Every aspect of life on the wards was considered in detailed minutiae. This consideration included the practical, e.g. we tried feeding each other, we used the hoist, but nothing is just practical; food and feeding also has nutritional/health aspects, social aspects, it will trigger memories and inevitably involve psychological factors back to the earliest of experiences.

The length of a chapter is insufficient to report in detail all the topics discussed. A full list of our considerations is in Appendix II.

Although a list of contents may look as if they were separate and contained subjects, clearly they could not be, e.g. privacy and dignity, engagement, falls, non-pharmacological management of problem behaviour and all the rest are interlinked. This chapter will give a summary of some of the topics covered.

Experience of the patient on the ward

We can only imagine what it is like, informed by empathy, careful attention to communication and behaviour and by reflecting on the way the patient makes us feel. The presentation of dementia and the experience of the patient is a complex interaction of neuropsychiatric pathology into which is added personality, personal and emotional history and the reaction of others – staff and patients. Kitwood (1990) has written of the social psychology which surrounds the patient. He introduced the idea that the patient's abilities, skills and mood are contingent on the attitudes and behaviour of those around them, in this case the staff. The social psychology need not be 'malignant' if thought and feeling are put into the interaction. This is a brain disease, but its expression is mediated by the inner world/mind and the reaction of the outer world. The patient is likely to have grief at previous and current losses and anxiety at potential future losses, fearing perhaps the loss of the self, in an existential terror, in a strange place away from the familiar. The patient may be consumed by the fear involved in a sense of abandonment. Insight as a heading on the Mental State Examination may seem to prompt a 'yes/no' answer but it is rarely so simple and often fluctuating. We all have patients in mind who cannot say 'what' is wrong but in a state of distress know 'something' is wrong.

For some incontinence is a humiliation. Misinterpretation of care as persecution is a difficulty for both patient and staff. Thought needs to be given to the best way to approach each person. Often it will be moving slowly, approaching directly and speaking in a soft, explanatory manner. For others it will be different, e.g. the male charge nurse addressing the patient who had a military history in a polite but firm and authoritative manner 'Major . . .'.

Choice for the patient is disappearing, it is limited by illness, but our institutional timetable and pressures may limit it further without thought. We need to respect the patient and their wishes even if they do not fit in with our routine. The patient is unlikely to be able to express all/any of this verbally. Feelings will be internalised, perhaps causing depression, physical illness or being expressed in frustrated aggression towards staff trying to care.

Not every experience will be negative, there may be something positive in the quality of relationships. It may be possible to appreciate the moment. One may get a temporary feeling of success in activities. Events and activities may bring to mind forgotten pleasures. Visitors may bring moments of pleasure, recognition and affection. The wife's perfume may bring a sense of joy at familiarity and remembrance. There may be satisfaction in feeling clean after the struggle to get in the bath/shower. There may also be a sense of relief to be in hospital, to feel contained with someone else to absorb the anxiety.

Personal identity

'Who is it that can tell me who I am?' asks King Lear (1:1V) on his way to personal and familial exile. 'Can I have become a different being while I still remain myself?' questions Simone de Beauvoir (1972, p. 283) on her increasing age.

A dementing illness with progressive deterioration in memory, language, skills prompts us to consider the meaning of personhood and identity. Institutionalising someone may further strip them of layers of identity. We need to acknowledge that the sense 'I AM', that non-trivial existential knowledge, persists throughout life until death (Garner, 2004). Although the notion of a concrete identity may be constraining for a philosophical discussion, clinical intuition suggests understanding social context, history, personal commitments and values is essential for addressing real human concerns and the identity of the person in front of you (Hughes, 2001). Practical activities and reminiscence groups on the ward may encourage identity consolidation. Psychotherapists recognise that even in the late stages of the disease the ability to make a relationship is retained so a therapeutic attachment may develop quickly. Personhood will be held within life history and experience, in relationships and in engagement with others. The person with dementia is no less a person than their neighbour or themselves when well. Staff need to behave in acknowledgement of that. Social constructionism (Sabat, 2001) argues that dementia is dually constituted of psychobiological pathologies and social processes. Part of our identity when well and also with dementia is contingent on social relationships. The ward needs information about the person's life history and experiences, preferences for name, day-to-day things, how they express their gender, what clothes they prefer, colour, style, etc. If we do not know these things then staff put their own imprimatur on the patient.

There is the concept of 'retrogenesis' (Reisberg et al., 1999) and a tendency even in some academic circles to describe dementia as a second childhood. However the patient is still an adult and needs to be so treated; it is not helpful to think of them as a child. The patient will be supported in thinking of themselves as an adult of worth and value if they are given respectful, understanding care.

There are also identity considerations for staff who are likely to be stigmatised by association with patients. There are different identities in staff along the continuum powerful-powerless. Those who visit the ward occasionally, doctors, psychologists, social workers etc., may be seen and see themselves as 'experts' (see Chapter 2) although they are likely to know less about the patients as people.

Identity considerations for family members/carers are complex. The phrase 'patients and carers' is often used as if they were one unit but there are two (at least two) identities, two people involved with different needs. All cope in different ways. The identity as a carer (Opie, 1992) may have emerged in the context of a long and positive relationship or taken on due to feelings of obligation and duty, for some taken on with resentment and anger. These different positions will persist beyond the patient's admission to the unit.

Dependency

Dementia by its nature is associated with increasing dependency. Being dependent brings a greater need for trust. For Erikson (1959) the first task/polarity for the baby is to negotiate *basic trust vs mistrust*. Will mother and food be available reliably for the baby, not in terms of quantity but of quality? In later life this becomes a question of whether to trust others or not, of whether they will be sufficient for one's needs. How one deals psychologically with dependency for basic care needs in old age will be dependent on how this phase in infancy was negotiated (Martindale, 1989). Staff need to be reliable, dependable, accepting and understanding. The pseudo-independent patient eschewing all attempts to help despite obvious need presents a difficult task for the staff. The patient feels the pain and possible humiliation of not managing. Earlier it could be the pain of giving up driving or household management. Now the pain maybe of not being able to attend to elimination and personal care needs. Staff need to support and facilitate, trying not to take over. This takes time and understanding and will inevitably fail if the patient feels under pressure. Judgement of the causes of distress is difficult. Is it physical pain, psychological pain or depression, psychosis, personality or an overwhelming sense of loss? We expect these judgements of poorly paid, not necessarily well-trained, carers.

Sexuality

Some referrals to Old Age Psychiatry departments indicate the strength of furious feeling, engendered at expressions of sexuality in older people, particularly those with a dementia. It is not useful to deny sexuality. We need to appropriately acknowledge gender, the manhood, womanhood, sexuality of the patient in ordinary human ways while recognising that subtle, sophisticated comprehension is lost. One's gender, even if one is no longer sexually active, may be an enduring source of gratification and self-knowledge. People with dementia have the same rights as anyone to express sexual feelings, but at a legal and ethical level the patient's capacity is central. Others may need to be protected from what can be seen as unacceptable behaviour. Some behaviours may not be harmful but are distressing to relatives, e.g. kissing and hugging another patient. This needs to be discussed sensitively with visitors, perhaps it is seen as yet another loss. Sexual behaviours often decrease in dementia, but sexually disinhibited behaviours are not uncommon (prevalence 2–17%, Series and Degano, 2005) in both men and women. There may be a number of reasons for this – disease related factors, social and psychological factors and drugs producing disinhibition or hyper-sexuality.

Professionals are not immune to the widespread negative socio-cultural attitudes of old age sexuality, but it is clear that sexuality is an important aspect of life throughout the lifespan (Garner and Bacelle, 2016). Particular issues arise in institutional care, but as the ward may be the patient's home for the rest of their life, sexuality needs to be considered and accommodated. Management of problems needs clear assessment, staff training, a low key approach to management the mainstay being distraction and understanding and a private space for the patient. Staff and patients need to be managed in a calm and contained way. Many drugs have been tried often with significant adverse events. No medication has a license for this use (Series and Degano, 2005).

Non-pharmacological management of 'problem' behaviour

There were frequent and lengthy discussions about the word 'problem' in relation to behaviour. To whom is it a problem? Staff attitudes are important, changing caregivers' behaviour changes patients' behaviour. The manner in which information is communicated at the shift handover meeting will influence the way the next shift views the behaviour. Behaviour is to be understood not necessarily stopped. Once understood the problem may have resolved. The genesis of the behaviour may be neurobiological, psychological (past experience, thoughts, belief and meaning) environmental and interplay between the three. The retired clerical worker may now sort through papers in the ward office, the retired removal man may move furniture about the ward. There may be an alternative way of engaging in a similar but less disruptive activity to give some meaning. It will be important to understand any perceptual/visual field defects. A patient who does not see someone or an object they are offering until they are close may hit out in fear. If the patient has one-sided inattention, approach needs to be from the unaffected side also during feeding, dressing and washing. The staff approach needs always to be friendly, calm, reassuring and empathetic.

Not everything that happens to a person with dementia is organically determined. Even though verbal skills and conscious memories diminish, the emphasis of psychoanalytic understanding on the unconscious and on non-verbal communication makes it a particularly useful paradigm to address these difficulties (Garner, 2013). Using these ideas and ways of working may make it easier for patients to accept other aspects of care that they were resisting. Patients may find some alleviation of terror, a sense of containment and continuity for a more peaceful end.

What I would like as a member of staff

The quality of working life for staff is intimately related to the quality of life for patients. Working on a continuing care ward may be thought, by those who have not really considered it, to be an easy option for staff who need little training to do it. However in reality it calls for personal capacities, particular training, skills in communication and relating with patients with major cognitive impairment also in the management of behavioural problems in someone who will probably not be able to explain their difficulties. 'I' would like managers, other staff and relatives to recognise that the work is skilled, often heavy physically and always hard psychologically. 'I' would like there to be adequate staff levels so I may work safely and well with sufficient rest breaks. 'I' would like to feel a positive affective atmosphere on the ward with staff from all disciplines, at all levels of responsibility, acknowledging, respecting and valuing each other. 'I' would like to feel that I am working as a member of a team both within my own discipline and also with other professionals. When I know a patient well, I would like my views about their care to be available to other disciplines and to the care review. 'I' would like to do my best for patients but recognise that there will be occasions when I find that difficult to accomplish. When feeling that I am having difficulties in a situation, 'I' would like to be free to ask for help from my colleagues and manager without it being deemed as a failure. When 'I' make a mistake which I have not recognised I would like to be told in a sensitive manner such that I may learn from it.

'I' would like to be treated respectfully by patients. However, I am cognisant that some patients may not always understand the nature or consequences of their behaviour. I need to be able to spend time with patients in order to get to know them better, to improve relationships and to be able to exercise patience when engaging in personal care. Pressure to complete a task quickly will result in poorer care for the patient and more stress for me.

'I' should be treated respectfully by relatives. I know that sometimes relatives will be upset and I will try to understand. However I will not expect to be shouted at or abused in any way.

For support with my development and training 'I' need regular supervision in an atmosphere where it is possible to really express my thoughts and feelings, positive and negative, about my work without evoking criticism. I need access to training so it is available frequently and regularly to introduce me to new ideas and skills and to modify or consolidate old ones.

'I' would like occasionally to be involved in other aspects of the work of the Department of Old Age Psychiatry, e.g. by visiting a patient at home or spending time in the day hospital so I may see how my ward and my work fit into the whole service.

Communication

This was a major and lengthy topic for the review. It involves practical aspects such as understanding the deteriorating speech and language difficulties as the illness progresses; making sure hearing aids, glasses and dentures are in place and work and distractions are at a minimum and making sure the patient can see the speaker's face and maintaining eye contact, much information is conveyed by facial expression. It is not helpful to modify speech in the singsong way in which adults speak to infants. This not infrequently happens when speaking with older people with and without dementia although they are adults. 'Elderspeak' (Kemper et al., 1998) is high pitched and patronising, using inappropriate terms of endearment and tends to make people feel more helpless. It will be helpful to explain clearly in short sentences and to avoid open-ended questions.

Although the patient may not understand everything that is said, communication will provide some valuable contact and reassurance. Communication is not only practical and directly verbal, there is a major emotional component. At an everyday level we can infer when a friend says that they are 'fine' whether or not that is the case; we understand non-verbal cues and body language. That skill needs to be refined and extended as a vital way of understanding what the patient is feeling and really saying. Staff need then to feedback their comprehension to see if they have understood correctly. If they have, then they are involved in real communication rather than what may be a pointless exchange. In the later stages the patient may have few or no words and body language will be the only way they communicate their feelings and needs. If staff know the patient well, they may be able to tell from the smallest movement or fleeting expression whether they feel discomfort, sadness, irritation and so on or feel pleasure at the contact. Mirroring the patient's movements may give a sense of recognition. Feeling understood may be of immense comfort to the patient.

Communication between staff involved in a patient's care is vital, particularly when caring for those not necessarily able to express needs or preferences themselves. It is likely that by the time a patient is admitted to a continuing care ward they will have been known to other staff within the wider organisation. Community nurses, social workers, day hospital and day centre staff, domiciliary carers will have a wealth of knowledge about the patient's personal circumstances, likes/ dislikes, anxieties. Also knowledge about how to approach the patient in order to complete care activities with the minimum of upset and distress, how the person copes with new environments and effective ways of dealing with behavioural disturbances are examples for an information base that is likely to have been accrued by others known to the patient. Effective communication of this will help smooth the transition between different areas of the service. Community staff are likely to have information about family carers and any differences that are present between relatives. Building up a picture of personal and psychosocial circumstances leads to a more person-centred approach, seeing the patient as an individual. Communication between staff on the ward is equally important; this included the communication of information and also of attitudes.

The other major aspect of communication on the ward is with relatives. Patient care will always be at its best if staff and relatives can be in a collaborative relationship. Staff are likely to know more about the neuropsychiatric condition. Relatives will know more about the patient and may help in compiling a 'life-review' book. Ideally there needs to be a cooperative pooling of information appropriate to the situation and the individuals. Some relatives greet the admission with unrealistic expectations, others with guilt that managing at home was not possible.

The ward environment and the condition of other patients may be unexpected and distressing. The relative may be coping with a type of bereavement, grieving for many aspects of the patient which are lost and fearing future losses (Garner, 1997 and see Chapters 5 and 10 of this volume). It is particularly upsetting when the relative is not remembered by the patient. However, although the patient may not recall the name or details of the relationship, they are likely to recognise and acknowledge internally that the close relative is someone for whom there is great familiarity, warmth, affection or love. Some intimate relatives wish to be involved still in the practical caring tasks. Some need help in recognising that just 'being there' in an active sense is not 'doing nothing'.

Staff are in a privileged position of trust, holding private and sensitive information about patients. The general principles of confidentiality are no different for older adults with a dementing illness than for any other adult. Family and friends who share thoughts and feelings also have a right to confidentiality. Difficulties may arise when family ask for information. It is usually in the best interests of the patient to share in this partnership of care. Staff must always act in the best interests of the patient and so occasionally need to question visitors' motives, e.g. for being interested in the patient's ability to sign their name perhaps on a cheque, will or other document.

Relatives should be invited to regular reviews which may provide a space to think and a way to talk about the patient.

What relatives may contribute to the ward

They bring detailed and intimate information and may literally bring in favourite things – clothes, objects, toiletries, photographs. They may be able to speak to other relatives, individually or in a group, for mutual support. They can assist practically if that is agreed. Sometimes they offer other talents, craft skills, playing a musical instrument etc. It is helpful if they apprehend the difficulties staff can face and acknowledge those who undertake the task of caring sensitively and well.

Relatives will bring into the situation their own personality and life experience, their particular relationship with the patient, their previous relationships with health care professionals whom they have encountered and their personal understanding of the patient's illness. Staff need to have an understanding of the wishes and fears of the relatives, those that seem to be general to the situation and those specific to the relative or relationship. They may be angry that this has happened to the patient. Understandable emotions may be displaced and worked out in hostility and complaints about staff. Sometimes these complaints will be fair but not always. They will be expressing their own pain, loss and guilt – a sensitive and listening ear can diffuse most situations, but one 'difficult' relative can have a powerful and negative effect on the ward. However this 'difficult' relative may sometimes also have a good point and make staff aware of something on the ward not previously known or perhaps previously ignored. Changes could be made to the benefit also of other patients.

End of life care

Patients admitted to a continuing care ward are towards the end of their life. Staff have guidance for themselves and relatives with regard to future care options (resuscitation and active medical intervention) for patients who do not have the capacity to make decisions themselves. This must account for previously expressed views of the patient, any lasting power of attorney in place and having regard that these decisions maybe too burdensome for some relatives. Cardiopulmonary resuscitation (CPR) is likely to be unsuccessful and may deprive the dying person of dignity. Nor is there evidence that percutaneous endoscopic gastrostomy (PEG) improves the quality of life of people with advanced dementia – maybe the opposite (Monteleoni and Clark, 2004).

Patients dying with dementia have been shown to have health care needs comparable to those with cancer but often with inadequate pain control (McCarthy et al., 1997). The palliative approach definition by the WHO (1990) although nearly thirty years old is still relevant also for patients with dementia; 'the active total care of patients whose disease is not responsive to curative treatment. Control of pain, of other symptoms and of psychological, social and spiritual problems is paramount'. The team need to think about what interventions are necessary and what is merely disturbing for the patient. They need to manage complex physical and psychiatric symptoms in the face of the patient's severely diminished ability to communicate. Staff need to be particularly alert to non-verbal cues and to make the patient feel safe and secure by letting them know they will not be left on their own (see Chapter 17).

Apart from appropriate control of symptoms there must be emphasis on quality of life with attention to psychological, social and spiritual needs, involving the family in decisions, facilitating important others to be at the bedside and fostering supportive communication between all involved (Hughes et al., 2005). Competent clinical assessments should not ignore subjective factors of love, human contact, hope and fear. Spiritual care needs to be understood in its broadest sense including whatever gives a person meaning, value and worth in life; for some this will have a religious element and it may be appropriate to contact a member of the patient's faith community.

The person with dementia experiences/suffers a chronic trauma related to separation, loss, powerlessness, displacement and hopelessness (Miesen, 1997). There is a pressing human need for interconnectedness. Life has to do with chronological time and simultaneously lies outside that dimension – a few minutes at the end of one's life can change the meaning of the whole of that life. One small second may be enough to give a feeling of eternity (Quinodoz, 2010). The presence of a caring person next to the patient who is about to die can help the patient feel that their internal objects are good and the world benevolent – the importance of not being alone. Staff need to have come to terms with the precariousness of life and their own end.

The emotional impact of working in end of life care needs to be acknowledged with time given to attend the funeral enabling a sense of completeness for the nurse and further support for the family.

Conclusion

Caring for patients with a dementing illness and meeting their family is traditionally and currently not seen as skilled work but to do it well requires skill, patience, imagination and understanding. The review aimed to balance the uniqueness of the individuals, patients and staff with commonality. Lipinska (2009) reports correspondence from the renowned neuropsychologist A.R. Luria (1975) to Oliver Sacks the neurologist who had a personal touch. It was advice on treating a patient with severe memory loss. Luria wrote

> Do whatever your ingenuity and your heart suggest. . . . a man does not consist of memory alone. He has feeling, will, sensibilities, moral being – matters of which neuropsychology cannot speak and it is beyond the realm of an impersonal psychology that you may find ways to touch him and change him. . . . Neuropsychologically there is little or nothing one can do; but in the realm of the individual there may be much you can do.

Freud's theory informs us, applicable to patients and to staff, that we act out what we cannot think about. The theme of all the sections of the review is the need to think, to think more and to think carefully about the continuing care patient and about ourselves in relation to the patient. What goes on inside people and what goes on between people. Working with someone with an irreversible illness may upset our unconscious determinants of our choice of profession – we want patients to recover or we feel the same sense of their helplessness (Main, 1957). We cannot spend all of our working lives in identification and anguish, we need some clinical detachment but to achieve that without emotional detachment, so that we are open to patients, to understand and to convey to them that understanding which we may also contain for them. The way the work is presented in sections is because the contributors did not feel they had a monopoly of ideas on the days it was written, and updating could be done easily.

None of the issues is straightforward. Engagement is about staff knowing they have more in common with patients than differences of health and illness between them. Clinical decisions are often ethical decisions (Hughes, 2013). The ethical imperative is to maintain or improve the quality of life, even at its end. That quality must not be circumscribed in addition to the damage of the disease. Fulford (1989) writes of 'values based medicine' which needs to be complementary to 'evidence based medicine'. The essential identity of the person persists throughout the dementing illness and we all should act with that in mind, maintaining as broad and as deep an identity as possible, endeavouring to 'be with' the patient at relational depth. There is a need for empathetic and understanding relationships with the inner world of the patients, the family and with staff.

Additional information

The multi-disciplinary group was pleased with the report produced, of which this is a summary. Unfortunately political pettiness in the NHS, an institution which is usually able to do wonderful work, intervened at the end. On the day the Review was to be sent to the printers with the cover to be a relief picture (not possible to publish it) by a group of four patients in art therapy, managers decided that it could not be presented as the Primary Care Trust (PCT) would not be funding continuing care in the future. Some years later PCTs no longer exist, but the continuing care patients remain. This decision was distressing to people who had really put their personal and professional selves into this discussion/task and it missed the obvious point that the work would be applicable whoever the provider. We can only appreciate the irony that this shortsighted decision emphasises the main point of the review which was about the importance of 'thinking'.

References

De Beauvoir, S. (1972[1970]). *Old Age*. Translated by Patrick O'Brian. London: Andre Deutsch, Weidenfeld and Nicholson.

Erikson, E. (1959). *Identity and the Life Cycle: Psychological Issues Monograph 1*. New York: International Universities Press.

Fulford, K.W.M. (1989). *Moral Theory and Medical Practice*. Cambridge: Cambridge University Press.

Garner, J. (1997). Dementia: An intimate death. *British Journal of Medical Psychology*, 70, 177–184.

Garner, J. (2004). Identity and Alzheimer's disease. In G. Leavey and D. Kelleher (eds.) *Identity and Health*. Hove: Brunner Routledge.

Garner, J. (2005). *Understanding Institutional Abuse of Older Patients: Some Reflections*. Mental Health NHS Trust (available from the author).

Garner, J. (2008). WOT! No psychotherapist. *APP Newsletter. Psychoanalytic Psychotherapy*, 38, 16–18.

Garner, J. (2013). Psychodynamic psychotherapy, chapter 19 In T. Dening and A. Thomas (eds.) *Oxford Textbook of Old Age Psychiatry*, 2nd ed. Oxford: Oxford University Press.

Garner, J., and Bacelle, L. (2016). Intimacy and sexuality in old age. In C.G. Fenieux and R. Rojas (eds.) *Sexo y Psicoanálisis: Una mirada a la intimidad adulta*. Santiago: Pólvora Editorial.

Hughes, J. (2001). Views of the person with dementia. *Journal of Medical Ethics*, 27, 86–91.

Hughes, J. (2013). Ethics and old age psychiatry, chapter 55 In T. Dening and A. Thomas (eds.) *Oxford Textbook of Old Age Psychiatry*, 2nd ed. Oxford: Oxford University Press.

Hughes, J., Robinson, L., and Volicer, L. (2005). Specialist palliative care in dementia. *British Medical Journal*, 330, 57–58.

Kemper, S., Ferrell, P., Harden, T., Finter-Urczuk, A., and Billington, C. (1998). Use of elderspeak by young and older adults to impaired and unimpaired listeners. *Aging, Neuropsychology, and Cognition: Journal on Normal and Dysfunctional Development*, 5, 43–55.

Kitwood, T. (1990). The dialectics of dementia: With particular reference to Alzheimer's disease. *Ageing and Society*, 10, 177–196.

Lipinska, D. (2009). *Person-Centred Counselling for People with Dementia*. London, Jessica Kingsley.

Luria, A.R. (1975) in Sacks, O. (1988). *The Man Who Mistook his Wife for a Hat*. New York: Harper & Row. pp. 34

Main, T. (1957). The ailment. *Medical Psychology*, 30, 129–145.

Martindale, B. (1989). Becoming dependent again: The fears of some elderly persons and their younger therapists. *Psychoanalytic Psychotherapy*, 4, 167–175.

McCarthy, M., Addington-Hall, J., and Altmann, D. (1997). The experience of dying with dementia: A retrospective study. *International Journal of Geriatric Psychiatry*, 12, 404–409.

Miesen, B.M.L. (1997). Awareness and family grieving: A practical perspective. In B. Miesen and G. Jones (eds.) *Caregiving in Dementia: Research and Applications*, Vol. 2. London: Routledge, 67–79.

Monteleoni, C., and Clark, E. (2004). Using rapid quality improvement methodology to reduce feeding tubes in patients with advanced dementia: Before and after study. *British Medical Journal*, 329, 491–494.

Opie, A. (1992). *There's Nobody There*. Oxford: Oxford University Press.

Quinodoz, D. (2010). *Growing Old a Journey of Self-discovery*. London: Routledge.

Reisberg, B., Kenowsky, S., Franssen, E.H., et al. (1999). Towards a science of Alzheimer's disease management: A model based on current knowledge of retrogenesis. *International Psychogeriatrics*, 11, 7–23.

Sabat, S.R. (2001). *The Experience of Alzheimer's Disease: Life Through a Tangled Veil*. Oxford and Malden, MA: Blackwell.

Series, H., and Degano, P. (2005). Hypersexuality in dementia. *Advances in Psychiatric Treatment*, 11, 424–431.

World Health Organisation (1990). Definition of Palliative Care, Geneva.

Appendix 1

Contents of continuing care review

Introduction.

Executive summary.

Experience of the patient on the ward: i Experience of the patient, ii What I would like as a patient, iii Improving patients experience within continuing care wards.

Engagement: i Engagement on a continuing care ward, ii Practical engagement on the ward.

Confidentiality.

Admission to the ward.

Staff, patients and carers working together.

Personal identity: i Maintaining personal identity, ii Personal identity, iii Ten things you should know about me.

Spiritual needs of patients and religious observance.

Dependency.

Slips, trips and falls.

Food.

Privacy and dignity.

Sexuality.

Management of incontinence.

Non-pharmacological management of 'problem' behaviour.

Aromatherapy.

Sensory stimulation.

Medication on a continuing care ward.

What I would like as a member of staff working on a continuing care ward.

Communication: i Communication and dementia, ii Emotional communication with patients, iii Communication between staff, iv Communication with relatives.

What I may contribute as a relative visiting the ward.

End of life decisions: i Guidance for staff and relatives on the physical care of those patients who lack capacity to make decisions for themselves, ii Reaching decisions on resuscitation.

End of life care: a palliative approach.

Assessment of pain.

Care for the dying patient and the family.

Discharge planning and follow up.

Roles and responsibilities of different disciplines contributing to care on a long stay ward: Nurses, Doctors, Occupational therapists, Social workers, Community psychiatric nurses, Chaplain, Clinical psychologists, Art therapists, Music therapists, Speech and language therapists, Managers and clinical leaders, Dieticians, Pharmacists, Physiotherapists, Dentists, Podiatrists, Estates and hotel services [*the list of disciplines looks as if the ward was well staffed. It was often a struggle to get services for the patients*].

Appendix II

Participants from different disciplines made important contributions to the review also putting their ideas into practice.

Chapter 17

Negotiating the border

Music therapy for people in the last hours of dementia

Adrienne Freeman

He often would ask us
That, when he died,
After playing so many
To their last rest,
If out of us any
Should here abide,
And it would not task us,
We would with our lutes
Play over him

Hardy (1917)

Introduction

Death and dying in Western culture generally remain somewhat removed from everyday life, frequently taking place out of the home environment. Our encounters with death may therefore be infrequent, thereby reinforcing an enduring taboo around dying.

Thinking about death can be frightening, with associated fears of suffering, indignity, dependence, loss and the unknown. The busy-ness of a modern lifestyle perhaps aids us in avoiding this topic. It may not be until we are first confronted with the death of a loved one that we start to wrestle with the implications of our mortality.

Hardy opens his poem 'The Choirmaster's Burial' with the epigraph to this chapter, encapsulating the idea that music can be an important accompanying factor both through life and at its end. This passage reflects my hopes as a clinician that I may discover and be able to bring meaningful music into the space occupied by a patient and their immediate family or friends at this time of transition. My hope is that, despite my own fears, through coming alongside the patient as a Music Therapist, I might be able to alleviate any loneliness and fear and bring some sense of peace and comfort through what I can offer.

The death of a person with dementia usually comes at the end of a protracted illness (often lasting many years), during which the patient, family members and loved ones have already sustained great losses. Death may then perhaps be experienced as a release from a ravaging illness. Sometimes family members are present at this time, but for some people with dementia they are accompanied only by the staff of their care setting. By the late stages of dementia, patients are usually unable to articulate their awareness of impending death so any living will or advance directive will be helpful in fulfilling their wishes.

The material for this chapter has been drawn from my work on a ward for people with advanced dementia, situated on a large general hospital site and run under the auspices of a NHS Mental Health Trust. The unit (at the time of the clinical work here described) had 23 beds, eight being for men whose dementia caused challenging behaviours. The remaining beds were for men and women, including a varying number of shorter admissions for assessment purposes.

This chapter is specifically concerned with needs arising in the arena of advanced dementia, a topic not always considered in publications on specialised therapeutic work. Features of advanced dementia as encountered at end of life include a lack of 'capacity', with the inability to exercise judgement and decision-making. Late stage dementia brings with it total dependence, with care being given that includes washing, dressing and toileting for double incontinence. Meals will consist of appropriately textured food being fed in ways that accord with swallowing ability. Deteriorating mobility will progressively require use of aids such as walking stick, frame, wheelchair and hoist. This may then lead to being nursed in bed (with associated pressure care). Language skills (both expressive and receptive) will have gradually become lost, although usually some vocal sounds remain. These, together with facial expression and gesture, allow for the person with dementia to communicate non-verbally to a certain extent.

The level of functioning is not dissimilar to that of a newborn infant, although the person with dementia has a lifetime's experience behind them.

T.S. Eliot both commences and concludes 'East Coker', the second poem of *Four Quartets* (1944, pp. 21–27), by blending the start and finish of life. Bunt (1994, pp. 157–158) links these life stages, reflecting on the connecting spiral of 'life-span development' as seen in Beethoven's string quartets, which were written in three collections between youth and old age. He describes the late quartets as:

> works full of the wisdom and spiritual insight of old age. Yet this wisdom also has the feel of the rapt innocence of childhood, with song-like melodies of the utmost simplicity. In later years we may find the youthful energy of the early quartets invigorating and inspiring. The very fact that people with dementia can often recall more of their childhood than of recent events may be part of this whole cyclical process of the interconnections between beginnings and

endings. Long-term memory still remains intact. Our sense of hearing is both the first to develop and, very often, the last to leave us.

(1994, p. 158)

For Music Therapists it is significant that hearing usually remains functional until death, rendering music a relevant tool for remaining present alongside the dying person. Weber comments:

Hearing is the sensory organ which usually functions until the end . . . so I know they can still hear me, even when they can no longer see or speak. I feel that whatever may be happening 'on the other side', it is important that the patient feel the presence of someone here with them – that they are not alone.

(1999, p. 102)

Sisson (1990) and Tapson et al. (2015), respectively researching and working with comatose patients, found that aural stimuli caused varied responses such as movement, opening of the eyes and so on, thus evidencing their hypothesis that hearing continues to function after other senses have been lost.

In order for the clinician to accompany and respond sensitively, attentive *'listening to'* the patient is required. As is widely known (Cueva, 2006; Jia and Liu, 2010), the Chinese manuscript character *'to listen'* assists here (Figure 17.1), for the symbol includes multiple aspects (such as seeing, focussing, thinking and feeling), implying listening with one's whole being. Alongside the undivided attention given to the dying patient, an instinctive and intuitive sense of what is appropriate will also guide the clinician.

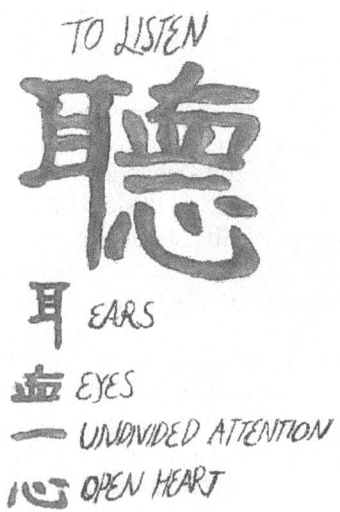

Figure 17.1 Chinese character 'To Listen'

Intimacy

Dying is a basic and inevitable human function involving intimacy, vulnerability and dependence. It is easy to assume that privacy may be preferred for such events, by both the patient and their loved ones. As advanced dementia care settings (and particularly hospital wards) can be difficult places in which to find privacy, it is important to consider who the dying patient might want to be with them and to facilitate ways in which they and their loved ones can find privacy together in a dignified manner.

Worth powerfully describes the border between life and death as unique territory. In a case description she presents this place of transition as follows:

> Frank was quietly slipping away into that mysterious border land between life and death where peace and rest and gentle sounds are the only needs. . . . More than anything else a dying person needs to have someone with them. . . . I disagree wholly with the notion that there is no point staying with an unconscious patient because he or she does not know you are there. I am perfectly certain, through years of experience and observation, that unconsciousness, as we define it, is not a state of unknowing. Rather, it is a state of knowing and understanding on a different level that is beyond our immediate experience.
>
> (2005, pp. 107–108)

Remaining alongside the dying person may provide an experience of company, this being all the more important for the fact that, as noted previously, hearing is the most likely of the senses to continue functioning in unconsciousness. This different level of operating, experienced at the border of life, introduces transcendent and spiritual qualities, explored by Mayne where he writes:

> to be human is to have a sense of the transcendent. To have a deep instinctive sense of mystery: of that which transcends us, that which is other and greater than we are and which we cannot account for or easily dismiss.
>
> (2002, p. 33)

Spirituality

Spirituality is intimately connected with identity: belief systems associated with spirituality (whether practised through a recognised faith or not) are usually exercised and developed over a period of many years and are often embedded in cultural and family traditions. Such traditions frequently carry with them particularly associated music. In my experience, I have found that people with dementia sometimes sing songs from their childhood, often learned in the family, community and spiritual context of their upbringing. People frequently find music of their own country and language to be highly meaningful, more readily responding to this when their dementia is advanced. As dementia progresses, if English is not their first language, people frequently revert to using their mother tongue.

It is vital to acknowledge, accept and respect that spiritual stances widely vary, with each person bringing their own unique experience to this realm.

The advantage of working in music is that it is possible for the patient and therapist to transcend cognitive processes and to function without words, thus continuing to offer connection for those with advanced dementia. We know from the experience of people with dementia that its impact leads to feelings of fragmentation and disintegration, for both the patient and those around them. A patient of mine, formerly a health professional and struggling to articulate his thoughts, recently commented on how his brain felt 'discombobulated'. Presenting features of the illness contribute towards this, particularly its effects on thought processes, language and mobility (together with other features described earlier in this chapter). Music is able to continue to be received throughout the course of dementia. While music provides a non-verbal and sensory means of connection, its organisational systems are able to offer a more coherent sound world. Being deeply expressive, it can non-verbally articulate multiple realms, including the spiritual, as seen in myriad compositions penned over the years. It is a key task of the Music Therapist to provide music, whether improvised or pre-composed, that meets the spiritual needs of the patient. Sensitivity is required: spiritual material can unexpectedly hold negative connotations for some patients. On a ward for those with advanced dementia, one person reacted to the communal singing of hymns with horror, cowering alone in the foyer with his hands over his ears. Upon gentle exploration it was discovered that the music reminded him of time spent in prisoner-of-war camps, causing much distress which was perhaps only partially alleviated by one-to-one conversation and alternative activity.

Professional boundaries require the personal life of the therapist to be kept separate from the patient, resulting in their being unaware of the clinician's own spiritual perspective. However, the Music Therapist can musically and verbally support whatever spiritual material the patient and their family brings, whether this represents any faith or none. Hymns and prayers may be included as appropriate with additional spiritual support being requested from the relevant chaplain as required.

Clinical approach

It is helpful to think of this field of work as requiring an extended palliative approach. Cicely Saunders (the founder of the hospice movement), a patient in her own hospice, found 'that dying took a very long time, and was harder work than she had expected' (du Boulay and Rankin, 2007, p. 227). At her funeral, her approach was noted:

> taking time and sometimes simply sitting quietly at the bedside without saying anything . . . it's the individual person that counts. It's the paying of attention to the individual's needs, symptoms, fears and pain, which matters.
>
> (2007, p. 230)

The clinician in the dementia setting will usually have some period of time in which to work with the patient, due to the longer prognosis. Patients' own insight and ability to acknowledge a terminal diagnosis, although more commonly occurring at early stages of dementia, may still occur fleetingly at a later stage.

Mayne describes the process of affirmation:

> When people are sick or hurting or in the shadow-lands of grief they need affirming. . . . When I am sick, and especially when I am dying, I need to bring some kind of order and design to what feels like chaos and a falling apart of my whole familiar world. At such moments we may need someone beside us who will listen to our stories and help us interpret them. And without music, we lack one of the most important vocabularies in which the spirit can speak.
>
> (2002, pp. 38–39)

Music therapy for someone in their last hours usually takes place at the bedside where the therapist perhaps may not feel immediately comfortable working. This more intimate space, occupied by the patient, is entered by the therapist who starts from the position of not having the room prepared in advance, as opposed to the pre-prepared therapy room into which the patient enters for a session. The vulnerability and varied new symptoms of the dying patient may add to the discomfort of the therapist.

However, here the therapist brings an acutely observing stance, offering a slowly paced watching and listening presence which informs their contribution of music, in turn assisting in countering the isolation people may experience when being nursed in bed. The therapist's music, gently and sensitively provided in a manner tailored to each individual, can promote relaxation, thereby decreasing agitation and contributing to enhanced quality of care.

As music takes place, I have found myself looking for physical signs from the patient which indicate response and aid connection. Changes in facial expression are important to observe and may indicate relaxation, discomfort, increased pain levels and so on. In their final hours, people's eyes often become unfocussed but I have noticed that music sometimes results in brief focussing of eyes and an alteration in direction of gaze towards the sound source. Alteration in breathing rates can be responded to by the therapist timing the playing of their music to fit the breathing rhythm (unless contraindicated by difficulties breathing, in which case I avoid this technique in order not to emphasise any distress of the patient). Vocal sounds or body movements made by the patient, together with alterations in levels of consciousness also inform the therapist's contributions.

Vigilant attention to the nature of such non-verbal responses informs the therapist. Accordingly their music can be adapted to interact with such bodily functions in order to fulfil the aim of offering 'alongside-ness' with a relaxing effect. If it is sensed that the music may be in any way over-stimulating or invasive, it is important to quickly withdraw and offer less musically. Any evidence of physical distress calls for immediate nursing assistance as maintaining the patient's comfort is of paramount importance (Krout, 2003, p. 130).

Clinical illustration

The Music Therapist first noticed Alex responding to her violin playing in the lounge, where he sat in his wheelchair. He usually appeared withdrawn and sleepy but his gaze became alert and intently focussed on the therapist as she played. So she soon started individual work with him. Six months before his death, Alex opened his eyes wide when the wind-chimes touched his hand. He appeared alert and engaged, his response being chiefly in his eyes as he looked at the instrument and orientated his head towards the sound source; he sometimes moved his fingers too. Upon returning to the lounge, the nursing staff commented in surprise, 'You've woken him up!' for Alex usually appeared less alert.

Only six days before he died, Alex re-orientated his head very slightly towards the sound source as the therapist played the Sounding Bowl (Figure 17.2). Then, as she gently moved the wind-chimes from side to side in front of him, he used his eyes to track the instrument's movement and made a few small vocal sounds in response.

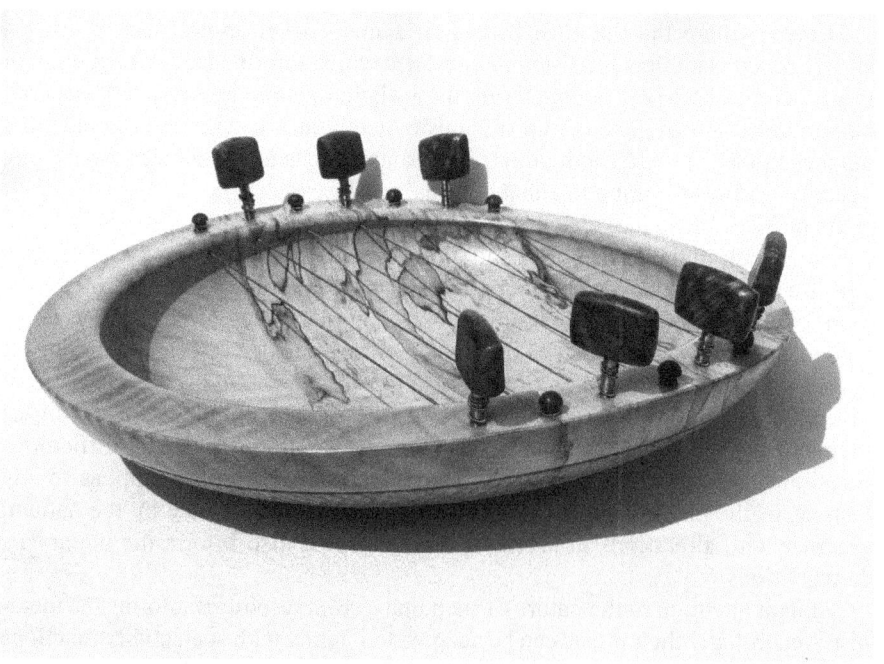

Figure 17.2 Sounding Bowl

Identity

Multiple aspects of the self comprise identity, as I have written about elsewhere (Freeman, 2017):

> Identity is conferred and affirmed in many ways, including culture and ethnicity, family/life context, sexuality, spirituality and so on. All contribute towards personal history, which when included in our work as Music Therapists deepens the sense of meaningful connection for those we are working with, be they people with dementia or their families.
>
> (2017, p. 45)

Bunt (1994, pp. 158–159) reflects on how music expresses identity: 'We express both our personal and our group identity through music at different stages in our lives. This is very clear when we look back and connect various pieces of music with significant life events'.

He exemplifies the music of adolescence as helping to create peer group identity, whilst identifying song as expressing life and community experience such as war. He also points to ways in which particular music becomes associated with loved ones. All such aspects become significant at end-of-life review.

Such a review will not usually be possible for the person in the late stages of dementia, unless family members are involved and can contribute information about life history (Freeman, 2017). Here, I have found it helpful to imagine holding for each patient an artist's palette, to which one gradually adds colours that represent each technique or approach that has enabled response and engagement, however minimal. This palette is not purely a musical one: it will include aspects of both personal history and that of the clinical work carried out together. This can be thought of as a *'Palette of Possibilities'*.

Liaison with carers and relatives greatly assists in building understanding of what is important for each person. Dementia UK's Template, 'My Life Story', is useful for gathering such information (Thompson, 2011). As the patient nears death, they may become unable to clearly indicate their wishes as to therapy processes: here the clinician can draw on the palette already established in prior clinical work. Deterioration of any client requires constant adjustment in approach, so this is simply a continuation.

Music therapy as an accompaniment

It may be daunting to work with the dying dementia patient, perhaps in part due to the irregularity and unpredictability of such work, making it unfamiliar for the therapist. For various reasons, clinicians may seldom experience their patients' transition from life to death.

A multi-disciplinary approach is vital: when it is evident that someone is in their last hours, I have found it to be crucial to effectively liaise with multi-disciplinary colleagues (particularly those nursing the patient) and receive adequate supervision.

When I find I can no longer rely on direct interaction with the patient, I largely switch to using receptive techniques, gently introducing music for the patient to listen to. In the patient's last hours, tactile methods (as used in a sensory approach at prior stages) may be too invasive. The focus now shifts to an auditory one (with an occasional visual aspect), drawing on the history of previous work if this is available.

Several musical instruments, specifically selected due to their having been positively responded to by the patient in previous clinical work, can be taken to the bedside. Resonant instruments such as harp/cimbala or Sounding Bowl provide a beautiful, gentle and relevant presence at such times and can be played in ways which have in earlier sessions been found to be effective.

My own experience in end-of-life work has mostly been to use live music, both pre-composed and improvised, which has the advantage of being able to be instantly adjusted. One seeks to achieve an accompanying and relaxing effect by playing music that feels, in the moment, to be the most emotionally appropriate.

The therapist cannot expect to proceed as in more usual therapy sessions, for at this stage the care of basic bodily functions (such as breathing, oral care, positioning, vomiting and so on) usually requires regular nursing interventions. Clinical work now needs a more flexible boundary enabling nurses to come and go as required. I have found it useful to think of this final stage of the work as *'start-stop-start-stop Music Therapy'*, allowing for various interventions to be taking place in close succession or even simultaneously. There have been instances where there has been enough trust from nursing staff for me to be able to make required practical interventions myself, for example repositioning a slipped oxygen mask (as seen in a subsequent clinical illustration).

Simplifying one's approach becomes important. People with dementia are often no longer able to comprehend more complex music that they formerly appreciated, a fact attested to by their relatives. Weber, writing in the context of hospice care, underlines the importance of simplicity in approach:

> As a patient gets closer to death, the music becomes simpler – like a mother singing lullabies. . . . Although patients may have loved listening to Mozart or similar music when they first arrived, for many it has become too complicated. I play a lot of . . . folk songs because of their gentleness and simple melodies. . . . This is a time when I also sing more.
>
> (1999, p. 102)

Song offers a relevant means of relating. Clair concludes:

> singing provides desirable emotional contact and intimacy that gives comfort and alleviates fear without speaking. . . . At some level persons in late stage dementia know that singing is associated with tenderness and that someone who is singing to them is not harmful or hurtful.
>
> (2000, pp. 90 and 97)

Songs can be wordless or may incorporate improvised/pre-composed lyrics that are relevant to the person's life. Personal items, such as family photographs and other articles that have been placed in the room by family members, can be incorporated into a simple improvised song and may also be briefly spoken about, thus linking with the patient's personal history. The names of the patient and their loved ones may be sung or their rhythms incorporated into an improvisation. Musical styles can be used as relevant to the individual's culture and personal preference. I was once surprised to observe someone in their last hours moving one finger in time to the live music being played – a song about family members that we had composed together in much earlier sessions.

Levels of consciousness fluctuate: when a person appears more deeply unconscious, music can retreat and be gentler in order to 'fit'. If physical signs indicate an increased level of alertness, music can become more prominent to match. This can be thought of as a tide advancing and retreating although in a somewhat unpredictable manner. The immediacy of improvisation is very relevant here. There is value in waiting, for sometimes a person can seem as if they will never regain a higher level of consciousness and then most unexpectedly they do so.

Clinical illustration

Violet had been engaging in individual music therapy for a number of years. Her last session took place three weeks before she died. She slept for the first 20 minutes of the session as the therapist gently played the Sounding Bowl, Violet's favourite instrument. Violet appeared to briefly surface as her name was sung and its rhythm hummed. When she woke up fully, the therapist moved nearer then placed the Bowl in the bed near Violet's hand – Violet held onto the rim with one finger, retaining her grip when the therapist later tried to move the Bowl away. The therapist therefore continued to play. Violet laughed as she listened and then as she was shown some of her family photographs which had been regularly used in their work together. When the beaded cabasa was held still against her hand, Violet moved her fingers in response, making vocal sounds and laughing. The therapist noted the value of waiting and slowly persisting, thus allowing time for Violet to respond.

Families

Each family will approach death and dying in different ways according to particular circumstances, culture and established family patterns around death and dying. Therapeutic approach will inevitably be determined according to the differing needs of each family (Krout, 2003, p. 130) and usually involves sensitive negotiation.

It is both important and difficult for the clinician to judge whether they would be intruding if they advance into a room with relatives in attendance and (in the case of music therapy) start playing music. The therapist cannot assume that their prior relationship with the patient gives them this right. The family could experience this as an invasion of privacy, seen as being insensitive, inappropriate, distracting and so on. Sometimes families need to be on their own (Krout, 2003, p. 133). A better alternative may be to provide an accompanying presence when the family are not there. Clinical judgement is aided by drawing on one's prior relationship with the patient and their relatives, also using instinct and intuition.

Clinical illustration

The Music Therapist started individual work with Fleur five months before she died. She was completely immobile and had lost language, as is usual at this stage. In Fleur's first session, she reached out for the therapist's violin, holding it for a long time. She plucked the strings and examined the wood, seeming fascinated by its materials and construction. She looked animated, making eye contact and smiling. Pausing to 'just look' at what was in her hands enabled meaningful connection.

In later work, she frequently became more alert when wind-chimes or finger cymbals gently touched her hand. She sometimes intentionally reached out to touch or take hold of the metal parts. Only a few weeks before she died, as the therapist attempted to retrieve the wind-chimes, Fleur made one or two vocalisations that resembled speech.

Ten days before her death, Fleur's family surrounded her at her bedside – this instinctively felt too private a moment for the therapist to enter the room as usual. Later that day, she returned after the family had left and when Fleur was alone. She placed the familiar Sounding Bowl sideways into the bed, with the 'acoustic bud' facing Fleur. As she played and sang Fleur's name, Fleur opened her eyes in response.

Enabling the therapist

Clinical illustration

In her very early years of clinical practice, the Music Therapist encountered a dying dementia patient for the first time. Ben had engaged in one-to-one music therapy for an extended period. One week the therapist arrived on the ward to be told that Ben was in bed dying. She instinctively wanted to see him, but had no idea what to do clinically. She decided to simply go and say good-bye without the help of music. The experience left her feeling rather at a loss and wondering what else could have been done.

One can easily wonder where to start and feel extremely uncertain (perhaps fearful, exposed and even foolish) when attempting to undertake clinical work at the bedside of a dying person. Various factors contribute towards enabling the therapist to manage the challenges of such work. As diverse experience is gathered (both clinical and personal) the clinician gains maturity in approach and greater confidence in new situations. Clinical judgements draw on such experience.

Personal experience of bereavement perhaps brings a corresponding acceptance of one's own mortality, easing the ability to sit alongside a dying person.
Nevertheless, it is important to hold boundaries around the therapist's personal
loss experience in order to keep this separate from the clinical situation.

It is uncomfortable being with the dying. The therapist's feeling of 'being able
to manage' may be variable and relies to some extent on an ability to tolerate the
unknown. Multi-disciplinary Liaison is vital and one is strengthened by drawing
on a team approach. Additional supervision sought on an ad hoc basis can provide
further support with opportunities to debrief and explore counter-transference
issues.

The patient's powerlessness and dependency often strongly manifests itself in
the counter-transference, making the therapist *in that moment* feel disempowered
and unable to clearly think what to do. This can occur even when the therapist has
worked for a considerable time with the patient and has established many prior
successful techniques, perhaps underlining the tendency for end-of-life work to
feel intense and overwhelming. The additional physical symptoms seen in the
dying patient can also be disturbing, adding to the therapist's feeling of disem-
powerment. An ability to manage such feelings is important and greatly assisted
by supervision and Liaison with colleagues.

For Music Therapists it is standard practice to make audio recordings of clinical work. However, in order to protect privacy and avoid any sense of voyeurism,
I refrain from recording sessions when someone is in their last hours. This may
also lessen any feelings of self-consciousness on the part of the therapist.

Clinical illustration

*Brian had worked as a nurse specialising in the area of dementia. He was
admitted to hospital when his residential care home placement became unsus-
tainable. The Music Therapist worked with him for almost a year.*

*Despite his illness, Brian conveyed much character, dignity and politeness.
As the Music Therapist worked with him, she gradually discovered Brian's
'Palette of Possibilities'.*

*Instruments such as the cimbala (Figure 17.3) became prominent in the
work. Brian seemed to find this relaxing to listen to and would reach out
for it, sometimes holding onto the strings then transferring his grip to the
therapist's hand as she moved the instrument away. Brian would also hold
onto the therapist's fingers as she strummed the guitar with her thumb.
Occasionally he would nod and interject 'yes' and 'I like it'. The bass string
on the guitar stimulated the comment 'nice and lovely', so the therapist
would place the instrument across his lap and play this note whilst singing
to him. He once appeared to comment, 'I've got the guitar'. Sometimes
Brian pulled and pushed these instruments as if operating a machine – the
therapist later discovered from his niece Jane that Brian was enthusiastic
and skilled at DIY and enjoyed using many different types of tools.*

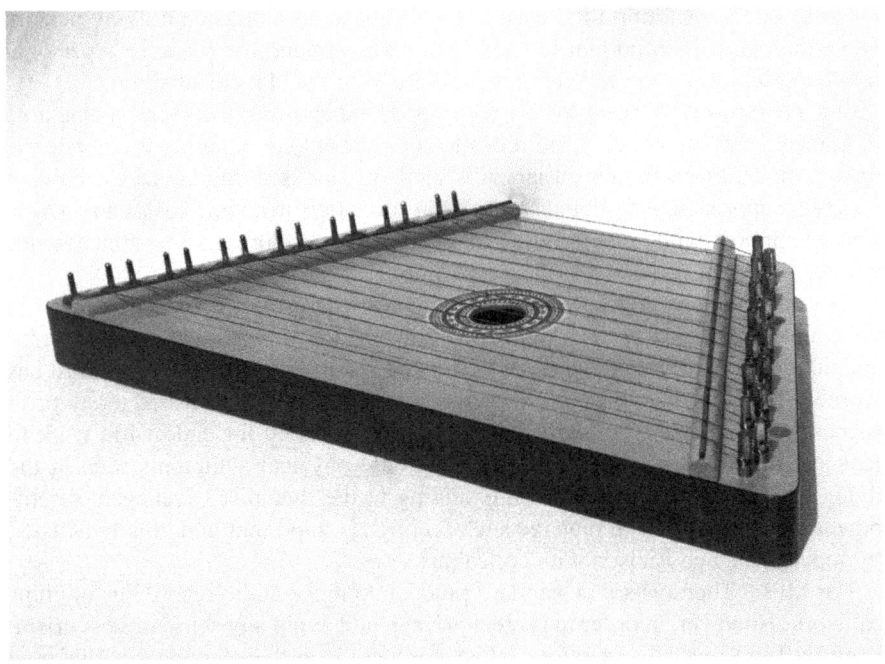

Figure 17.3 Cimbala

Using Brian's name in sung improvisations resulted in more sustained eye contact from him towards the therapist who observed that his facial expression appeared more relaxed when she sang. He once appeared to respond 'good afternoon' to her sung greeting. Brian often vocalised, almost in a conversational manner, with song-like sounds at distinct pitches which the therapist mirrored in her music. In the second session, as she sang with Brian's non-verbal vocalisations, he suddenly said 'that's right'.

When presented with a new instrument, Brian would look at the therapist alertly, once clearly saying 'hello' when another instrument was brought to him. His facial expression, as he laughed, seemed to be saying 'oh, it's you again, what **have** *you got now?' Brian retained his sense of humour – instruments such as the walking xylophone and energy chimes (Figure 17.4) he always found very funny. Sometimes he indicated he had had enough by withdrawing from the interaction.*

Wind-chimes and finger cymbals were used in a sensory manner, touched to Brian's hands. As the therapist held the instruments still, Brian would move his hand to feel or hold them. A week before he died, when the finger cymbals gently touched his hand, he said 'cold' (the metal of the instrument would have felt cold).

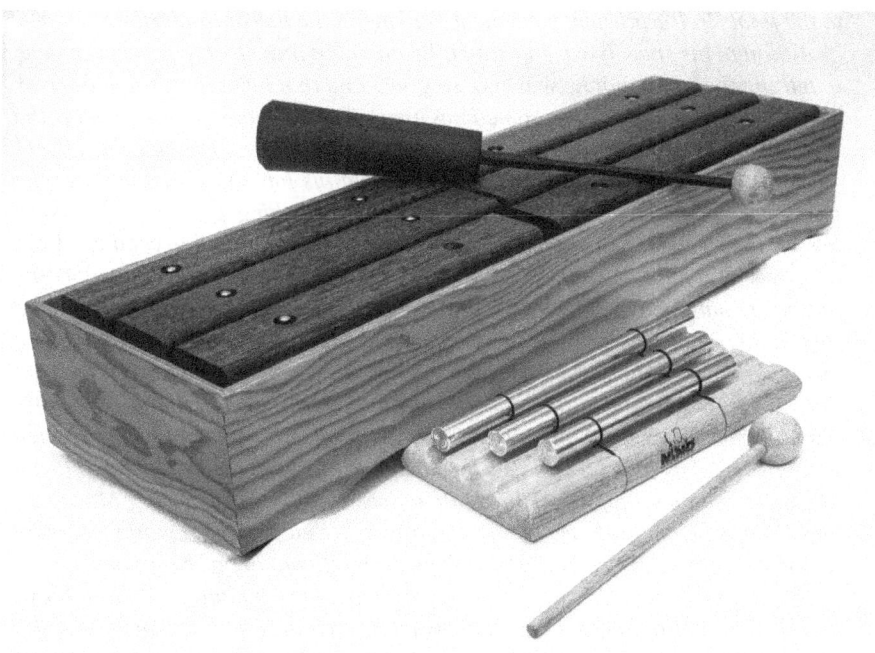

Figure 17.4 Walking xylophone and energy chimes

*Two weeks before Brian's death, the therapist (by chance or instinct) played the tune 'English Country Garden' on her violin. Brian seemed to acknowledge the song, becoming alert and attentively still – the therapist sensed that something important had been touched. She subsequently was informed by Jane that Brian had done other people's gardening as well as his own because he loved it so much! The therapist reflected how gardening can be a way of **taking care of things** and how through this song she was perhaps connecting with Brian's life and work.*

Brian's hobbies included driving at speed in his car and doing courses in other motorised vehicles such as racing cars and light aircraft. The therapist included such aspects in song, either pre-composed (such as 'Those Magnificent Men in their Flying Machines') or improvised. Jane commented that she felt the therapist's approach to the work reflected some of Brian's own thinking about this client group.

Music and concert-going had been important to Brian. Jane pointed out that he liked listening to solo instruments and that Fauré's 'Requiem' was a favourite work – Brian responded 'yes' when the therapist suggested to him that they listen to parts of this. Whilst listening, Brian vocalised the same note as the singers at various points. Fifteen days before he died, Brian attentively responded 'yes' to the final 'In Paradisum' movement, looking at the therapist alertly.

Although his speech was indistinct, Brian did in these last few weeks appear to tell the therapist that he was 'not so good' and that he had a cough. In prior weeks, Brian's vocalisations sometimes exacerbated his cough, which made the therapist wonder how to alter her music-making in order to reduce this effect.

On his last day, Brian was on oxygen to aid his laboured breathing, so the therapist avoided working musically with his breathing patterns. She found herself interweaving music-making with repositioning Brian's oxygen mask (as agreed with nursing staff), which his mouth movements kept dislodging. As the therapist continued playing gentle music, particularly on the cimbala, it seemed that Brian relaxed a little for he stopped making such strong mouthing movements and seemed to settle. The therapist therefore carried on playing for some time, improvising music that incorporated the rhythm and sound of Brian's name in various ways. Staff coming into his room commented that he seemed more peaceful as a result of music therapy. The therapist talked briefly to Brian about his hobbies, singing 'Those Magnificent Men in their Flying Machines' and 'English Country Garden'. She also improvised gently on violin, recorder and walking xylophone, which had all been significant in prior sessions.

Several familiar CD tracks were interspersed, including Julian Lloyd Webber on 'cello then the 'In Paradisum' from Fauré's Requiem. The lyrics seemed apt: **'may the angels lead you into paradise . . . may you have eternal rest'**. *A few hours later, Brian died.*

Afterwards, Jane told the therapist:

> *I continue to be so grateful to everyone on the ward for the care they gave Brian and also the way they looked after him at the end. . . . It was very important to me at the time that you sat with him.*

Finding appropriate ways of spending time with Brian on his last day took up all the therapist's clinical time. Her line manager was validating of this shortly afterwards when she went to debrief, feeling remiss about not seeing other patients that day. She wrote in her personal reflections: 'I really do not know much about working with the actual dying. I worked instinctively'. Such an instinctive approach was generally encouraged by her clinical supervisor.

Involvement in funerals

Clinicians may be invited to be involved in their patient's funeral especially after clinical work which has included the patient's spouse. This can be difficult, for one is entering a very personal family space at a highly sensitive time. On such an occasion the therapist's role may be somewhat altered, for they are no longer within the clinical session. Their role here could perhaps now be seen as a specialised extension and ending to the relationship that has already been established with families on the ward outside (and sometimes within) sessions. After a lengthy piece of clinical engagement, funeral involvement can represent a fitting end to the work. The clinician also represents their employing organisation.

For the therapist each occasion differs according to the wishes of next-of-kin. On occasion the therapist might be asked to contribute in a particular way: I have experienced being requested by next-of-kin to give a short tribute, prepared with their specific guidance and approval. At one funeral, I was informed by the patient's wife that music therapy had helped her to say good-bye to her husband. She had been surprised to find that music therapy had enabled them both to enjoy renewed intimacy through dance and shared music-making. She had also been able to use sessions to reflect upon her husband's deteriorating condition together with gradually acknowledging his imminent passing and its implications for her (for further description of this case see Freeman, 2017, p. 48) .

Conclusion

It is unsurprising that the effects of music therapy for people in the final stages of dementia comply with National Institute for Health and Care Excellence (NICE) Guidelines (2006) and the Department of Health's Dementia Strategy (2009) which aim to improve the quality of care for people with dementia, both throughout their illness and at end of life. Spiro et al. (2017) investigated how music therapy contributes towards the aims of the Dementia Strategy, sampling family members, staff, managers and Music Therapists. Their findings (2017, p. 259) showed that 'the Dementia Strategy . . . objectives that are related to direct activity of the music therapists (such as care and understanding of the condition) were seen as most fulfilled by music therapy'. One suggestion of this study's findings was that the sampled Music Therapists possibly had little experience of work at end-of-life and in a hospital setting (2017, p. 268), both of which are the remit of this chapter. The allocation of Music Therapists to settings for later stages of dementia can be somewhat random and to some extent relies on the therapist being in the right place at the right time in order to carry out such work.

This chapter has explored the role of music therapy in accompanying the dying person with dementia. Factors that equip the therapist for this task have included drawing on the strength of the multi-disciplinary team and receiving good supervision. Consideration has been given to influences upon clinical judgement executed in undertaking final clinical interventions. Both the patient's personal history and their music therapy history are significant at such times. Clinical illustrations have demonstrated that music therapy can affect levels of alertness and aid relaxation, serving to underline its impact at end-of-life.

Acknowledgements

Special thanks go to all who enabled this work, particularly patients and their loved ones; multi-disciplinary colleagues; Dr Julia Brownlie and Dr Rachel Darnley-Smith for supervision; and my family, especially for their assistance with images and proof-reading.

References

Bunt, L. (1994). *Music Therapy: An Art Beyond Words*. London: Routledge.

Chinese character 'To Listen' together with photographs: provided by Ejay Freeman, Interior Design student at The University of Edinburgh.

Clair, A. (2000). The importance of singing with elderly patients. In D. Aldridge (ed.) *Music Therapy in Dementia Care*. London: Jessica Kingsley Publishers.

Cueva, M. (2006). Moving beyond edutainment to engagement. *Journal of Cancer Education*, 21(3), 141.

Department of Health. (2009). *Living Well with Dementia: A National Dementia Strategy* (online). Available at www.gov.uk/government/uploads/system/uploads/attachment_data/file/168220/dh_094051.pdf [accessed 21 January 2017].

Du Boulay, S., and Rankin, M. (2007). *Cicely Saunders: The Founder of the Modern Hospice Movement*. London: SPCK.

Eliot, T.S. (1944). *Four Quartets*. London: Faber and Faber.

Freeman, A. (2017). Fathoming the constellations: Ways of working with families in music therapy for people with advanced dementia. *British Journal of Music Therapy*, 31(1), 43–49.

Hardy, T. (1917/2005). The choirmaster's burial. In J. Gibson (ed.) *Chosen Poems of Thomas Hardy*. Cerne Abbas: Casterbridge Books, p.104.

Jia, Y., and Liu, C. (2010). Listening as an indispensable access to dialogues among cultures. *Intercultural Communication Studies*, 19(2), 104–110.

Krout, R. (2003). Music therapy with imminently dying hospice patients and their families: Facilitating release near the time of death. *American Journal of Hospice & Palliative Care*, 20(2), 129–134.

Mayne, M. (2002). Music, spirituality, healing: This intimate stranger. Keynote presentation at the 10th World Congress of Music Therapy, Oxford. *BSMT Bulletin*, 44/45(Summer/Autumn double issue), 31–40.

National Institute for Health and Care Excellence (NICE). (2006). *Dementia: Supporting People with Dementia and their Carers in Health and Social Care* (online). Available at www.nice.org.uk/guidance/cg42/chapter/1-Guidance [accessed 21 January 2017].

Sisson, R. (1990). Effects of auditory stimuli on comatose patients with head injury. *Heart & Lung: The Journal of Critical Care*, 19(4), 373–378. Available at http://europepmc.org/abstract/med/2370168 [accessed 22 October 2017].

Spiro, N., Farrant, C.L., and Pavlicevic, M. (2017). Between practice, policy and politics: Music therapy and the Dementia Strategy, 2009. *Dementia*, 16(3), 259–281.

Tapson, K., Sierotowicz, W., Marks-Maran, D., and Thompson, T.M. (2015). 'It's the hearing that is last to go': A case of traumatic head injury. *British Journal of Nursing*, 24(5), 277–281. Available at www.ncbi.nlm.nih.gov/pubmed/25757582 [accessed 22 October 2017].

Thompson, R. (2011). Using life story work to enhance care. *Nursing Older People*, 23(8), 16–21. Available at www.dementiauk.org/for-healthcare-professionals/free-resources/life-story-work/ [accessed 15 September 2016].

Weber, S. (1999). Music: A means of comfort. In D. Aldridge (ed.) *Music Therapy in Palliative Care: New Voices*. London: Jessica Kingsley Publishers.

Worth, J. (2005). *Shadows of the Workhouse*. London: Phoenix, Orion Books.

Chapter 18

Can anything good be born of a dementia

Potential for reparation?

Jane Garner

'*The heart has its reason, which reason knows nothing of*'
(*Pensées, Blaise Pascal 1670*)

Introduction

The term 'dementia' has had various meanings over the years, once synonymous with 'madness', 'insanity' and 'lunacy'. Even a modern OED defines it as a 'species of insanity characterised by failure or loss of the mental powers'. Whatever the definition the connotations of the word are almost exclusively negative. Health professionals concentrate on the disabilities occasioned by the condition the dysmnesias, dysphasias, dyspraxias, discontents, incontinence, neurological fits, flexion and rigidity, negative changes in personality and behaviour. The common opinion of the destructive horror of dementia is reasonable and understandable but also omits greater consideration of aspects of the person, the self unaffected by the disease process, thinking beyond the medical model. One may come to learn what about the self is being lost and what will always remain (Bryden, 2005). This chapter is an attempt to think about possible positive changes in relational aspects of the illness despite the overtly negative ones.

A biopsychosociocultural process

The patient with dementia may have the experience of witnessing their own decline in abilities and as skills are lost may come the existential terror of anticipating loss of self. Not only the patient but also informal and professional carers will witness the loss of ego functions in the sufferer. Spouse and family carers have varied reactions depending on the type and quality of the prior relationship and experiences. Often the feeling is of intense loss with consequent grief (Garner, 1997) at losing aspects of the relationship, the loss of aspects of the self and of memories invested in the patient. Professionals too are affected by the disease process feeling deskilled by the vulnerability and apparent helplessness of the patient (no doubt accounting for the over prescription of major tranquillisers to this group as the helplessness is projected onto the staff and then acted out) (Garner, 2004a). Main (1957) reminds us that in spite of professional ideals ordinary human feelings are inevitable and also that we need to recognise and examine them. The underdeveloped space between our cognitive and emotional understanding gives us more in common with our patients than we may wish to think. Undoubtedly there are organic determinants to a dementing illness, but it is possible to be taken up by biological explanations and treatments to the exclusion of other aspects. The presentation of the illness will be biopsychosociocultural and needs to be understood in all the parts of that term. We know the interaction of psychosocial conditions and organic changes when considering the brain effects of abuse on children. Advances in neuroscience research have led to a more integrated and sophisticated understanding of not only mind changes but also brain changes following psychotherapy and environmental impact on gene expression (Gabbard, 2000). We understandably emphasise cognitive factors and disabilities in dementia. Neuropsychological testing emphasises left hemisphere functions, but non cognitive factors play an important part in the presentation. It is easy to have expectations and assumptions about people with dementia, for us to appear demeaning and disregarding. Kitwood (1990) terms this 'malignant social psychology' – it can affect family as well as staff. Attitudes of those around the patient can mean that they function in a more disabled way than the degree of illness would determine alone. Meisen (1998) writes of the 'metaphorical decapitation' to which it is easy to subject dementia patients by not taking their emotional needs seriously. Solms (1995) who is both a neuropsychologist and a psychoanalyst regrets that within mental health services the brain is getting bigger and the mind smaller. However, we know that psychological symptoms cannot be reduced to only organic lesions. In such reductionism we lose what we are looking at. We used to think dichotomously of depression being endogenous or reactive, aetiologically biological or psychological, organically determined psychoses and psychologically determined neuroses, now we consider conditions rather more broadly. The early theories of Freud, the neurologist, had a biological basis. When he later departed from this theme it was with the thought that psychoanalysis, biochemistry and neurology would rejoin. A century and more later this conjunction is still awaited. Perhaps it is in work with patients with dementia that biological, psychological and social research and clinical work can develop together. Evans (2008) in writing of how psychoanalytic ideas can help us understand the experience of patients with dementia reminds us that although some forgetting is undoubtedly due to organic brain damage, some may also be a defence as in us all.

Some more positive aspects of age

Old age and dementia are not synonymous, but part of the stigma and neglect inflicted on patients with dementia are associated with the demography of the disease – the majority of sufferers are over 65 and it forms a caricature of old age. We live in an ageist society which values youth, physical prowess, independence, enterprise and productivity (Garner, 2004c). Dartington (2010) questions the acceptability of vulnerability in our society. Bell (1996) suggests that the introduction of the ideology of the market into socialised medicine is an attack upon human values with dependency and vulnerability regarded as despicable weakness. We are fascinated/obsessed by how to stay young rather than how to age well and some spend a financial and perhaps emotional fortune having bits of their bodies removed and other bits pumped up to maintain or regain a youthful face and silhouette. However, there are advantages to being older (Garner, 2009) and seeing it as part of life's ongoing adventure. There is good evidence that older people have outcomes from different types of psychotherapy, including psychodynamic, that are at least equal to those for younger people (Knight, 1996; Woods and Roth, 1996; Garner, 2013). Many do not wish to repeat being younger but appreciate the maturity which may develop in working through the depressive position – one may develop a basic benevolent attitude with the ability to love oneself and others as whole objects (Quinodoz, 2010). This change can also apply to objects in the internal world who died long ago or for other reasons cannot currently respond to reconciliation. Improving relationships in the internal world may give order also to the external world. Psychosocial development does not stop when we are young but continues until we die, change is inevitable but is not necessarily synonymous with decline (Garner, 2004b). There is the potential to view life through the lens of experience and from a perspective informed by decades of acquired knowledge and having managed sorrows, joys, failures, disappointments and losses. We take into the senium the possibility of growth in response to adversity, character strengths and coping skills developed earlier in life along with an increased capacity for delayed gratification and for getting on with things. Brains do decrease in weight and volume by 2% per decade, but normal ageing is not a straightforward decline in cognitive function. Verbal and numeric ability is usually preserved, well-practised skills show little decline, vocabulary and semantic tasks tend to be stable. There tends to be life-long stability in autobiographical memory, theory of mind tasks and implicit memory. Some creative individuals continue working into late life, e.g. Hokusai, Picasso, Verdi, some embarking on new ideas and techniques. Goya experimented in his 70s with the newly discovered medium of lithography. Matisse, when bedridden in his final years, invented a new art form, gouaches découpées, in which he instructed his assistant in the meticulous arrangement of brightly coloured cut-out shapes into patterns.

Retirement from paid work for some is difficult 'laboro ergo sum' (I work therefore I am): identity and self-esteem, libidinal investments, false self-identities and a sense of social inclusion are tied up with professional identities. Work may be a denial of ageing and death. For others who can afford it, casting off the burden of work comes as a great relief and release and they are able to use the increased time available to realise new skills and put their energies into making and keeping relationships. Ageing itself, for those with sufficient internal resources, can be a creative process in developmental adaptation. Salzberger-Wittenberg (1970) thinks even the negative experiences can be a source of growth, strengthening the individual.

A sexless old age is the dominant societal myth (Garner and Bacelle, 2004) and health professionals tend to go along with that being reluctant to embark on conversations about sexuality with older patients. However, the reality for those older individuals who have not allowed themselves to be taken up by these negative attitudes may be very different (Garner and Bacelle, 2016). Sexuality may be no longer 'driven' but more sensual and in the service of a tender and affectionate object relationship. Gender response may be better synchronised with the requirement for longer foreplay and delay in male orgasm. There is no reason in age per se why a sexual life should not continue into old age for both the psychological and physical benefit of older people.

At a societal and political level older people tend to be lumped together in thought and policy documents as a homogenous mass, whereas diversity actually increases with age. At 70 there are seven decades of individualised experience to make a difference between one and the next 70 year old and all of the others.

Although older people are characterised as the 'demographic time bomb', as a burden on the younger taxpayer, as passive recipients of care, they are more often providers of care. Older people are a resource for their families, for communities and for society. In Africa it is older people who provide most of the care for Aids patients and orphans. In the UK most of the care for sufferers of dementia is provided by older people who are therefore part of the solution to the so-called ageing problem.

Some more positive aspects of dementia and relationship with the other

Despite the horror and suffering involved in a dementing illness there may also be aspects which are less negative, all of us are more than any diagnosis we attract. Positive psychology uses the idea of affect-balance, the relative balance between positive and negative emotions on a daily basis – the positive needs to outweigh the negative (Clarke and Wolverson, 2016). Alzheimer Scotland has a publication 'Remember I am still me'. Self-help books for patients and carers (Garner, 2007) can present a way of thinking and managing. They are written in different styles which would suit different readers. If the book is couched in too positive a manner the reader, either patient or carer, may feel a failure by contrast that they have not managed as well as the author. However, in *Dancing with Dementia* Christine Bryden (2005) tells us that people can still live well, can still maintain old relationships and make new ones – including marrying after the diagnosis.

The creative process may persist in dementia. William de Kooning's (1904–1997) later works caused great controversy in the world of art. Espinel (2007) wrote of creating in the midst of dementia, others saw a falling off of mastery, or were the works removed from the studio unfinished? During the late 1940s early 1950s, de Kooning became an acknowledged leader of American progressive painting, an abstract expressionist also known as 'action painting'. He was diagnosed in 1989 with Alzheimer's Disease complicated by alcoholism. Although the court proclaimed him unfit to manage his affairs, he continued to paint. His wife Elaine an art critic, who had supported him until her death in 1989, had said 30 years earlier 'a painting to me is primarily a verb, not a noun, an event first and only secondarily an image'. This fits in with his label of 'action painter'. His view of art perhaps explains why painters continue even when experiencing a dementia 'the attitude that nature is chaotic and that the artist puts order into it is a very absurd point of view, I think. All that we can hope for is to put some order into ourselves' (William de Kooning from Hess [2005, p. 15]). Continuing creative work may be aimed at battling against psychic disorganisation (Polini, 2007). Polini writes of William Utermohlen (1933–2007) charting his work before, at the time of and after his diagnosis of Alzheimer's Disease in 1985 age 62. He painted his daily life and routines, anchoring him in the world. As the disease progressed, the domestic world tended to lose perspective seeming disorganised and unstable. Following the diagnosis his self-portraits conveyed pain, waiting for death. There was an asymmetry sometimes with half the face ageing and decaying the other half lively and vivacious. He was seeing his deterioration but was maintaining a sense of self. He communicates through art what it feels like inside of the disease.

Creativity is not only about artistry and continuing to express through previously held imaginative skills but it is about being alive. All of us even when suffering from a dementia may have creativity in human contact and relationships.

We take into old age and also into dementia much more than neuropathology, we take our personality and attachment development, life history and experience, relationship history and experience and may draw on all of this. Some, although fearful, see the illness as a challenge and are determined to do their best in the face of it. The disease is no respecter of persons, anyone of us may develop it, 'in his old age, Sophocles was accused of being weak minded' (Cicero 44 BCE). Terry Pratchett the novelist who publicly shared his diagnosis of posterior cortical atrophy had wanted it to be known 'I'm not dead yet'. We are aware of existing at many levels – the social constructivists describe layers of personae. The external selves may change, deteriorate, but the singularity of the person, the interiority, 'I AM', persists until death (Garner, 2004c). Due to this persisting affective self the acceptance and empathy which is required of the staff or carer may unexpectedly also be found in the patient (Lipinska, 2009). The patient while living in the minute, in the present, will have emotional memories if not cognitive ones. As the patient loses cognitive strengths they rely more on external relationships and internal representations of earlier ones, of those aspects of the self unaffected by the disease process. As the false self dissolves perhaps a more authentic self emerges over time. Many losses occur but in part some losses maybe the uncovering of something previously buried, qualities which had not been able to be expressed adequately before. (Jung, 1960) writes of 'glowing coals under grey ashes'. Perhaps we need to look harder for the glow. For and from the patient concrete detail goes but affective memory and self remain. Communication continues, it will not only be verbal, but will rely on the 'other' listening not necessarily to the lack of coherence but to the manner of expression, the non-verbal cues, feelings evoked in the listener. Communications may be disjointed and need piecing together. This requires either training and psychological sophistication or warmth for and intimate knowledge of the patient. The attitude of the other is a crucial factor in the enabling of the patient to feel understood and to have back some control. If the other is able to understand, without retaliation, without expectation, the patient is given a sense that there is a containing mind. Waddell (2007) writes a moving account of family interactions – the elderly mother has a dementing illness, father some forgetfulness, daughter and son recognise the healing properties of listening, of entering the inner world taking time to see the mother as unique in a unique situation. They also see that the terror of dementia needs containment. No patient is beyond hope, there is always something that can be done – that something is *thinking*. Bion (1970) spoke of containment and that there was a 'thinker' in a therapeutic relationship. Much is expected of the other, never to be frightened nor confident but accepting. Bion wrote of the 'reverie' of the mother managing the emotional states of the infant and giving them meaning. In dementia the more the mind is lost, the more the patient is dependent on the thinking of the other and for receiving a sense of containment. The state of mind of the carer/relative is vital in influencing the experience of the patient and how fragmented they feel. This seems to put yet another burden on the relative but if they are able to manage any of this the reward is felt within the relational world of the patient who will be less disintegrated, more of themselves. Waddell (1998) writes of 'windows of clarity' if it has been possible to make emotional contact with the patient's inner world. For Sinason (1992) strong emotion in the patient or the sense of being understood produces integration for them albeit temporarily. The illness trajectory of the patient is not solely determined by the neurophysiology of the dementia. It is the interaction between the married couple and the emotional commitment of the carer, the quality of the relationship determines which patients will not only be at home but also be alive two years later (Wright, 1994). Patients within a sexually active couple are less likely to be admitted to a home (Wright, 1998). Positive attitudes, behaviour and understanding in the other clearly affect attitudes, behaviour and understanding in the patient. Shifts in power and dependency which can be disturbing in the constellation of some families, for others may be a resolution to previous anxieties.

Development

The relationship with the 'care giver' in adulthood seems as important as security and understanding in the relationship with the earliest caregiver. The way in which early experiences of physical and emotional dependency are remembered greatly determines the capacity to face the dependency of dementia (Martindale, 1989). The capacity for trust which is the first stage for the baby to negotiate (Erikson, 1959) is once more to the fore. This link between early experience and later life dependency can determine how negative (or positive) the experience of dementia is both for the patient and for the other. Not everyone with a dementing illness uses paranoid defences or becomes deluded or aggressive (when they do this may have a protective function). Different states of mind from different stages of development shift and oscillate in relation to each other however young or old the patient (Waddell, 1998). If basic trust has been a hallmark of early experience and dementia develops later the patient will be open to caring attention and not feel the other will be disgusted by them and hate them. The other will feel acknowledged in terms of loving trust. It is not only psychologists/analysts who have an understanding of the human experience being eternally present in our past, present and future, it has been a theme also for poets and writers over the years. *'Eternity was in that moment'*, *Wm Congreve, The Old Bachelor, 1693*.

Reparation and understanding

As the patient continues to be an emotional being with their developmental history internalised despite the disease, then resolution, forgiveness and reconciliation may be possible between those involved – higher cognitive skills are not necessary for these affective tasks. Reparation is possible. Reparation according to the OED is the act of repairing or mending, the action of making amends for a wrong done. In *A critical dictionary of psychoanalysis* (1968) it is 'the process of reducing guilt by action designed to make good the harm imagined to have been done to an ambivalently invested object'. Klein (1930) regards all creative activity as reparative with reparation a normal process by which one resolves inherent ambivalence to objects, the love and hate we feel for the same person. Reparative work may still be done by the patient with dementia who retains an affective interior self as well as by the other in the relationship who may also be engaged in the creative process of caring.

Occasionally the development of dementia may be used as a reason/excuse for abandoning the spouse in a couple who were anyway living in emotional alienation. Some take on the caring role because they feel they should, as an obligation. Others take it on more willingly as evidence of love and commitment. Some see it as a way of acknowledging and paying back for previous positive aspects in the relationship. A lot is expected of the one who takes on care, not only the physical tasks but also psychosocial ones. Our daily management of patients in which we are deficient in emotional understanding (Evans, 2008) extends also to the family and carers – they can feel emotionally isolated or out of their depth. Behaviour in dementia may be seen as a symptom without meaning. When one is non-demented it is possible to step back from one's own behaviour, wonder about it and give it meaning; when the patient has dementia it is up to others to give meaning and understanding and to help the patient make sense of the current moment. In return the person with dementia may help us appreciate or teach us how to live in the moment, capture the moment which is difficult for many who are ostensibly 'well' but are dashing around *doing* rather than *being* and putting off *life* until this particular important project is over . . . and the next and the next.

In a BBC interview (02.05.2015) a daughter commented that she took her father with dementia for a drive. 'We had a lovely time – he can no longer remember the standards I don't live up to'. A humorous way of reporting the change in the relationship, however the change in Father's attitude may not be just dysmnesia.

Clinical illustration

Ella Jones was diagnosed with Alzheimer's Disease in her 70s a few months before her husband died. They had been in a loving marriage of traditional roles for 50 years. There were two children, Marie and her younger brother. Marie's life was overtly different from her mother's. Ella was bright but not particularly well educated. She encouraged and supported education for her children and decided from an early age that her daughter should be a doctor, and so she became. Marie disliked being a medical student and would have given up if she could summon the courage to tell her parents but once qualified things were better and she departed from Ella's ideas that she would be a paediatrician or GP and chose medicine for the elderly. Her work with older patients was initially motivated by politico-philosophical considerations about supporting the least well off, most stigmatised in society. It did not seem then to be about remaking relationships with older family members. She had good memories and feelings about her maternal grandparents; grandfather was endlessly patient and seemed to possess some maternal qualities, grandmother was glamorous and witty. Her relationship with her mother felt less than ideal. Ella was assiduous, even perfect, in her physical care of the children. Every domestic task was undertaken: biscuits, cakes and most clothes were homemade, she cared well for the children when they were ill, she was always at home when they returned from school with tea on the table the moment father's key was in the door. This housewifely perfection irritated Marie immensely as it was not accompanied by the possibility of discussion of anything but positive feelings about life. She complained about her mother to her school friends, but for them it was difficult to understand as they found Ella a delight when they met her. Marie as 'aspiring intellectual' in adolescence continued to react to her mother's 'niceness', practicality and efficiency by being contradictory and contrary. These negative feelings about mother continued far into adult life along with a painful guilt because of them. Ella herself could never miss an opportunity to criticise her daughter (not others) in what felt like every utterance – there was always something wrong with her hairstyle, her makeup, her clothes, the fact that she lived in Birmingham having moved away from the small town to attend university and not having returned – all this despite her also being proud of Marie and her qualifications. When Marie tried to take up the criticisms it was laughed off and she was further criticised for not being able to take a joke.

The death of her father was a difficult time for Marie, along with her personal grief was guilt about her widowed mother living alone at considerable distance and now with Alzheimer's Disease. The role of direct, practical care giving can be an immense trial and strain particularly in the context of

preceding ambivalence in the relationship. Marie knew she could not under-
take that but maybe there were things she could do. In middle age with some
maturity she had begun at last to really appreciate all she owed to her par-
ents, including her mother. She had thought that in these circumstances she
would be ruthless and uncaring and felt a degree of self-loathing and guilt
about that – instead she was surprised to find that as well as recalling her
negative feelings she also felt 'ruth': pity, compassion and concern. From
her professional work she knew how to negotiate her way round health and
social services. Using enduring power of attorney which had been organised
by father many years earlier, she arranged care for Ella via direct payments,
employing carers eventually for 24 hours per day. Although she was at a
distance she was involved frequently and regularly, feeling pleased to use the
education, training and skills which her parents had made possible.

The characteristics of her mother which Marie had previously disliked now
proved themselves capable of sustaining Ella and others in these new and dif-
ficult circumstances. Although initially anxious about her state and not want-
ing to hear a diagnosis Ella took well to receiving care considering the carers
her friends and the carers in turn found much to like even love about her.

Ella's habit of always leaving the bathroom door ajar which had disgusted
and infuriated Marie in earlier times now helped Ella bear the dependence
of having others perform intimate personal care tasks for her in apparent
comfort. Perhaps early trust was being enacted. Throughout her life, also
into illness, Ella had described her own mother as particularly beautiful and
she saw beauty also in the natural world, the countryside where she and her
husband had moved after his retirement. Aesthetic considerations play an
important role in development. Intense appreciation of beauty is perhaps the
same as the reaction of the newborn to the first sight of its mother and her
breast, the perception of beauty as the idealised good object in the passions
of intimate relationship. It is rare in development 'for the original passionate
response to the beauty of the world and of the mother, her breast and her face
as the objects of its passion to remain undiminished' (Meltzer and Williams,
1988, p. 159). However, that seemed the case for Ella, she only rarely men-
tioned that her mother could be domineering and a snob, rather talk was all
about her beauty which she also saw reflected in the world – at least in her
part of it. In illness when still mobile she walked around the house indicating
objects 'my mother gave me that' whether or not that was actually the case.
The family of origin takes on increasing importance in the mind of the patient
with dementia. Parent fixation is unlikely to be purely a dysmnesic problem
but an equivalent of attachment behaviour in response to the fear and feeling
of loss evoked by the disease. At times she had said that she saw aspects of
her mother in her daughter. Perhaps Marie had received the criticisms infre-
quently voiced about Ella's mother who had endured the dependency and
pain of immobilising arthritis with great stoicism. Often older people identify
with the fate of their own parents in the last part of their lives.

Ella had never engaged in gossip nor speaking badly of others, she was never overtly angry nor depressed but only expressed attitudes of thanks and gratitude – all of which had exasperated Marie previously but which now helped Ella and her carers. Marie no longer took the automatic contrarian views she had taken in adolescence and for many years beyond. She was pleased to be mindful of her mother's needs, to think about 'best interests' and the relationship between philosophical theory, ethics and actual human practice. She was an involved participant in the care despite geographical distance and reflected on her mother's and her own conscious and unconscious processes. Lipinska (2009) reflects that one may have a new, real and refreshingly unencumbered relationship with the person with dementia. When Marie was able to visit the warmth and pleasure in her mother's greeting was fantastical to her. There was no criticism of her at all. Any criticism, albeit limited, was directed to the carers who because of greater emotional distance were able to laugh it off. To Marie, arms were outstretched with exclamations of 'Oh you are so lovely, I do love you' and many kisses. This could be repeated many times and Marie did not tire of it.

Ella clearly retained good internal objects and fleeting hallucinations were benign, her father or auntie Lucy. When people in her presence were laughing, she too laughed not having any paranoid interpretation but enjoying the contact and togetherness. She did not seem to have conscious or unconscious preoccupations with the possibility of future losses which for some cause psychopathology and suffering (Martindale, 2007).

Marie often wondered how the relationship would have been if Ella had remained cognitively well. As it was, although late, reparation was achieved for Marie, perhaps also for Ella. Harm done to the ambivalently invested object was made good – and it felt if not good because of the disease, certainly much better.

Conclusion

Much that old age brings can be difficult and unpleasant but along with greater likelihood of loss, bereavement and ill health may also come some advantages: experience and knowledge, the ability to make and remake relationships – external and internal – and the possibility of review and acceptance of one's own life.

Developing dementia may be seen as one of the worst things that can happen in life. It is reported to be the most feared illness among the general public (Brunet et al., 2012). It will happen to 25% of the over 80s. Although dementia has neurobiological determinants it occurs to the patient in the context of a human life, a personal history and development, relationships and personality. Paradoxically, more positive aspects of the person previously hidden may be revealed and available. These aspects of personality and previous experience will provide the possibility of coping with the dementia for the patient and their partner/family; perhaps also for setting things right in relationships, for reparation.

Our expectations of someone with a dementia are limited, we tend to have rather nihilistic assumptions about what is possible. However, the ability to make relationships is retained, some memories can be laid down (Williams and Garner, 1998) and psychotherapeutic work is possible. Person-centred counselling (Lipinska, 2009) encourages empathy, unconditional positive regard and congruence as ways of relating to a patient. These concepts can be explained and taught both to professional staff and also to the family. If the informal carer can use any of these ideas and tolerate 'not knowing' then there will be positive effects in the relationship. Dementia powerfully evokes feelings in the 'other' love, hate, compassion and disgust. If the positive of these emotions are available with an understanding that each of us is more than any diagnosis then changes may occur in the relationship. It is difficult to be in sustained contact with the disturbed state of mind (Waddell, 1998) which dementia produces – the other may become irritated, frustrated, bored. Attentiveness on the relationship using thoughtful mind and feeling heart can produce a different experience and positive early experiences/trust internalised by the patient may come to the fore.

The clinical illustration given suggests it is possible to repair relationships, find aspects long forgotten – the daughter was, with compassion, able to see positive aspects of mother previously hidden to her, mother was able to use a good early care receiving experience and to express warmth and love assumed to have lain under the previously critical attitude. For the daughter, attentive thinking was important, for the mother retaining good internal objects – using experience in the past for the future.

Acknowledgement

Part of the clinical illustration (993 words) was published under the title "The Daughter's Tale" on the website of the community interest company "Innovations in Dementia" 2014. It was written by the chapter author, permission has been given to reproduce the information here www.innovationsindementia.org.uk

References

Bell, D. (1996). Primitive mind of state. *Psychoanalytic Psychotherapy*, 10(1), 45–47.

Bion, W.R. (1970). *Attention and Interpretation*. London: Tavistock Publications.

Brunet, M.D., McCartney, M., Heath, I., Tomlinson, J., et al. (2012). There is no evidence base for proposed dementia screening. *BMJ*, 345, e8588.

Bryden, C. (2005). *Dancing With Dementia*. London: Jessica Kingsley.

Clarke, C., and Wolverson, E. (eds.). (2016). *Positive Psychology Approaches to Dementia*. London: Jessica Kingsley.

Dartington, T. (2010). *Managing Vulnerability: The Underlying Dynamics of Systems of Care*. London: Karnac.

Erikson, E. (1959). *Identity and the Life Cycle Psychological Issues Monograph No 1*. New York: International Universities Press.

Espinel, C. (2007). Memory and the creation of art: The syndrome, as in de Kooning, of 'creating in the midst of dementia'. *Frontiers of Neurology and Neuroscience*, 22, 150–168.

Evans, S. (2008). Beyond forgetfulness: How psychoanalytic ideas can help us to understand the experience of patients with dementia. *Psychoanalytic Psychotherapy*, 22(3), 155–176.

Gabbard, G. (2000). A neurologically informed perspective on psychotherapy. *British Journal of Psychiatry*, 177, 117–122.

Garner, J. (1997). Dementia: An intimate death. *British Journal of Medical Psychology*, 70, 177–184.

Garner, J. (2004a). Dementia, chapter 15 in S. Evans and J. Garner (eds.) *Talking Over the Years: A Handbook of Psychoanalytic Psychotherapy With Older People*. Hove: Brunner-Routledge.

Garner, J. (2004b). Growing into old age: Erikson and others, chapter 6 in S. Evans and J. Garner (eds.) *Talking Over the Years: A Handbook of Dynamic Psychotherapy With Older Adults*. Hove: Brunner-Routledge.

Garner, J. (2004c). 'Identity and Alzheimer's' disease, chapter 4 in D. Kelleher and G. Leavey (eds.) *Identity and Health*. London: Routledge.

Garner, J. (2007). Reading about self-help books on dementia. *Psychiatric Bulletin*, 31(3), 118–119.

Garner, J. (2009). Considerably better than the alternative: Positive aspects of getting older. *Quality in Ageing*, 10(1), 5–8.

Garner, J. (2013). Psychodynamic psychotherapy, chapter 19 in T. Dening and A. Thomas (eds.) *Oxford Textbook of Old Age Psychiatry*, 2nd ed. Oxford: Oxford University Press.

Garner, J., and Bacelle, L. (2004). Sexuality, chapter 17 in S. Evans and J. Garner (eds.) *Talking Over the Years: A Handbook of Psychodynamic Psychotherapy with Older Adults*. Hove: Brunner-Routledge.

Garner, J., & Bacelle, L. (2016). Intimacy and sexuality in old age. In C. Fenieux & R.Rojas (eds.), Sexo y psicoanálisis. *Una mirada a la Intimidad Adulta, Santiago: La Pólvora Editorial* pp. 141–58.

Hess, B. (2005). *Abstract Expressionism*. Los Angeles: Taschen.

Jung, C.G. (1960). The stages of life. In *CW* 8.

Kitwood, T. (1990). The dialectics of dementia: With particular reference to Alzheimer's Disease. *Ageing & Society*, 10, 177–196.

Klein, M. (1930). *Love, Guilt and Reparation and other works*. London, Routledge.

Knight, B.G. (1996). Psychodynamic therapy with older adults: Lessons from scientific gerontology. In R. Woods (ed.) *Handbook of the Clinical Psychology of Ageing*. Chichester: Wiley.

Lipinska, D. (2009). *Person Centred Counselling for People With Dementia: Making Sense of Self*. London: Jessica Kingsley.

Main, T. (1957). The ailment. *Medical Psychology*, 30, 129–145.

Martindale, B. (1989). Becoming dependent again: The fears of some elderly persons and their younger therapists. *Psychoanalytic Psychotherapy*, 4(1), 67–75.

Martindale, B. (2007). Resilience and vulnerablity in later life. *British Journal of Psychotherapy*, 23(2), 205–216.

Meisen, B. (1998). *Dementia in Close Up*. London: Routledge.

Meltzer, D., and Williams, M.H. (1988). *The Apprehension of Beauty: The Role of Aesthetic Conflict in Development, Art and Violence*. Strath Tay, Scotland: Clunie Press.

Polini, P. (2007). Conveying the experience of Alzheimer's Disease throughout: The later paintings of William Utermohlen', chapter 17 in R. Davenhill (ed.) *Looking Into Later Life: A Psychoanalytic Approach to Depression and Dementia in Old Age*. London: Karnac.

Quinodoz, D. (2010). *Growing Old: A Journey of Self Discovery*. Hove: Routledge.

Salzberger-Wittenberg, L. (1970). *Psychoanalytic Insight and Relationships*. London: Routledge and Kegan Paul.

Sinason, V. (1992). The man who was losing his brain, chapter 4 in *Mental Handicap and the Human Condition*. London: Free Assoc Books.

Solms, M. (1995). Is the brain more real than the mind? *Psychoanalytic Psychotherapy*, 9(2), 107–120.

Waddell, M. (1998). *Inside Lives: Psychoanalysis and the Growth of the Personality*. London: Duckwork.

Waddell, M. (2007). Only connect – The links between early and later life, chapter 11 in R. Davenhill (ed.) *Looking Into Later Life: A Psychoanalytic Approach to Depression and Dementia in Old Age*. London: Karnac.

Williams, D.D.R., and Garner, J. (1998). People with dementia can remember. *British Journal of Psychiatry*, 172, 379–380.

Woods, R.T., and Roth, A. (1996). Effectiveness of pychological interventions with older people. In A.D. Roth and P. Fonagy (eds.) *What Works for Whom? A Critical Review of Psychotherapy Research*, 2nd ed. New York: Guildford.

World at One. BBC R4 02.05.2016.

Wright, L.K. (1994). Alzheimer's disease afflicted spouses who remain at home: Can human dialectics explain the findings? *Social Science Medicine*, 38(8), 1037–1046.

Wright, L.K. (1998). Affection and sexuality in the presence of Alzheimer's disease. A longitudinal study. *Sexuality and Disability*, 16(3), 167–179.

Index

Note: page numbers in *italic* indicate a figure and page numbers in **bold** indicate a table.

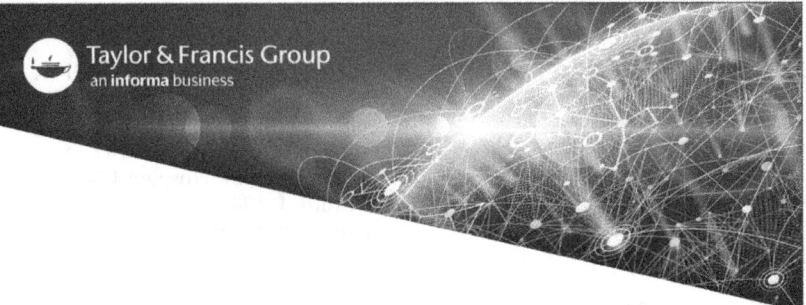
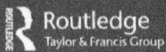
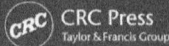